Drug Development
for Women

To Cure, Sometimes
To Relieve, Often
To Comfort, Always

Anon

Drug Development for Women

Edited by

Vanaja V. Ragavan

FemmePharma Inc.,
Wynnewood, Pennsylvania, USA

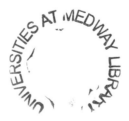

JOHN WILEY & SONS

Chichester • New York • Weinheim • Brisbane • Singapore • Toronto

Other Wiley Editorial Offices

John Wiley & Sons, Inc., 605 Third Avenue,
New York, NY 10158-0012, USA

WILEY-VCH Verlag GmbH, Pappelallee 3,
D-69469 Weinheim, Germany

Jacaranda Wiley Ltd, 33 Park Road, Milton,
Queensland 4064, Australia

John Wiley & Sons (Asia) Pte Ltd, 2 Clementi Loop #02-01,
Jin Xing Distripark, Singapore 129809

John Wiley & Sons (Canada) Ltd, 22 Worcester Road,
Rexdale, Ontario M9W 1L1, Canada

Library of Congress Cataloging-in-Publication Data

Drug development for women / edited by Vanaja V. Ragavan.
    p. cm.
  Includes bibliographical references and index.
  ISBN 0-471-96850-1 (cased)
  1. Drug development. 2. Gynecologic drugs—Development.
3. Women—Diseases—Chemotherapy—Research. 4. Women—Health and
hygiene—Research. I. Ragavan, Vanaja V.
  [DNLM: 1. Clinical Trials. 2. Reproduction. 3. Women's Health.
QV 771 D79385 1998]
RM301.25.D765 1998
362.1'782'082—dc21
DNLM/DLC
for Library of Congress   97–42810
                                                                        CIP

British Library Cataloguing in Publication Data

A catalogue record for this book is available from the British Library

ISBN 0-471-96850-1

Typeset in 10/12pt Baskerville from the author's disks by Mayhew Typesetting, Rhayader, Powys
Printed and bound in Great Britain by Bookcraft (Bath) Ltd, Midsomer Norton, Somerset
This book is printed on acid-free paper responsibly manufactured from sustainable forestry, in which at least two trees are planted for each one used for paper production.

This book is dedicated to

Justin Vikram Berrier and
Loren Anand Berrier
my children, for making it all worthwhile

Robert Jim Berrier
my husband, whose encouragement and love
made this book happen

Vimala Ragavan and
Vijay Ragavan
my parents, for their enduring faith and love

Contents

Contributors

Julia Amadio *Global Marketing Director, Women's Health, Rhone-Poulenc Rorer, Collegeville, PA 19426, USA*

Barbara Barnett *Senior Science Writer/Editor, Policy and Research Utilization Division, Women's Studies Division, Family Health International, PO Box 13950, Research Triangle Park, NC 27709, USA*

Pirow J. Bekker *Director, Clinical Research, Amgen Inc., 1840 DeHavilland Drive, Thousand Oaks, CA 91320-1789, USA*

Ridgely C. Bennett *Medical Officer, Food and Drug Administration, HFD 510, 5600 Fishers Lane, Rockville, MD 20857, USA*

Russell T. Burge *Director, Proctor and Gamble Company, Sharon Woods Technical Center, 11450 Grooms Road, Cincinnati, OH 45242-1434, USA*

Aman U. Buzdar *Professor of Medicine, Deputy Chairman, Department of Breast and Medical Oncology, University of Texas, Anderson Cancer Center, 1515 Holcombe Boulevard, Box 56, Houston, TX 77030, USA*

Gautum Chaudhuri *Professor, Department of Obstetrics and Gynecology and Pharmacology, 22-184 CHS, UCLA School of Medicine, Los Angeles, CA 90095-1740, USA*

Eleni Diamandidou *Anderson Cancer Center, The University of Texas, Houston, TX 77030, USA*

Samarendra N. Dutta *Medical Officer, Food and Drug Administration, HFD 510, 5600 Fishers Lane, Rockville, MD 20857, USA*

Michael J. Gast *Vice-President, Wyeth-Ayerst Research, PO Box 8299, Philadelphia, PA 19101, USA*

George P. Giacoia *Special Expert, Endocrinology, Nutrition and Growth Branch, Center for Research for Mothers and Children, National Institute of Child Health and Human Development, National Institutes of Health, Executive Building Room 4B11, 6100 Executive Boulevard MSC 7510, Bethesda, MD 20892-7510, USA*

Karen Hardee *Director of Research, Policy Projects, Futures Group, 100 Capitola Drive, Suite 306, Durham, NC 27713, USA*

David Juan *Medical Director, Clinical and Medical Affairs, Proctor and Gamble Company, Sharon Woods Technical Center, 11450 Grooms Road, Cincinnati, OH 45242-1434, USA*

Christine Mauck   *Research Coordinator, CONRAD Program, 1611 North Kent Street, Suite 806, Arlington, VA 22209, USA*

Martha J. Morrell   *Associate Professor of Neurology and Neurological Sciences, Stanford University Medical School, Director, Stanford Comprehensive Epilepsy Center, Stanford, CA 94305-5235, USA*

Paul V. Pluorde   *Executive Medical Director, Zeneca Pharmaceuticals Group, Wilmington, DE 19897, USA*

Vanaja V. Ragavan   *Founder, FemmePharma, Inc., 1121 Remington Road, Wynnewood, PA 19096, USA*

Philip N. Rauk   *Assistant Professor, Department of Obstetrics, Gynecology and Reproductive Sciences, University of Pittsburgh School of Medicine; and Assistant Investigator, Magee Women's Hospital, 300 Halket Street, Pittsburgh, PA 15213, USA*

Veronica Ravnikar   *Professor, Department of Obstetrics and Gynecology, University of Massachusetts Medical Center, 55 Lake Avenue North, Worcester, MA 01655, USA*

Roberto Rivera   *Corporate Director, International Medical Affairs, Family Health International, PO Box 13950, Research Triangle Park, NC 27709, USA*

Marlene Tandy   *Director and Counsel, Health Industries Manufacturing Association, 1200 G Street NW, Suite 400, Washington, DC 20005, USA*

Lian Ulrich   *Senior Registrar, Department of Gynecology and Obstetrics, Copenhagen University Hospital, Gentofte, Copenhagen, Denmark*

Brinda Wiita   *Director, Medical Affairs, Solvay Pharmaceuticals, 901 Sawyer Road, Marietta, GA 30062, USA*

Sumner Y. Yaffe   *Director, Center for Research for Mothers and Children, National Institute of Child Health and Human Development, National Institutes of Health, Executive Building Room 4B11, 6100 Executive Boulevard MSC 7510, Bethesda, MD 20892-7510, USA*

Preface

The purpose of this book is to provide a comprehensive review and analyze the scientific and social environment associated with developing drugs for women, relating to all aspects of their reproductive life cycle, from puberty to old age. It is hoped that a book such as this, which identifies the need for developing new drugs for women and analyzes the critical paths for their development, will lead to an understanding of multiple issues which play a role in this process and will furthermore provide the basis for finding solutions.

The book will present these issues by following a logical sequence. In Part A, the book outlines the historical events which have played an important role in this area, describes the demographic and social environment today and identifies factors other than scientific which have a critical bearing on the development of drugs for women. In Parts B and C, special areas of clinical need are evaluated and divided by the reproductive and postreproductive years. The emphasis in these sections is on conditions/diseases related to the reproductive cycle and/or hormones. These Parts examine drug development issues and identify ongoing clinical and research efforts which could lead to drugs in the near and long term.

Because of the special nature of childbearing and of the cessation of reproduction with the onset of menopause, women have unique needs related to their normal life cycle. Drug development for these conditions/life cycle management require special considerations. Often, perfectly normal women must take potent drugs for many years and undergo daily analysis of the risk of taking such products or suffering the consequences, such as pregnancy in early life or menopause-induced diseases later. Because these drugs are taken for so long in normal women, the risk/benefit ratios require different analyses than do acute treatments of serious illnesses.

In spite of much effort in the past to provide effective contraceptives and other such drugs for women, there continues to be a great need to keep women healthy and provide for acceptable alternatives to present-day choices. It is important, then, to examine the present state of drug development and to examine those issues which must be considered for future drug development in order to maintain the well-being of women.

Many lessons have been learned along the path of drugs developed for women. The collective wisdom from historical developments provide an important precedence for any future development. The book examines historic trends and factors which have affected drug development, considerations for developing drugs in women, evaluates efficacy and safety issues and identifies areas of need requiring special considerations in women. The book also, in its appendices, includes a list of drugs in present development for women set out in a logical and useful fashion.

This field is very dynamic: the complex set of issues which often affect development of drugs for women is changing. The editor understands that the book will capture a moment in history and hopes in future editions to keep the interested reader updated on any developments.

Vanaja V. Ragavan
Founder, FemmePharma, Inc.

Acknowledgments

First and foremost, I thank Dr Michael J. Gast for all his contributions, help, encouragement, patience and faith in the book. Without his help, I could never have completed this book.

It has been an immense pleasure to work with all the stellar authors who have contributed to the book. Although these authors come from many segments in the field of women's health-academia, pharmaceutical companies, regulatory agencies and non-profit public organizations, they have devoted their careers, one and all, to promoting the health and well-being of women.

I am deeply indebted to the Externship Program at Radcliffe College, Harvard University, Cambridge, Massachusetts. Three very talented young women from this program helped in compiling and completing the Appendix of the book, as part of their externship conducted under my guidance. Mayssam Ali, Ang Shi and Susan Yeh, all students at Harvard University, contributed their intelligence, hard work and dedication to making the Appendix a comprehensive and useful part of this book. The Externship Program at Radcliffe College is a program which brings working alumni together with undergraduate women for one week every year and is one of those inspirations that make a difference to both sets of participants. I have been lucky in finding three such outstanding women who have helped me with the book.

In addition to the Radcliffe women, I also wish to thank Melissa Pachikara for her contributions while a student at Bryn Mawr College, and Marcia Tolliferreo RN for her help and assistance in managing this project.

I wish to thank Dr Judith Jones for helping me start the concept of the book and for her contributions and assistance. I wish to thank my business partner, Gerianne M. DiPiano MBA for her encouragement and ideas generated through many, many discussions and time spent together at work.

I am very grateful to Hilary Rowe, Michael Davis, and Deborah Reece, my publishers, who have been very patient, kind and encouraging, and always available and helpful, through the sometimes difficult process of pulling this book together.

Finally, I would like to thank my husband, Dr Robert J. Berrier, who gave me the idea to compile this book, and provided innumerable hours of encouragement and advice throughout the process.

Issues Confronting Drug Development for Women

1

Introduction

Vanaja V. Ragavan

OVERVIEW OF THE BOOK

The health and well-being of a woman have implications far beyond the individual involved and have profound influences on the health of her children, her husband, her family, and ultimately on society in general. Throughout her adult life, a woman is often primarily responsible for the health and well-being of all those around her, from her immediate to her extended families. Preserving her in health will mean that others around her will benefit greatly.

Yet, given the various stressors in her life, a woman is more likely to ignore her own health in preference to her family's health and well-being. In addition, in many societies she remains a second-class citizen, given less education, health resources, access to services and financial security than the men around her. This tide is slowly turning in some societies. In some countries such as the USA, a woman's critical role in the well-being of her family and society has become more importantly recognized and resources are now being found to evaluate her well-being. However, in most of the world this is not the situation. Even in the USA, this is a very recent trend and it is not clear how long the momentum will be carried forward.

Throughout her life, a woman needs certain drugs to maintain her good health, prevent disease and improve her well-being, along with treating certain diseases. The common theme of this group of drugs and diseases is their close relationship to her reproductive system or their relationship, in some way, to the sex steroid hormones secreted by her reproductive system and the diseases or conditions related to them. This book will primarily discuss the present status of treatment and describe possible future development of these drugs for the woman as she evolves in her reproductive life, from young girlhood when she requires contraceptives to her later years when more complex medical issues will surface. This book will also focus on diseases and conditions intimately related to her reproductive system and the drugs used in such conditions as pregnancy, infertility, menopause or osteoporosis. A much broader scope of diseases which occur more frequently but not uniquely in women, such as autoimmune diseases, are not discussed in this book.

Drug Development for Women. Edited by V.V. Ragavan. © 1998 John Wiley & Sons Ltd.

Part A discusses the many non-scientific factors that necessarily influence the development of drugs for women, which have played critical roles in this field, both positive and negative. Public and private policy issues, legal, ethical and market factors are discussed at length as they relate, in association with science, to drug development.

Historically, there has been considerable hesitancy in including women in clinical drug trials because of fear of harm to a potential fetus. This has led to an absence of critical data on gender factors which may affect drug use and metabolism in women but, as Morrell describes in *Chapter 2*, not including women in drug trials can lead to significant problems for health care providers. In Chapter 2, Morrell leads us through this history and how this particular situation is now slowly being remedied. An important characteristic of many of the drugs developed for women is the chronicity of drug intake. Contraceptives, for instance, are used by perfectly normal young women, who are in good health, for many years. The threshold for risk/benefit must necessarily be very different from, for instance, drugs developed for the treatment of women terminally ill with breast cancer. In fact, as Bennett discusses so well in *Chapter 3*, the US Food and Drug Administration, like other regulatory and policy-making bodies, have always deliberated carefully on these issues prior to approval of drugs and have, furthermore, followed ongoing safety issues carefully through the years, making appropriate changes as needed. Bennett's discussions also provide invaluable insight into the review of drugs from an individual regulator's important point of view.

Careful evaluation of risk/benefit balance must be considered very early in the development of drugs, for although a drug may be the most effective drug ever developed, understanding the end user's needs for a drug taken chronically or primarily for prevention is critical to ensure that its use will in fact benefit the woman. These issues are discussed by Amadio & Ragavan in *Chapter 4*. Scientific and medical issues are paramount in drug development, but a pharmaceutical company will only at its own peril ignore the critical information provided by market research and market analysis. The changing climate of reimbursement for drugs, or an understanding of the financial burden on the patient of taking drugs for many decades, must be weighed carefully in the drug development process. Just as pharmaceutical companies deliberate on the commercial success of companies, many public health agencies and organizations must also often champion the public health effects of drug development. In an unique approach, Rivera, Hardee & Barnett discuss the critical role of public health agencies in *Chapter 5*, but examine the issue from a centrifugal point of view, i.e. the way in which government agencies often form policy and then implement it. It is perhaps necessary to change this paradigm. Let us examine what a woman needs to preserve her health and create policies that assure her needs are fulfilled. Such a radical approach may be necessary, as governmental agencies continue to feel increasing pressure to solve problems with smaller and smaller purses. Allocation of resources often means that the woman will end up at the bottom of the totem-pole.

This first Part is well concluded by Tandy in *Chapter 6* in a careful and thoughtful discussion of the legal issues which may be the final arbiter of a drug's fate: indeed, the legal system may resolve problems in ways not anticipated by drug developers. Tandy provides a clear and critical discourse on the role of the legal system in ensuring that women's health gets top priority and a fair share of the resources allocated to health.

Part B captures the present status of drug development for women during their reproductive years. In *Chapter 7*, Mauck describes in great detail the historical development of contraceptives, but brings us rapidly up to date on the nature and utility of products under testing. Although many contraceptives are available and their efficacy is superb, there are still many women who are at risk of pregnancy who do not use contraceptives. Perhaps, at this 50-year crossroads of the contraceptive story, it is necessary to take stock of where we need to go next. In *Chapter 8*, Ragavan and Gast discuss the many diseases of the reproductive system which a woman must face during her reproductive and early peri-menopausal years. At the present time, although these diseases or conditions have varied etiologies, there are only a few therapeutic options, and almost all of them revert to suppression of the menstrual cycle. This chapter reminds us of the great work that lies ahead to understand and appropriately treat the underlying diseases, which, although not life-threatening, certainly cause prolonged pain and suffering.

Pre-term labor remains a serious problem in almost 10% of pregnancies and Rauck describes the present state of drug availability and potential research in this vital area in *Chapter 9*. Many factors, including litigation, have kept manufacturers from investigating this area and bringing to the marketplace innovative new treatments that assure the normal development and well-being of the unborn child and its mother. In *Chapter 10* by Chaudhuri, Giacoia and Yaffe, we learn about the considerable progress made in the understanding of drug metabolism in pregnancy, but this knowledge of pharmacokinetics has been matched by adequate studies addressing the various drugs and their pharmacology during pregnancy. It is a matter of fact that pregnancy can result in medical problems for the pregnant woman. Lack of knowledge of drug dosing, the drug's effects on the mother's disease and potential effects on the fetus cannot be known without a careful but systematic study of drugs in pregnancy. The authors very clearly define the boundaries of what is known and what information still needs to be gathered in this field.

Part C continues with the discussion of disease therapeutics but with the emphasis on the older woman. Her reproductive years completed, a woman still has at least half a life-time left in which quality of life and fulfillment of new roles in her life become important. Preserving her overall health through the menopausal years is discussed by Wiita, Gast & Ravnikar in *Chapter 11*, which outlines succinctly the various organ systems affected by menopause. Although estrogen loss is the underlying problem, its manifestations in the various systems are profoundly different. The focus of this chapter is treating the whole woman, helping her cope with a changing life-style and providing the medical practitioner with a unique opportunity to emphasize preventive measures and ensure her good health.

Cardiovascular disease, discussed by Ulrich in *Chapter 12*, and osteoporosis, discussed by Bekker, Juan, Burge, Dutta & Gast in *Chapter 13*, are treated separately because these diseases have significant mortality and morbidity. Scientific research has considerable potential to prevent and treat these common diseases of the older woman. Ulrich takes a superb perspective on cardiovascular diseases; while estrogen was long thought to have a negative effect on cardiovascular health, due to its noted effects in oral contraceptives, it has become abundantly clear that estrogen, in the menopause, plays a critical role in the prevention of heart disease. Ulrich clearly states the controversies and resolutions and looks forward to new theories, such as direct vascular effect, which could, in the future, change our understanding of the nature of cardiovascular disease. Osteoporosis, the silent killer, is discussed in Chapter 13. Recent advances in this field make this chapter interesting reading and we will continue to see rapid advances in this field, leading to new modes of therapy with direct focus on the pathophysiology of bone and drugs targeted at this process.

Part C concludes with a thorough and very well laid out *Chapter 14*, which is a careful treatise on breast cancer by Diamandidou, Buzdar and Pluorde. Breast cancer is included in this book because of the intimate relationship between cancer of the breast and sex steroid hormones. Estrogen receptor status plays a critical role in management of breast cancer, as do anti-estrogens. In the pre-menopausal years, this is a deadly disease with poor prognosis. Many advances have been made in menopausal breast cancer, but the rapid increase in the incidence of this cancer is indeed very worrisome to both oncologists and epidemiologists. Recent ground-breaking studies, including the discovery of the breast cancer oncogene, the prevention of disease using anti-estrogens, and understanding disease etiologies through initiatives such as the Women's Health Initiative, will be critical to the future decrease in the mortality associated with breast cancer and controlling the growing incidence of this deadly disease. The authors provide a well thought-out summary of the whole issue.

THE DRUG DEVELOPMENT PROCESS

At first glance, the universality of the human condition can be presumed to make the development of drugs available for diseases worldwide a uniquely global process. Yet, in a world approaching globalization of many processes and products, and in spite of attempts by responsible national regulatory authorities to harmonize the process of drug development, approval of a new drug into the marketplace still remains the primary responsibility of individual countries. An exception to this general rule is the attempt by the nations of the European Union to provide a central process for drug approval. But even this process often only attempts to incorporate the varied and not often coordinated agendas of the individual member countries.

This state of affairs makes the development of a drug for worldwide use a difficult and cumbersome process for many pharmaceutical companies, which

TABLE 1.1 Drugs—from discovery to marketing: an average yield

Phase/stage of development	Number of compounds	Number of patients tested	Length	Purpose
Discovery	5000	–	2–10 years	Experimental drug
Pre-clinical testing	250	–	1–3 years	Understand mechanism of action and toxicity
Phase I	100	20–100	<1 year	Mainly safety
Phase II	70	Up to several hundred	<2 years	Short-term safety, mainly efficacy
Phase III	25–33	Several hundred to several thousand	1–4 years	Safety, efficacy, dosage
FDA review	20		2 months to 7 years	

Adapted from FDA, 1985.

themselves have become more and more a global phenomenon. As will be seen in later sections of this book, local social, religious, ethnic and governmental processes play a critical role in the development and availability of many drugs, especially those needed by women to control fertility and other similar conditions. Pharmaceutical companies considering the global availability of drugs must plan this process very early in the process of drug development. Expenditures then must be added early on to consider the global availability of drugs. In spite of such attempts, many countries may require specific studies on their own populations prior to a drug's approval.

Various aspects of the drug development process are addressed throughout the book, with a special emphasis on the drug development process in the USA. This Part will present a very brief overview of the drug development process as a primer. Several excellent textbooks have been written on this topic and some of these are referenced. Drug development, in many ways similar to clinical medicine, is both a science and an art. Practitioners of this science understand that within the very general guidelines developed by regulatory agencies lie many variations and opportunities for both innovation and frustration which must be addressed along the way.

The process from discovery of a potential compound to its launch in the marketplace can be long, tedious and fraught with many pitfalls. In fact, as shown in Table 1.1, the potential yield from the laboratory to the market is in fact very small.

FROM THE TEST TUBE TO THE MARKET

The path to the market for any particular drug does not necessarily follow a strict sequence of research, development and study. The seed idea for a particular type of drug is often initiated in the published literature regarding the nature of a particular disease process. Bench scientists then may take the basic concepts, often studied in animal models, and try to synthesize chemical entities to address the basic pathophysiology. Although this was a typical model for any number of neuroactive or cardiovascular drugs, we are now staunchly immersed in new concepts of drug syntheses. The organic and synthetic chemists have given lead places to the gene researchers and computer programmers. Designer molecules, designed by computer programs to bind to known receptors, often lead the way before any actual syntheses of chemicals have been attempted. Furthermore, gene studies have isolated genes associated with many diseases. Gene products associated with these genes may form the basis of new drug development.

Traditionally, the chemist will synthesize a whole 'library' of new chemical entities (NCEs). These are then screened for efficacy and safety. In the past, this first screen was often conducted in biological systems, but may often now be first conducted in a test tube, using specific enzyme pathways or other molecular mechanisms to identify products with specific desired characteristics. Those NCEs then that make the grade are next tested simultaneously for safety and efficacy in toxicity and pharmacology studies in animals. If a specific animal model is available, potency and duration of effect are often determined. Further chronic studies such as carcinogenicity are conducted in parallel to human studies for final market application.

With the short- and medium-term safety of a drug tested in animals, the company will embark on an initial study of a single, ascending dose in a Phase Ia study in normal volunteers. Pharmacokinetics and safety will be tested in a closely monitored setting in these 'First in Man' studies. Doses below the safety limits will then be tested in a longer-term Phase Ib study. Once the acute and sub-acute toxicity of a drug is known, then the drug will be introduced in a series of studies to patients with the disease, in this Phase II of development. At the end of Phase II, there should be considerable knowledge on the safety and toxicity of the drug in patients with a target disease, appropriate dose and timing of drug delivery and knowledge of its metabolism. Phase II must be viewed as a critical phase in a drug's development and a manufacturer must be comfortable that the drug works well before embarking on an expensive and committed Phase III path. Recent guidelines have also mandated or suggested specific studies as appropriate, in gender-, age- or race-based populations, to round out a drug's effect on these various sub-populations.

Phase III then concludes these extensive analyses and is a pre-market, well-controlled study of a drug's efficacy and safety. Phase III is a very large commitment in time and expense and its success must be improved and risk minimized by appropriate Phase II studies. The percentage of failure must be decreased before Phase III. At the end of Phase III, the entire data package is submitted to the regulatory agencies for review and approval to market.

After approval, the drug now enters the wide marketplace. Safety of the drug is often monitored closely for the first few years after launch, for then data about real use (as opposed to clinical trials) are gathered, as are rare safety events. In addition,

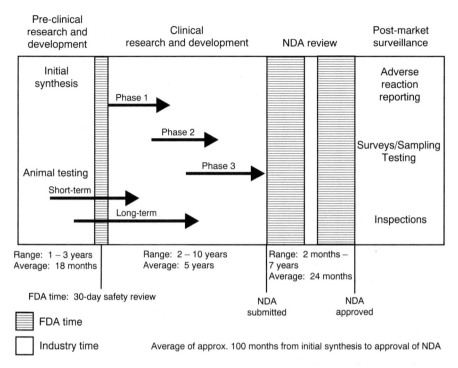

Pre-clinical research and development | Clinical research and development | NDA review | Post-market surveillance

Initial synthesis

Phase 1

Phase 2

Phase 3

Animal testing
Short-term

Long-term

Adverse reaction reporting

Surveys/Sampling Testing

Inspections

Range: 1 – 3 years
Average: 18 months

Range: 2 – 10 years
Average: 5 years

Range: 2 months – 7 years
Average: 24 months

FDA time: 30-day safety review

NDA submitted

NDA approved

FDA time

Industry time   Average of approx. 100 months from initial synthesis to approval of NDA

FIGURE 1.1   New drug development. Reproduced by permission from FDA (1988)

the manufacturers may wish to continue to study further indications, doses, formulations and sub-populations. Recent changes related to the User Fee Act have drastically reduced the review times, as the FDA continues to make major inroads. In some high priority cases, review times have been halved.

PATENTS, PATENT RIGHTS, AND DRUG DEVELOPMENT

It is well recognized that intellectual property must be preserved for the inventors in order to nurture creativity. For pharmaceutical companies, this issue is of tremendous importance because of the time, effort and cost of drug development. Traditionally, US Patent Laws have allowed a 17 year term for a new invention. As can be seen in Figure 1.1, an average time to develop a drug can indeed encompass many of these 17 years, leaving the inventor a mere few years of exclusivity to gain back its development costs and generate a profit.

In the USA, as can be seen from Figure 1.1, the time at the FDA is usually credited to the patent holder.

Furthermore, the Waxman–Hatch Act of 1984 (Drug Competition and Patent Term Restoration Act of 1984) allowed into the marketplace the generic equivalent of marketed drugs, thus creating, virtually overnight, a sophisticated industry quite capable of imitating innovator drugs and placing enormous pressure on innovator companies, especially those with block-buster drugs. However, this Act did extend exclusivity of the marketplace for a few more years, as a concession to the innovator companies. Recent World Trade Organization rules have resulted in slight modification of the 17 year rule. Patent life can be based on countries where the patent is first filed.

Worldwide patent protection has sometimes been contentious among international trade bodies. Given the globalization of pharmaceutical markets, most companies will obtain worldwide patent protection at the same time or close to the time of US application and foreign companies will follow a similar suit.

HARMONIZATION ISSUES IN DRUG DEVELOPMENT

Harmonization of drug development between the regulatory bodies of the three major pharmaceutical markets—USA, Europe and Japan—continues to be a work in progress. The discussions and negotiations have had to account for positions that are very far apart. Even the best-intentioned scientists and regulators have a difficult time agreeing on certain criteria. In fact, several areas of harmonization have been successful. In particular, many pre-clinical issues have come close to harmonization. Issues regarding carcinogenicity studies and doses for such studies and toxicity studies are well under way.

Clinical issues, especially those relating to efficacy studies, appear to be the most difficult to harmonize. Clinical issues with regard to data management, international safety surveillance, etc. are also further along. Europe, as the European Union, is also attempting to harmonize and speed up its review process.

Details of all the above topics are beyond the scope of this chapter. Some critical reference materials are cited below for further review.

CONCLUSION

We have come a long way, but still have a long path to follow. This book will bring together the issues surrounding drug development in the hope that serious discussion will lead to a renewed interest in developing appropriate, safe and effective drugs.

BIBLIOGRAPHY

Ansel HC, Popovich NG, Allen LV. *Pharmaceutical Dosage Forms and Drug Delivery Systems*, 6th edn, 1995. Malvern, PA: Williams and Wilkins.

FDA. *From Test Tube to Patient: New Drug Development in the United States* 1988, Consumer Special Report. Rockwell, MD: FDA.

Foster FH, Shook RL. *Patents, Copyrights and Trademarks*, 2nd edn, 1993. New York: Wiley.

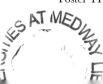

Guarino RA. *New Drug Approval Process* 1987. New York: Marcel Dekker.

Mann RD, Rawlins MD, Auty RM (eds). *A Textbook of Pharmaceutical Medicine* 1993. New York: Parthenon.

Mathieu M. *New Drug Development: A Regulatory Overview* 1990. Cambridge, MA: PAREXEL International Corporation.

Perun TJ, Propst CL (eds). *Computer-aided Drug Design: Methods and Applications* 1989. New York: Marcel Dekker.

Report of the FDA Task Force on International Harmonization 1993. Springfield, VA: National Technical Information Service, US Department of Commerce.

Silverman RB. *Drug Discovery, Design and Development. The Organic Chemistry of Drug Design and Drug Action* 1992. New York: Academic Press.

Smith W. *The Process of New Drug Discovery and Development* 1992. Boca Raton, FL: CRC Press.

Sneader W. *Drug Development: From Laboratory to Clinic* 1986. New York: Wiley.

Women in Clinical Drug Trials: Protection or Inclusion?*

Martha J. Morrell
Stanford University Medical School, Stanford, CA, USA

For many years, women of reproductive age were excluded from clinical trials of pharmaceuticals because of concerns of harm to a potential fetus, or because gender-specific evaluation was not believed to be important. Therefore, important information concerning gender-specific disease epidemiology and drug response has not been available. Although several recent initiatives are attempting to encourage investigation in gender-relevant areas, there continues to be a paucity of information, specifically on the safety of drugs used during pregnancy.

This chapter will examine the continued controversy surrounding inclusion of women in pharmaceutical trials and examine whether present policies allow for appropriate access to clinical drug trials, provide adequate safeguards against harm to the woman and to a potential fetus, and whether issues of concern to reproductive aged women are adequately addressed during the drug development process.

Issues associated with the preclinical development of drugs will be addressed separately from those arising in the post-marketing period. Particular attention will be directed towards areas in which the drug development process is perceived to address the concerns of women inadequately.

PRE-MARKETING ISSUES

Access to Trials

Inclusion of Women of Child-bearing Potential

The extent to which women have been involved in clinical drug trials has reflected societal beliefs concerning the status of women. In the 1950s–1980s, regulations

---

* Adapted from Morrell (1998), by permission of Lippincott-Raven Publishers..

Drug Development for Women. Edited by V.V. Ragavan. © 1998 John Wiley & Sons Ltd.

were developed to protect individuals against research subject abuse (Tuskegee Syphilis Project) and to protect potential fetuses from adverse morphological outcomes after exposure to drugs in utero (thalidomide). Post World War II attitudes about the role of women in society and a woman's ability to make an informed choice also reinforced the belief that women of child-bearing potential, and pregnant and lactating women, formed a vulnerable population in need of special protection.

These assumptions were evident in the FDA's 1977 guidelines, which directed that women of child-bearing potential be excluded from Phase I and early Phase II trials (FDA, 1977). Once data had been obtained regarding the relative efficacy and safety of the pharmaceutical, and once preclinical data on fertility and teratogenesis in animals was available, then women of child-bearing potential could participate in later Phase II trials. In 1977, a woman of child-bearing potential was narrowly defined as any woman physiologically capable of becoming pregnant, regardless of sexual activity, sexual practices and contraceptive use. This policy did not address the manner in which safety and efficacy should be assessed in order to determine whether participation was appropriate, but left decisional authority to Institutional Review Boards (IRBs), investigators and research subjects.

In the past two decades, attitudes have evolved. Consumers, investigators and governmental agencies have expressed concerns that guidelines and regulations implemented to protect research subjects are overly restrictive and are, in fact, detrimental to the health of the groups denied access. This has led to a number of significant changes in regulatory policy, all of which are based on the assumption that patients included in clinical studies should reflect the population that will receive the drug (Merkatz et al, 1993).

In 1990, the NIH directed that women and minorities be included in clinical trials (NIH Guide, 1990). The 1993 NIH Revitalization Act directed the NIH to establish guidelines for the inclusion of women and minorities in federally funded biomedical and behavioral research involving human subjects, except where specific criteria for the exclusion of these groups can be satisfied (NIH, 1993).

In 1994, the NIH released guidelines on the inclusion of women and minorities as subjects in clinical research (NIH, 1994). These guidelines mandate that women and minorities be included in Phase II trials in sufficient numbers so that valid analyses of difference in intervention effect can be accomplished. The NIH acknowledged that the detection of significant gender-based differences in response might require large, time-consuming and expensive clinical studies. However, the guidelines emphasized that cost is not an acceptable criterion for exclusion and directed investigators to initiate programs and support outreach efforts to recruit under-represented groups.

In 1993–4, the FDA withdrew its restriction on participation of women of child-bearing potential in early clinical trials (FDA/DHHS, 1993, 1994). Three reasons were cited for reversing the 1977 FDA guidelines: the expectation that gender-specific data obtained early in a drug investigation would be used to make appropriate adjustments in larger clinical studies; to avoid unwarranted discrimination against women; and to not perpetuate the view of the male as the primary focus of drug development.

Inclusion of Pregnant or Lactating Women

Many drugs in the market place are likely to be used by women while pregnant or lactating. Although regulations now support and even demand the inclusion of women of child-bearing potential using effective contraception in clinical trials, there is still debate and discomfort regarding the participation of pregnant and lactating women. Concerns focus on how best to define the risks and benefits of any particular therapeutically needed drug in this population.

Although federal statutes, regulations, guidelines and policies have been enacted which encourage the inclusion of women of child-bearing potential in clinical trials, there has been no specific guidance on the inclusion of pregnant women. Federal policies and Health and Human Services Regulations have generally assumed that pregnant women would be excluded (DHHS, 1994). Constitutional, legislative and tort law have failed to provide a clear framework in which to clarify the appropriateness of inclusion of pregnant women in clinical drug trials.

Federal regulations have largely restricted access to clinical trials for pregnant and lactating women, but policies are being re-examined. In addition to the protections provided to volunteers in research studies by the Federal Policy for the Protection of Human Subjects (NIH/OPRR, 1991), DHHS regulations provide additional protections pertaining to research development and related activities involving pregnant women, fetuses, and human in vitro fertilization. DHHS regulation (DHHS, 1994, Subpart B) directs that pregnant women may not be research subjects except under two circumstances: the purpose of the activity is to meet the health needs of the mother and the fetus will be placed at risk only to the minimum extent necessary to meet such needs; or the risk to the fetus is minimal. This has been interpreted as supporting the inclusion of pregnant women with life-threatening illnesses in trials of antivirals and cancer chemotherapy after informed consent is obtained.

Consent requirements for pregnant women are very stringent. The DHHS specifies that

> . . . both mother and father (must give) . . . informed consent. The father's consent is (not necessary) if the purpose of the activity is to meet the health needs of the mother, his identity or whereabouts cannot be reasonably ascertained, he is not reasonably available, or the pregnancy results from rape (DHHS, 1994).

The NIH and FDA directed the Institute of Medicine (IOM) to examine policies regarding inclusion of pregnant and lactating women in clinical trials. The IOM Committee on Women in Research made a controversial recommendation in 1994 that pregnant and lactating women be considered eligible to be subjects in clinical research (Institute of Medicine, 1994). The IOM report stated that, '. . . the prevailing presumption regarding the participation of pregnant women in clinical trials . . . [should] be shifted from one of exclusion to one of inclusion'. The IOM felt that women who are, or may become, pregnant during the course of a research study should be viewed like any other competent adult who is a potential research subject.

The justification for the IOM's statement was as much ethical as medical, derived out of principles of respect for women's autonomy and capacity to act as responsible moral agents. Two principles cited included distributive justice, which implies that '. . . the benefits as well as the burdens of clinical research . . . should be equitably distributed among all individuals in society'; and respect for humans, which implies that men and women should share equally in the opportunity to serve as subjects in clinical research.

The IOM indicated that investigators and IRBs have the responsibility of ensuring that pregnant and lactating women are provided with adequate information about the risks and benefits to themselves and their potential offspring. When risks are not known, the determination of what constitutes acceptable risk to the fetus should be made by the woman as part of the consent process. Exclusion of women from the study by the IRB is warranted only if there is no prospect of benefit to the pregnant woman and there is a known or plausibly inferred risk of fetal harm. According to the IOM:

> . . . far from needing protection, the pregnant woman is the most motivated and in the best position to decide for the health of herself and the potential child.

Three levels of law, constitutional, legislative and tort, are relevant to this discussion. The Fourteenth Amendment is the equal protection clause of the US Constitution. This Amendment guarantees the protection of 'life, liberty and property' and has been interpreted to provide decisional privacy with respect to terminating life-sustaining treatment and obtaining an abortion. It also implies the right to assume the risk of experimental drugs. In addition, the Fourteenth Amendment states, '. . . no states shall . . . deny to any person within its jurisdiction equal protection of the laws'. This could be interpreted as contradicting DHHS Regulations that bar the inclusion of pregnant women in research. This amendment might be used as a constitutional challenge to consider the liberty and privacy interests of the woman vs. state interests concerning fetal protection and protection of the woman's health.

Legislative laws also address the participation of pregnant women in clinical trials. The Federal Pregnancy Discrimination Act of 1978 (Pregnancy Discrimination Act, 1978) bans discrimination on the basis of pregnancy, childbirth or related conditions. Title VII of the Civil Rights Act of 1964 (Civil Rights Act, 1964) forbids employers to discriminate on the basis of race, color, religion, sex or national origin.

The Supreme Court interpretation of Title VII has been somewhat contradictory. The Supreme Court has written that differential treatment of pregnancy does not represent a suspect gender classification in the context of a state disability insurance program. In general, however, the court has been consistent in its rulings that pregnant women cannot be discriminated against in the context of employment unless gender is a bona fide occupational qualification (Annas, 1991).

A Supreme Court case that is relevant to this issue is *United Automobile Workers v. Johnson Controls* (Annas, 1991; International Union vs. Johnson Controls, 1991). Johnson Controls, a manufacturer of batteries, established a fetal protection policy which excluded women capable of bearing children from jobs involving lead exposure. This policy was established after eight women became pregnant while maintaining critically high blood lead levels, as established by Occupational Safety and Health Administration (OSHA) guidelines. In 1984, a class action suit challenged the policy as a violation of Title VII. A Federal District Court and the US Court of Appeals upheld *Johnson* on the basis of medical evidence of potential harm to the fetus. The Supreme Court reversed these decisions, stating that it was wrongfully discriminatory to exclude women from a benefit on the grounds of fetal protection. The Court felt that the bias in this policy was obvious since 'fertile men but not fertile women are given a choice as to whether they wish to risk their reproductive health for a particular job'. The Court went on to note that the company did not seek to protect all unconceived children, only those of its female employees. The Court also felt that the act was in violation of the Pregnancy Discrimination Act once the company had chosen to treat all its female employees as potentially pregnant—a policy which evinces discrimination. While *Johnson Controls* argued that its policy was ethical, socially responsible, and medically defendable, the Court wrote, 'it is no more appropriate for physicians to attempt to control women's opportunities . . . on the basis of their reproductive role than it is for the courts or individual employers to do so'. The Court concluded, 'Decisions about the welfare of future children must be left to the parents who conceive, bear, support and raise them rather than to the employers who hire those parents'. These decisions may be relevant to issues concerning the exclusion of pregnant women in clinical trials.

Tort law may also address the interests of the woman and fetus. Tort liability is civil or private law that evolves from judge-made decisions in order to compensate individuals for injury resulting from the actions of a defendant. Tort law varies by state and each state may have a different variation of Tort law which applies to whether a woman's informed consent can bar independent action by a child harmed as a fetus. Although state tort liability usually holds that warnings may preclude claims by injured *parties*, warnings may not preclude claims by injured *children* because, in general, parents cannot waive action on behalf of their children, and the parent's negligence cannot be imputed to the children.

Two legal theories might be asserted against manufacturers of pharmaceuticals in a tort action: negligence and strict liability (Flannery, 1994). In a negligence action, the plaintive must prove that the defendant (the manufacturer or investigator) had a legal duty toward the plaintiff, the defendant breached that duty, the plaintiff suffered an injury and the defendant's breech of his duties was the cause of the plaintiff's injury. For example, in a drug product liability case, the plaintiff would show that they were not given the information that would permit a truly informed consent. Under strict liability, the manufacturer of a product that is 'in a defective condition unreasonably dangerous to the . . . consumer' is subject to liability for injury caused to the consumer without proof of fault by the manufacturer.

However, products deemed 'unavoidably unsafe' are exempted from this rule if the manufacturer has given proper directions and warnings for their products. Therefore, a prescription drug is not considered unreasonably dangerous if it is accompanied by adequate warnings of potential side effects. In many states, prescription drugs, prescription medical devices and vaccines are exempted from strict liability on a case-by-case basis. The manufacturers must bear the burden of proving that the benefits of their product outweigh the risks at the time of its release. Nevertheless, although these are realistic concerns regarding liability, manufacturers have not faced substantial litigation from participants in clinical trials (Reisman, 1992).

There are no case precedents which resolve whether informed consent from the pregnant woman is relevant to determine the likelihood of a successful tort action for injuries to offspring that may have been caused by inclusion of the pregnant women in a drug trial. The Supreme Court addressed tort liability for fetal injury in *Johnson Controls*. According to the Court, under Title VII, liability for fetal injury is remote if an employer has followed Federal guidelines and has fully informed its workers of the risks involved.

Other issues to consider concerning tort liability include the statute of limitations for research-related injury, and the parties who would be liable in a negligence action. At present, the fetus can sue to the age of majority for any adverse consequences related to exposure to a pharmaceutical agent. Whether liability in such a suit applies only to pharmaceutical companies or involves health care providers as well has not been established.

Excluding pregnant women from clinical trials has been viewed as a way to avoid liability for injuries, especially to potential offspring. However, there may also be liability related to exclusion, particularly for drugs that will subsequently be used to treat pregnant women. Pharmaceutical companies and health care providers may be liable for injuries that occur to pregnant women and their fetuses post-marketing, if there was a failure to test for a foreseeable risk. A pregnant woman or injured offspring might sue a manufacturer after a pharmaceutical is marketed because the pharmaceutical had not been tested in this population prior to release—particularly if pregnant women are expected users. Health care providers might also be liable for using drugs in pregnant women before they have been tested in controlled trials of pregnant women.

If pregnant women are to be included in investigational drug trials, then investigators must ensure that an adequate number of pregnant women can be recruited and retained in the study to allow valid and meaningful scientific conclusions to be drawn. If insufficient numbers are recruited, then the manu-facturer will not be allowed to provide any statement of the drug's appropriateness for use in this population. In this case, failure to include a sufficiently large number of pregnant women might be considered negligent.

Given these liability issues, inclusion of pregnant women will probably proceed only when adequate compensation mechanisms are established. These compensa-tion mechanisms could be contractual or legislative, such as with the Vaccine Compensation Act. The IOM (1994) recommended that NIH thoroughly review the area of compensation for research injury in general and that compensation mechanisms address prenatal and preconceptional injuries to children resulting from a parent's participation in a clinical study.

Although legal issues may appear to discourage inclusion of vulnerable popu-lations such as pregnant women and their fetuses in investigational drug trials, a rational and consistent application of legal and ethical principles can also be argued to prevent the arbitrary exclusion of any class of people from the benefits of research. The potential benefit of participating in the trial may be the most important factor in determining if participation is appropriate. Risk to the fetus may be acceptable if the study is likely to have important medical benefits for the mother. Women with life-threatening conditions such as cancer and AIDs have typically been included in the earliest phases of drug testing. Whether sufficient benefit is derived from participation in an investigational trial of a drug for a non-life-threatening illness, or for a condition for which alternative pharmaceutical agents exist, can be argued.

Inclusion of pregnant women is most appropriate when the woman is provided with sufficient information to allow informed consent. This includes information regarding the risks of alternative therapies and hypotheses regarding the terato-genic risks of the tested agent. Such hypotheses would be drawn from knowledge of the pharmacokinetics of the new agent as well as animal reproductive toxicology studies. This information would guide the design of appropriate trials to include pregnant and lactating women.

Clinical Issues

Contraceptive Use During Investigational Trials

The FDA 1977 guidelines on participation of women of child-bearing potential in Phase I and early Phase II trials excluded premenopausal women who were sexually active and using no contraception, as well as women using mechanical, oral or injectable contraceptives, women whose partners had vasectomies, women who were sexually inactive and homosexual women. The revised FDA guidelines in 1993 state:

> It is expected that, in accordance with good medical practice appropriate precautions against becoming pregnant and exposing the fetus to a potentially dangerous agent during the course of a study will be taken by women participating in clinical trials.

The FDA (1993) also indicated that it is expected that women will receive adequate counseling regarding the importance of taking precautions against becoming pregnant, and that efforts will be made to ensure that a woman is not pregnant when she enters a trial, as determined by a negative pregnancy test detecting the β-subunit of the human chorionic gonadotropin molecule. Reliable contraceptive methods include abstinence, homosexuality, barrier methods, hormonal contraception, and willingness to consider pregnancy interruption.

The IOM (1994) believes that the participant should be permitted to voluntarily select the contraceptive method of his/her choice where there are no relevant study-dependent, scientific reasons for excluding certain contraceptives, such as drug interactions:

> The investigator must have knowledge of interactions that might compromise the efficacy of certain contraceptives, such as failure of hormone based contraception in women on liver cytochrome P450-inducing drugs.

When an unintended pregnancy occurs in an investigational drug trial, the woman and her physician will need to consider whether termination is appropriate (FDA/DHHS, 1993). The IOM (1994) recommends that 'pregnancy termination options (should) be discussed as part of the consent process in clinical studies that pose unknown or foreseeable risks to potential offspring'.

Investigative Issues

Gender Specific Analysis

In 1993 the FDA released guidelines for the study and evaluation of gender differences in the clinical evaluation of drugs which called for careful characterization of drug effects by gender. This followed a 1988 FDA guideline which called for analyses of data to identify variations in efficacy and adverse effects of drugs among different age groups, races and by gender. In 1983 and 1989, the FDA examined the relative numbers of women in the database of new drug applications. In general, women were represented to the same extent that women were affected by the disease. The General Accounting Office conducted a larger study of drugs approved during 1988–1991 with similar results. Yet while women comprised an acceptable percentage of research subjects, gender-specific analyses were not necessarily conducted (FDA/DHHS, 1993).

In 1993 the FDA wrote:

> Over the past decade there has been a growing concern that the drug development process does not produce adequate information about the effects of drugs on women. For Phase III trials . . . women and minorities and their sub-populations must be included such that valid analysis of differences in intervention effect can be accomplished (FDA/DHHS, 1993).

In order to detect efficacy and safety differences related to physiological gender differences, such as the effects of hormones, substantial representation of both sexes is expected, as is analysis by gender of effectiveness, adverse-event rates and dose–response.

One rationale for gender-specific analysis comes from the increasing recognition of differences in pharmacokinetics in women and men. Gender-related differences in pharmacokinetics are partly due to variations in body size and composition—women are generally smaller, have higher body fat and lower body water. Hormones may also affect pharmacokinetics. Changes in pharmacokinetics might be expected at puberty, over the menstrual cycle, and at menopause. Pharmacokinetic variations could also occur due to interactions with steroid hormones taken for contraception or post-menopausal hormone replacement therapy.

The FDA encourages pharmacokinetics screening by gender (FDA/DHHS, 1993). A small number of steady-state concentration measurements are obtained in most Phase II and III subjects, then analyzed by gender to determine whether there are important differences. If such differences are detected, then formal pharmacokinetics studies are undertaken. The FDA also encourages that an evaluation be conducted of potential interactions between the test drug and contraceptive steroids.

Reproductive Toxicology

Reproductive toxicology studies must be completed before there is large-scale exposure of women of child-bearing potential to investigational drugs. The FDA guidelines for reproductive toxicology (FDA/DHHS, 1994) call for a three-segment design which evaluates fertility and general reproductive performance, teratology, and perinatal and postnatal evaluation in rodents and other non-primate mammals.

Reproductive toxicology studies, as currently utilized, may not be specific predictors of human teratogenic potential. Animals may be more sensitive to the teratogenic effects of new drugs because of differences in metabolism and because dose exposures usually substantially exceed the expected dose range in humans. In vitro techniques might permit a more accurate and specific analysis of mechanisms of teratogenesis. For example, properties of a drug that could promote teratogenesis include the propensity to form arene oxide metabolites or to have antifolate effects. Cell culture techniques could identify drug effects on specific organ formation, such as the palate (Mino, Mizusawa & Shiota, 1994) and the neural tube (Regan et al, 1990).

POST-MARKETING ISSUES

Define Appropriate Use in Women of Child-bearing Potential

Effects of Contraception

Any pharmaceutical which will be used in reproductive-aged women must be evaluated for potential interactions with therapeutic steroid hormones (e.g. contraceptives and hormone replacement therapy). Hormone-dependent contraception—including oral contraceptive pills, long acting depot hormone preparations and hormone-impregnated intrauterine devices—represents the most effective family-planning method. However, these methods may fail if interactions with other drugs increase steroid metabolism or protein binding. Some examples are drugs that induce the cytochrome P450 system of the liver, such as many serotonin uptake inhibitors, antibiotics and antiepileptic drugs known to have each of these effects.

Effects on Reproductive Health

Several drugs can disrupt reproductive health. Disturbances in the menstrual cycle and in the hypothalamic–pituitary–ovarian axis may arise with drugs that alter steroid hormone metabolism. Disruption of sexual desire and arousal can also be disturbed by many drugs. These issues may need to be addressed in post-marketing studies.

Use in Pregnant and Lactating Women

Post-conception Management

Traditionally, FDA's labeling of every approved drug carries a reproductive risk category (see Table 2.1). In most instances, this information is derived from pre-clinical reproductive studies. If a new product is selected for a woman of child-bearing potential, she must be informed of what is understood to be the risk should she become pregnant.

Pregnancy risk categories were established by the FDA to assist the clinician in the decision towards using drugs for women in pregnancy. But the FDA has

TABLE 2.1   FDA Use-in-Pregnancy drug categories (FDA 211 CFR, etc.). The categories are based in the degree to which available information has ruled out risk to the fetus, balanced against the drug's potential benefits to the patient

Category A: Controlled studies show no risk
Adequate, well-controlled studies in pregnant women have failed to demonstrate risk to fetus

Category B: No evidence of risk to human fetus
Either animal findings show risk but human findings do not, or, if no adequate studies have been done, animal findings are negative

Category C: Risk can not be ruled out
Human studies are lacking and animal studies are either positive for fetal risk, or lacking as well. However, potential benefits may justify the potential risk

Category D: Positive evidence of risk
Investigational or post-marketing data show risk to the fetus. Nevertheless, potential benefits may outweigh the potential risk

Category X: Contraindicated in pregnancy
Studies in animals or humans, or investigational or postmarketing reports have shown fetal risk that clearly outweighs any possible benefits to the patient

received numerous complaints from physicians who treat pregnant women, academic and specialty medical organizations and women's health groups about the vagueness of these categories (Federal Register Notice, July 31, 1997). The FDA holds that:

> The confusion concerning gradation of risk across categories is believed to be due, in part, to the fact that criteria for inclusion in categories A, B, and to a certain extent, C are based primarily on risk with risk increasing from A to C while criteria for inclusion in categories D and X, and to a certain extent, C, are based on risk weighed against potential benefit. In addition, category C may be provided to drugs with known reproductive toxicities and to drugs with no knowledge.

The present categories do not provide direction or guidance for the clinician, who must make a decision that is most beneficial to the patient.

In fact, clinicians have long held that these risk categories are not sufficiently specific or directive to be of clinical benefit. Based on these comments, the FDA convened an advisory meeting in 1997. This meeting may well be the first of several which will result in changing the pregnancy category designation.

In particular, the above quoted Federal Register notice mentions:

> The task force will also consider other possible actions that may be necessary to make pregnancy labeling content more consistent, informative and accessible, including: (1) Changing or creating categories to the pregnancy labeling categories; (2) Clearly distinguishing in labeling between information that addresses whether to prescribe a therapeutic option during pregnancy, whether to prescribe a therapeutic option in a woman of childbearing potential and the consequences of inadvertent fetal exposure;

and (3) attempting to better delineate the different types of reproductive and developmental risks associated with a product.

Appropriate risk counselling requires that all information regarding outcome after human pregnancy exposures be available to physician and patient; including pregnancy complications, incidence of fetal malformations and anomalies and potential cognitive development. A review of the animal reproductive toxicology studies is appropriate. The physician must also know the most effective means to evaluate for abnormal morphogenesis, including appropriate use of level II fetal ultrasound, maternal serum α-fetoprotein and amniocentesis.

Folate supplementation has been conclusively shown to prevent the occurrence (Czeizel & Dudas, 1992) and recurrence (MRC Vitamin Group, 1991) of risks of neural tube defects and other congenital malformations. All women of childbearing potential should receive folate supplementation of at least 0.4 mg/day, with women at risk for folate deficiency receiving more. Some drugs, such as antiepileptic drugs, interfere with folate absorption or folate-mediated biochemical processes. If it is not known whether a new drug has antifolate properties, then folate supplementation in excess of 0.4 mg/day should be considered.

In order to best manage drug therapy in the pregnant woman with a disease condition requiring medication, the physician must be able to anticipate pharmacokinetic changes of the drugs through pregnancy. Changes in drug absorption, protein binding, volume of distribution, metabolism and clearance must be defined. Pharmacodynamic changes may also occur as a result of hormones secreted in pregnancy.

Postconception Surveillance

Whether women are included or excluded from preclinical trials, it is clear that postmarketing data regarding outcome after pregnancy exposures to a new pharmaceutical must be pursued aggressively.

Observational methods have typically been employed to monitor marketed medications for the risk of birth defects (Andrew, 1994). Adequate clinical surveillance also requires that the exposed group be identified and that timing of fetal exposure to a drug and the extent of exposure be documented. With the present surveillance systems, these goals are not always possible. Also, observational databases have limited sensitivity and specificity. It is unlikely that a medication can be determined to be free of risk to the fetus because of the extremely large sample sizes needed to rule out an increased risk of a specific defect.

Surveillance has traditionally been conducted by governmental agencies. The FDA relies on postmarketing surveillance of voluntarily reported adverse events. However, only 10% of these adverse outcomes are likely to be reported. The FDA, CDC and industry have engaged in other surveillance activities as well. The CDC administers a birth defects program, which includes the National Birth Defects

Monitoring Program, and the International Clearing House on Birth Defects. These and other large observational databases, such as Medicaid, provide clues regarding adverse outcomes in an epidemiologically diverse population. Industry can assist in establishing registries to evaluate pregnancy and fetal outcomes after exposure to their drug products. Other methods which can be utilized to capture pregnancy exposures to a drug include use of automated medication databases and case-control surveillance of birth defects, so that hypotheses can be generated regarding associations between medications and specific birth defects. Ultimately only mandatory postmarketing epidemiological safety monitoring can be expected to permit rapid and thorough accumulation of information regarding human exposure to a new drug. Postmarketing pregnancy registries that are easily accessible to health care providers will permit medication-related adverse outcomes to be identified in an appropriately short period of time. Information should be obtained regarding time and duration of exposure, maternal dose, exposure to polytherapy and identification of other variables affecting fetal outcome, including adequacy of prenatal care.

Postconception Counseling

A discussion of the advisability of breastfeeding is part of postconception counseling in the woman receiving a drug. Pharmaceutical compounds concentrate in breast milk in inverse relation to their degree of protein-binding. The higher the protein-bound fraction, the lower the transmission into breast milk. Knowledge of the extent of protein-binding of a new drug permits an estimate of breast milk concentration. Other necessary information needed to provide adequate counseling concerns the concentration of the pharmaceutical in the neonate and the effects of the pharmaceutical in the neonate. Neonatal pharmacokinetics are likely to differ from maternal pharmacokinetics, so that the effective concentration in the neonate will vary depending on the neonate's capacity to metabolize and clear the drug. Finally, any acute or chronic effects on development and behavior after neonatal exposure should be defined. This information would enable the woman to make an informed choice regarding breastfeeding.

Conclusion

New drug development will ideally consider issues relevant to the women who will use that drug. These are likely to include the effects of female physiology on efficacy, tolerability and pharmacokinetics; interactions with steroid hormones and the effects of the drug on reproductive health, including fertility and sexuality; and the consequences of exposing a fetus to the new drug.

These valid scientific concerns must be balanced by society's wish to protect individuals from the potential harm of an untested compound. For women of childbearing potential, these concerns have led to decades of restriction from participation in investigational drug trials. Regulatory agencies have recently revised guidelines to correct what is now viewed as excessive past restrictions. For pregnant and lactating women with any diseases, the proper course of action does not seem clear. Although pregnant and lactating women with disease are likely to take a new drug after release, at present this population is prohibited from inclusion in new drug trials. This policy is currently being re-examined, prompted by input from consumers, regulatory agencies and the Courts.

With the release of a new drug, health care providers begin to define the optimal use in special populations. The more a drug's efficacy and tolerability can be defined in special populations, such as women, the more effectively that drug will be used. This provides the greatest benefit to the pharmaceutical company, the health care provider and, especially, the patient.

REFERENCES

Andrew EB. Use of observational methods to monitor the safety of marketed medications for risks of birth defects. Presented at the Regulated Products and Pregnant Women Workshop, FDA, Crystal City, VA, November 8, 1994.

Annas G. Fetal protection and employment discrimination—the Johnson Controls Case. *N Engl J Med* 1991; **325**: 740–43.

Civil Rights Act of 1964 (as amended), 42 USC section 2000d, *et seq*.

Czeizel AE, Dudas I. Prevention of the first occurrence of neural-tube defects by periconceptional vitamin supplementation. *N Engl J Med* 1992; **327**: 1832–5.

NIH/OPRR (Office for Protection from Research Risks). Protection for human subjects. Title 45: Code of Federal Regulations, part 46, 1991. 46.

DHHS. Additional DHHS protections pertaining to research, development, and related activities involving fetuses, pregnant women, and human in vitro fertilization. Title 45: Code of Federal Regulations, part 46, sub-part B, March 15, 1994.

FDA. *Use-in-pregnancy Drug Categories*, undated. Title 21: Code of Federal Regulations, part 57, (f)(6)(i)(a)–(e).

FDA/DHHS. International Conference on Harmonization; guideline on detection of toxicity to reproduction for medicinal products; availability. *Federal Register* 1994; **59**(183): 48746–52.

FDA/DHHS. Guidelines for the study of and evaluation of gender differences in the clinical evaluation of drugs. *Federal Register* 1993; **58**(139): 39406–16.

FDA. *General Considerations for the Clinical Evaluation of Drugs* 1977; Washington, DC: Government Printing Office (Publication No: HEW(FDA)77-3040).

Flannery EJ. Confronting legal concerns in pregnancy research—the perspective of the company. Presented at the Regulated Products and Pregnant Women Workshop. FDA, Crystal City, VA, November 8, 1994.

Institute of Medicine. *Women and Health Research: Ethical and Legal Issues of Including Women in Clinical Studies* 1994, pp 1–25; Washington, DC: National Academy Press.

International Union, United Automobile, Aerospace and Agricultural Implement Workers. *UAW v. Johnson Controls* 1991; Inc. 111S. Ct. 1196.

MRC (Medical Research Council) Vitamin Research Group. Prevention of neural tube defects: results of the Medical Research Council Vitamin Study. *Lancet* 1991; **338**: 131–7.

Merkatz RB, Temple R, Sobel S, Feiden K. Working Group on Women in Clinical Trials.

Women in clinical trials of new drugs: a change in Food and Drug Administration policy. *N Engl J Med* 1993; **329**: 292–6.

Mino Y, Mizusawa H, Shiota K. Effects of anticonvulsant drugs on fetal mouse palates cultured in vitro. *Reprod Toxicol* 1994; **8**(3): 225–30.

Morrell MJ. Pregnancy and epilepsy. In Porter RJ, Chadwick D (eds) *Epilepsies II* 1996; Boston: Butterworth-Heinemann.

Morell MJ. Issues for women in antiepileptic drug development. In French JA, Leppick I, Dichter MA (eds) *Antiepileptic Drug Development. Advances in Neurology*, Volume 76; 1998, pp 149–60; New York: Lippincott-Raven.

NIH/ADAMHA. *Policy Concerning the Inclusion of Women in Study Populations. NIH Guide for Grants and Contracts* 1990. Washington, DC: ADAMHA.

NIH. NIH guidelines on the inclusion of women and minorities as subjects in clinical research. *Federal Register* 1994; **59**(59): 14508–13.

NIH. *NIH Revitalization Act* 1993. Public Law (Pub.L.) 103–43.

Pregnancy Discrimination Act 1978. 92 Stat. 2076, 42 U.S.C. Sec 2000e (k).

Reisman EK. Products liability—what is the current situation and will it change (and how) when more women are included in studies? Presented at the 'Women in Clinical Trials of FDA-Regulated Products' Workshop. Washington DC: Food and Drug Law Institute, October 5, 1992.

Regan CM, Gorman AMC, Larsson OM et al. In vitro screening for anticonvulsant induced teratogenesis in neural primary cultures and cell lines. *Int J Dev Neurosci* 1990; **8**(2): 143–50.

3

Historical Perspectives on the Development of Reproductive Drugs

Ridgely C. Bennett*

Food and Drug Administration, Rockville, MD, USA

INTRODUCTION

Drug development in the USA is regulated by the Food and Drug Administration (FDA). Prior to 1906 there were no effective laws regulating the use of drugs in the USA. The Pure Food and Drug Act of 1906 became the first legislation attempting to regulate both food and drugs in the USA. This gave the government authority to remove a drug from the market only if it could prove that the drug was misbranded or adulterated. All efforts to strengthen the law failed until a drug tragedy in 1937, the 'elixir of sulfanilamide' episode, in which 107 people died. Public outcry over this tragedy led to enactment of the Federal Food, Drug, and Cosmetic Act (FD&C) of 1938. An important aspect of the 1938 Act was the provision that a new drug could not be marketed until the FDA had received evidence of its safety for its proposed uses. Shortcomings of the 1938 law were apparent soon after its passage. The modern era of drug development for women was marred by the thalidomide tragedy of the 1950s in which serious birth defects occurred in newborn babies. In response to this devastating occurrence, the Kefauver–Harris Amendments to the FD&C Act were enacted in 1962, requiring that drugs must be found to be effective as well as safe for their intended uses before approval. The development of birth control pills and fertility drugs are good examples of the continuing development of drugs for women that are not only safe but highly effective and very beneficial. They are also good examples of the careful monitoring of new drugs that the FDA performs on an ongoing basis. These drugs have improved immensely the lives of millions of women worldwide.

---

* This chapter was written by Ridgely C. Bennett, MD, MPH, in his private capacity. No official support or endorsement by the Food and Drug Administration is intended or should be inferred.

Drug Development for Women. Edited by V.V. Ragavan. © 1998 John Wiley & Sons Ltd.

This chapter provides a perspective on some of the highlights of drug development for women in the USA, using as examples several drugs that have played critical roles in the regulatory process. The majority of the chapter uses the evolution of oral contraceptives as an important paradigm of drug development. For more than four decades, oral contraceptives have played a major role in control of the incredible growth of the world population. Basic science and clinical investigation now in progress will result in the development of many new and exciting drug therapies unique to women that will be marketed by the year 2000.

DRUG APPROVAL PROCESS

Drug development and approval are carefully regulated in the USA by the FDA, an agency of the Department of Health and Human Services. The FD&C Act and implementing regulations for the investigational use of new drugs require the FDA to regulate the clinical (human) testing of new drugs. Since 1962 the Act has required that before a new drug may be introduced into interstate commerce, the FDA must approve it for safety and efficacy. Before that time there was no requirement that the FDA be notified when drugs were tested on humans or that a new drug be proven effective for its intended use. The Act defines a new drug as any drug not generally recognized, among qualified experts, as safe and effective for use under the conditions prescribed and as recommended or suggested in the drug's labeling. A new drug may be an entirely new substance, a marketed drug in a new formulation, or a marketed drug being proposed for a new use (i.e. a use for which the drug is not approved).

The development of new drugs, which can be undertaken by a drug firm, a Federal agency, or an independent investigator (all referred to as sponsors), usually begins with the screening of large numbers of chemical compounds in laboratory animals for possible therapeutic activity. The sponsor then selects a few of the most promising compounds for further study and submits an investigational new drug (IND) application to the FDA to begin clinical testing of the compound in humans. The sponsor must demonstrate the safety and efficacy of a new drug product through closely controlled clinical tests. After completing the animal and clinical tests, the sponsor may file with the FDA a New Drug Application (NDA), which, if approved, permits the sponsor to market the drug. The NDA contains: (a) full reports of investigations, including animal and clinical investigations, that have been made to show whether the drug is safe and effective; (b) a statement of the drug's composition; (c) a description of the methods used in, and the facilities and controls for, the manufacturing, processing and packaging of the drug; (d) samples of the drug and components as may be required; and (e) a copy of the proposed labeling.

All NDAs are reviewed by scientists in the FDA's Center for Drug Evaluation and Research. This Center is composed of divisions which review NDAs. Each of the divisions is responsible for evaluating drugs in a particular therapeutic class or for use in a particular organ system. To review the data submitted, the FDA uses a team made up of: (a) a medical officer, who reviews the clinical test results; (b) a pharmacologist, who reviews the animal test results; and (c) a chemist, who reviews the chemistry and manufacturing controls and processes. The review team may also be supported by a biopharmaceutic specialist, a microbiologist and a statistician, and is coordinated administratively by a project manager. The medical officer is responsible for coordinating the team's activities as its scientific leader and assumes the demanding burden of evaluating the adequacy of the studies submitted by the sponsor. As required by the FD&C Act, within 180 days after a NDA is filed, the FDA must approve the application or give the applicant notice of an opportunity for a hearing on the deficiencies found. The FDA may take longer than 180 days to decide on an application if the applicant and the FDA agree to an additional period of time.

In the review and processing of a NDA the medical officer evaluating the submitted data must consider and face many problems. In the applications that are submitted it is expected that there will be presented full reports of adequate tests by all methods reasonably applicable, and they should contain detailed data derived from appropriate animal and other biological experiments in which the methods used and the results obtained are clearly set forth. Full reports of all clinical tests, by experts qualified by scientific training and experience to evaluate the safety and effectiveness of drugs, should be submitted and should include detailed information pertaining to each individual treated, including age, sex, conditions treated, dosage and frequency of administration, duration of administration of the drug, results of clinical and laboratory examinations made, and a full statement of any adverse effects and therapeutic results observed. The kind and extent of information that is required will depend on several factors, such as the nature of the drug and its indication for use. This must be determined individually for each new drug or class of drug.

A limited number of generic drug products have been available for many years (Nightingale & Morrison, 1987) The most recent piece of landmark legislation affecting the US drug review and approval process has been the Drug Competition and Patent Term Restoration Act of 1984 (Waxman–Hatch Act). These amendments to the FD&C Act were motivated almost entirely by economic considerations. The 1984 amendments created an abbreviated mechanism for the approval of generic copies of drug products first approved for safety and efficacy after 1962. The 1984 bill provided a clear regulatory mandate to allow generic substitution and publicly affirmed the FDA's position that duplicative, costly and ethically questionable preclinical and clinical tests did not have to be repeated for each generic product.

The 1984 Waxman–Hatch amendments to the FD&C Act required that a firm demonstrate to the FDA that its product is the same as that of the corresponding innovator drug (the listed drug) in terms of active ingredient(s), strength, dosage form, and route of administration. In addition, the applicant must demonstrate that the labeling of its proposed generic version is comparable to that of the innovator product and that the generic product is bioequivalent to the reference listed drug. For all requirements except those related to safety and efficacy, the regulatory requirements relative to the review and approval of a generic product in the USA are essentially the same as those of an innovator product.

Bioequivalence testing based on pharmacokinetic principles is a comparatively new and evolving science. Consequently, the current methodology employed in the design and evaluation of bioequivalence trials can be expected to continue to improve, as has been the case with safety and effectiveness trials. The FDA makes every effort to keep its procedures current with 'state-of-the-art' technology and knowledge.

All 50 states have now repealed the antisubstitution laws enacted in the 1940s and 1950s that prohibited alternative dispensing of prescription drug products. Approaches to generic substitution, called drug product selection in all of the state statutes, vary from state to state. No state, however, takes away from the physician the prerogative to limit or prohibit drug product selection.

DIETHYLSTILBESTROL (DES)

The modern era of drug development for women began over 60 years ago when estrogens were first prescribed for menopausal symptoms about 1932. They were administered intramuscularly. Orally effective estrogens became available later, ethinyl estradiol in 1940 and conjugated estrogens in 1942. Large doses of DES were prescribed to treat threatened abortion, habitual abortion, and pregnancy complicated by diabetes in the late 1940s, 1950s and 1960s. It is estimated that 3 million pregnant women in the USA received DES before a serious problem associated with its use was detected and reported for the first time in 1971 by Herbst, Ulfelder & Poskanzer (1971). From their studies the authors concluded that maternal ingestion of DES during pregnancy appears to increase the risk of vaginal adenocarcinoma developing years later in the offspring exposed. The authors studied eight cases of adenocarcinoma of the vagina in patients born between 1946 and 1951. The malignancies were identified and treated between 1966 and 1969. In seven of the eight cases, there was a history of maternal use of DES. Because this type of malignancy in young girls had rarely been reported previously, the authors conducted a retrospective investigation in an attempt to find factors that may be associated with such malignancy in this age group. Four matched controls were established for each patient and the data obtained were subjected to statistical analysis. A statistically significant relationship was observed for three variables: DES given during pregnancy ($p = 0.00001$); bleeding in that pregnancy ($p =$ less than 0.05); and prior pregnancy loss ($p =$ less than 0.01). It is obvious that the most significant of the variables is the exposure to DES in utero.

After publication of this study, five additional cases of this malignancy associated with the maternal use of DES were reported by Greenwald and associates (Greenwald, 1971). In 1971 a 'Registry of Clear Cell Adenocarcinoma of the

Genital Tract' was established by Herbst, Scully & Ulfelder. The Registry was renamed the 'Registry for the Research on Transplacental Carcinogenesis'. By January of 1979, 346 women with clear cell adenocarcinoma of the vagina and cervix had been registered. Two-thirds of the registered women gave a history of in utero exposure to a non-steroidal estrogen such as DES. However, the actual risk of clear cell adenocarcinoma occurring in exposed offspring is very slight (0.14–1.4 per 1000).

Several benign abnormalities of the vagina and cervix in offspring exposed in utero to DES have also been reported. The DES syndrome consists of a characteristic change in the vagina (adenosis), the cervix ('cockscomb', 'hood', or ectropion) and the uterus (T-shaped, hypoplastic cavity). An increased incidence of infertility, spontaneous abortion, and premature labor is associated with the DES syndrome. Offspring exposed in utero to DES should be examined periodically for evidence of clear cell adenocarcinoma of the vagina and cervix.

DES is no longer prescribed for use in pregnancy. Thus, this public health problem will eventually be completely eliminated. DES has, however, in the past been prescribed in large doses as a postcoital contraceptive. It is effective when administered within 72 hours after unprotected mid-cycle sexual exposure. Nausea and vomiting occur frequently with this regimen and may render the treatment ineffective. It is not a preferred postcoital contraceptive method.

THALIDOMIDE

Another drug of historical note is thalidomide. Clinical trials of thalidomide for spasmolytic, local anesthetic, and anticonvulsive effects started in 1954 in Europe. It was marketed under the tradename 'Grippex' in 1956 and 'Contergan' in 1957 in West Germany. The first known 'thalidomide child' was born on Christmas day, 1956 (Lenz, 1988). The female child had no ears. Another 'thalidomide child' was born in 1957 and 24 more in 1958—all in the Federal Republic of Germany. The thalidomide tragedy epidemic was now conspicuous, and it closely followed the monthly sales figures by a distance of about 7–8 months. Thalidomide was introduced in Sweden in September 1958 and the Swedish epidemic started in late 1959. It was introduced in Brazil in March 1959 and the Brazilian epidemic followed in 1960.

A NDA for thalidomide was submitted to the US Food and Drug Administration in September 1960 (Kelsey, 1988). Deficiencies were found in the original application and in several resubmissions. Of particular concern was the report of peripheral neuritis as a side effect, which was not always completely reversible. There was also a lack of data relative to safe use in pregnancy. Before these concerns were resolved, the sponsor notified the FDA in November 1961 that thalidomide had been withdrawn from the market in Germany because of reports that it had a teratogenic effect. It was also withdrawn from the market in Brazil and Japan in 1962.

The FDA received a very clear account in April 1962 of the association of thalidomide and birth defects from the late Dr Helen Taussig, of Johns Hopkins University, who had just returned from a trip to West Germany where she had studied the situation at first hand.

The FD&C Act of 1938 was adequate to prevent the marketing of thalidomide in the USA, but the thalidomide experience hastened its amendment in October 1962, when it was revealed that, rather than the 60 or so investigators that the FDA originally believed had received thalidomide for testing purposes, over 1200 physicians had actually received the drug. Ten cases of birth defects associated with the investigative use of thalidomide in the USA, as well as seven cases in which the drug had been obtained abroad, were discovered.

The 1962 amendments and the 1963 investigational drug regulations have not impeded well-designed and properly controlled clinical studies of thalidomide. In 1963 an IND was submitted for the use of thalidomide in the treatment of cancer. In 1965, investigational exemptions were requested to permit clinical trials in Hansen's disease. The US Public Health Service in Carville continues to sponsor studies with the drug for erythema nodosum leprosum. Individual sponsor–investigator INDs have also been submitted for the use of thalidomide in a number of rare dermatologic diseases unresponsive to alternative medication.

Every effort is made to preclude pregnancy in women receiving thalidomide and the consent form warns women of the teratologic potential of the drug. Thalidomide currently is being used to prevent graft vs. host disease and transplant rejection under an orphan drug designation.

BIRTH CONTROL PILLS

Much of this chapter is devoted to a discussion of the development of the birth control pill. This is because the development of the birth control pill is one of the major milestones in women's health improvements. It has had a profound effect on the control of the rate of growth of the human population which, if uncontrolled, has the potential to be the greatest danger to all mankind. Birth control is the most important problem that the medical profession has to solve. A prolonged discussion of the development of the birth control pill is used also to give the reader an example of how the FDA monitors a drug from its inception to the present—in this case a period of almost 50 years.

Birth control practice is today regarded by a substantial and influential majority of doctors as an important element in preventive medicine and the provision of contraceptive advice an appropriate activity for the medical practitioner. Millions of women throughout the world now take birth control pills, realizing that they are a safe, highly effective contraceptive method.

Contraception is far from being a new entity. In societies of antiquity contraceptive knowledge had a written basis in texts which formed a continuous medical tradition, beginning with the works of Aristotle in the fourth century BC.

Hippocrates is known to have had a recipe for an oral contraceptive. The modern history of oral contraceptives began in the early 1950s, when independent investigators began to develop new orally active steroids. In 1956 Drs Rock, Ramon-Garcia & Pincus published their paper demonstrating contraceptive effectiveness of an oral sex steroid. The first clinical trials of oral contraceptives were begun and in November 1959 the FDA approved the first oral contraceptive. For the first time in history, reversible contraception that was virtually 100% effective was made possible. The oral contraceptive pill thus became one of the most significant advances of modern science. The increasingly widespread use of these compounds has presented society with problems unique in the history of human therapeutics, since continuing use for periods of 20 years and more is commonplace. Never will so many people have taken such potent drugs voluntarily over such a protracted period for an objective other than for the control of disease.

In view of the widespread use of pills it is to be expected that many diseases, common as well as rare, to which women in general are subject, will also be encountered among oral contraceptive users. When, in a woman using oral contraceptives, such disease becomes manifest, there is naturally a tendency to assume that this is a consequence of the treatment. Unless the biological mechanism of a side effect has been established, it is essential when evaluating the possible harmfulness of oral contraceptives to take into account the incidence of the side effect in comparable women who do not use these agents. Thus, a cause-and-effect relationship should only be accepted when the side effect is encountered significantly more frequently among oral contraceptive users than among non-users, or when adequate experimental data confirm such a relationship. Failure to do this by either method has been all too conspicuous in many isolated reports of various side effects occurring among women using oral contraceptives, although the possible 'early warning' value of such reports is not denied. Perhaps it should be emphasized that epidemiological observations can provide evidence of associations, but can rarely prove causation. Three factors must always be borne in mind. First, many side effects that occur in pill users also occur in women who have never used an oral contraceptive. Second, in most instances the degree of risk can only be determined approximately, thus reducing the evidential value of the results. Third, the risks described in the results vary considerably in degree from one disease to another.

Whenever drugs are administered to healthy persons for experimental or prophylactic purposes, great concern is appropriately expressed about possible side effects. When such drugs are administered to millions of people, even a low incidence of serious side effects may become an important health problem. Such is the case with oral contraceptives. These agents, initially demonstrated in animal and human trials to be remarkably safe, have now after 3½ decades of use by patients been demonstrated to have many minor and a few serious, some of them life-threatening, side effects. It should be emphasized that the possible statistical increase in life-threatening side effects in women without predisposing risk factors is very low.

Probably the most talked-about side effect, the most serious side effect and the one with the longest history, is thromboembolism. To ensure virtually 100% efficacy, the first oral contraceptive pills, marketed in 1960, contained as much as 150 μg of estrogen and high doses of a progestational agent. It is interesting to know how the establishment of an increased risk of thromboembolic disorders with higher estrogen content of oral contraceptives came about, the regulatory steps the FDA enacted as new facts emerged, and the impact on public health subsequent progressively decreased usage of high-estrogen-dose oral contraceptives has had, so that oral contraceptives currently available on the market are remarkably safe as well as effective.

The first suspicion that oral contraceptives might predispose women toward vascular occlusive phenomena arose in 1961, when Dr W. M. Jordan, a general practitioner in Suffolk, England, published the first report in the medical literature of a patient developing a thromboembolic disorder while taking an oral contraceptive. Similar case reports followed. An ad hoc FDA Committee in 1963 found, as yet, no definite evidence to incriminate oral contraceptives with the production of thromboembolism. Isolated case reports continued to be reported. It became evident that an epidemiologic study was urgently needed to specifically study this possible link. The FDA awarded such a contract in 1965 to Dr Philip E. Sartwell of the Johns Hopkins University School of Hygiene and Public Health. The FDA also asked its newly established Obstetrics and Gynecology Advisory Committee, in 1965, to evaluate the available individual case reports. The Advisory Committee, in 1966, as well as a World Health Organization (WHO) Scientific Group, independently found no evidence incriminating oral contraceptives with the production of thromboembolism. Beginning in 1967, however, there appeared several reports, all from Britain, which strongly indicated a relationship between oral contraceptives and thromboembolism. The first of these was carried out by selected members of the Royal College of General Practitioners, who reported on 147 women from their practices with thromboembolic disease (mostly superficial venous thrombosis) and 294 controls. The risk of venous thrombosis was estimated to be increased nearly threefold among users of oral contraceptives (Royal College of General Practitioners, 1967).

Also, a study of women who had fatal attacks of pulmonary, cerebral and coronary thrombosis and embolism in the year 1966 was made by Inman & Vessey (1968). Among 26 idiopathic cases of pulmonary embolism, there was a clear excess of users of oral contraceptives over the number expected from the experience of control women. In 49 cases where predisposing conditions existed, there was a small, statistically insignificant excess. For cerebral thrombosis, there was again an association with oral contraceptives, limited to patients without predisposing conditions. Findings for coronary thrombosis were conflicting.

The most significant study was that of Vessey & Doll (1968). They interviewed 87 women with idiopathic deep vein thrombosis or pulmonary embolism, 19 of cerebral thrombosis, and 17 of coronary thrombosis. They interviewed two matched controls per case with other diseases. Large differences between cases and controls in the proportions having used oral contraceptives within one month before onset were found for the thromboembolism and cerebral thrombosis series, but none for the coronary thrombosis series.

Also, in 1967, the FDA Obstetrics and Gynecology Advisory Committee advised that prospective, as well as retrospective, studies of the side effects of oral contraceptives were needed. The FDA then helped provide the impetus to the National Institute of Child Health and Human Development (NICHD) to fund a long-term prospective study. Accordingly, in 1968, the Kaiser Foundation Research Institute contracted with the NICHD to set up this study, which came to be called the Walnut Creek Contraceptive Drug Study. On May 10 1968, the FDA declared that the results of the British studies demonstrating the relationship between the use of oral contraceptives and thromboembolic episodes must be included in labeling for all oral contraceptives.

Subsequently, in November 1969, Dr Sartwell published the results of his FDA sponsored study in the *American Journal of Epidemiology* (Sartwell et al, 1969). Cases were 175 women aged 15–44, discharged alive from the hospital after initial attacks of idiopathic thrombophlebitis, pulmonary embolism, or cerebral thrombosis or embolism. The 175 controls were matched pairwise with the cases. There were 57 case-control pairs in which only the cases had used an oral contraceptive within one month of admission compared to 13 in which only the control had done so. The relative risk of thromboembolism for oral contraceptive users was estimated to be 4.4 times that of non-users. In addition to reporting a positive association between oral contraceptives and thromboembolism, Dr Sartwell also reported that, in general, the results of his study supported the opinion that oral contraceptives of high estrogenic activity and low progestational activity were the most strongly associated with thromboembolism, while those with low estrogenic activity and high progestational activity were the least associated with thromboembolism.

On November 14 1969, the FDA revised its class labeling for oral contraceptives to include a sentence stating that, 'An increased risk of thromboembolic disease associated with the use of hormonal contraceptives has now been shown in studies conducted in both Great Britain and the United States'.

In early January 1970, the FDA was made aware of the fact that the British Committee on Safety of Drugs was recommending the use of oral contraceptives containing 50 μg or less of estrogen because, based on an analysis of data derived from national adverse reaction reporting systems in the UK, Sweden and Denmark, they had concluded that the risk of thromboembolism, including coronary thrombosis, was directly related to the dose of estrogen present in the oral contraceptive. Preparations containing 100 μg or more of estrogen were associated with a higher risk of thromboembolism than those containing 50–80 μg of estrogen. On January 12 1970, this information was transmitted to every physician in the USA in the form of a 'Dear Doctor' letter from the FDA. The article that provided the basis for this action was published in the *British Medical Journal* on April 25 1970 by Inman et al (1970). This information was also mandated for all oral contraceptive physician labeling and for the very first time ever, the FDA required patient labeling, in lay language, which informed patients of the risks of oral contraceptives.

The day before publication of the Inman et al (1970) article, the FDA issued a Current Drug Information bulletin to every practicing physician in the USA on the subject of 'Oral contraceptives and thromboembolic disorders'. Based on the various studies mentioned, as well as on studies and clinical experience implicating estrogen itself in causing an increase in the risk of thromboembolic disorders when used for purposes other than contraceptives, the FDA's position was summarized as follows:

1. Use of oral contraceptives increases the risk of thromboembolic disorders.
2. There is evidence that estrogens per se increase the risk of thromboembolic disorders.
3. Data are inadequate to delineate differences between specific products, but indicate a trend toward increased risk of thromboembolic disorders with higher estrogen dosage.
4. Good therapeutics would indicate the use of the lowest effective dose of estrogen that is otherwise acceptable.

In the bulletin, the FDA also mentioned that they and others were currently conducting studies to further elucidate and quantitate the risks involved with the use of various types of oral contraceptives. The studies referred to were the Walnut Creek Contraceptive Drug Study, which started recruiting subjects in December 1968, and the Stolley et al study, which began in 1970. In addition, the FDA had by now approved highly effective oral contraceptives containing only 35 μg or less of estrogen.

An interim report of the Walnut Creek study, entitled 'A prospective study of the side effects of oral contraceptives', was subsequently published in monograph form in January 1981, and the Stolley study was subsequently published in 1975 (Stolley et al, 1975).

In 1974, the Royal College of General Practitioners published an interim report of their ongoing prospective study involving 46 000 women. They reported that the attributable risk of deep thrombosis was 80/100 000 pill users/year with the 50 μg estrogen preparations, and was 112/100 000 users/year with preparations containing more than 50 μg of estrogen. Therefore, the attributable risk decreased 29% upon using a lower estrogen dose.

Stolley et al (1975) reported that the risk of thrombosis for women using oral contraceptives containing 100 μg or more of estrogen was higher than for users of lower doses. He reported a relative risk of 4.7 in women using oral contraceptives containing less than 100 μg of estrogen and a relative risk of 10.1 in women using higher doses.

Based on the Inman et al (1970) and Stolley et al (1975) reports, the FDA in early 1977 mandated that all oral contraceptive labeling contain a section entitled 'Dose-related risk of thromboembolism from oral contraceptives', which stated:

Two studies have shown a positive association between the dose of estrogens in oral contraceptives and the risk of thromboembolism. For this reason, it is prudent and in keeping with good principles of therapeutics to minimize exposure to estrogen. The oral contraceptive product prescribed for any given patient should be that product which contains the least amount of estrogen that is compatible with an acceptable pregnancy rate and patient acceptance. It is recommended that new acceptors of oral contraceptives be started on preparations containing 0.5 mg or less of estrogen.

At the same time the FDA also mandated that a statement appear in the Warnings section titled 'Risk of Dose', which stated:

In an analysis of data derived from several national adverse reaction reporting systems, British investigators concluded that the risk of thromboembolism including coronary thrombosis is directly related to the dose of estrogen used in oral contraceptives. Preparations containing 100 micrograms or more of estrogen were associated with a higher risk of thromboembolism than those containing 50–80 micrograms of estrogen. This finding has been confirmed in the United States.

In May 1980, two new papers appeared in the literature. Meade, Greenberg & Thompson (1980) reported that oral contraceptives with 30 μg of estrogen were associated with significantly fewer reports of venous death and ischemic heart disease than those with 50 μg of estrogen. Also, Bottiger et al (1980) reported that since the disappearance of high-dose oral contraceptives in Sweden, morbidity due to thromboembolism seemed to have fallen, and the number of thromboembolic incidents reported to the Swedish Adverse Drug Reaction Committee decreased dramatically.

Prescriptions for oral contraceptives containing more than 50 μg of estrogen decreased in the USA from 65% of the market in 1970 when the FDA first recommended use of the lowest effective dose, to 17% of the market in 1980. In October 1980, the FDA asked its Obstetrics and Gynecology Advisory Committee its views regarding the continued marketing of oral contraceptives containing higher amounts of estrogen. The Committee expressed its concern about the published reports suggesting an association between thromboembolism and estrogen dose. However, it was their opinion that the data were inconclusive to indicate that higher dose pills were less safe than those containing lesser amounts of estrogen. They recommended that all doses of oral contraceptives remain on the market, but that the labeling should indicate that four studies now had shown a possible association between the dose of estrogen in oral contraceptives and the risk of thromboembolism, and reaffirmed that the lowest effective dose should be used except when a higher dose was specifically indicated. The FDA followed the advice of its advisory committee.

In 1983, staff from the FDA Division of Drug Experience published an article in the *American Journal of Epidemiology* entitled, 'Relationship of oral contraceptive estrogen dose to age' (Van De Carr et al, 1983). The authors reported that women aged 35–39 were more than twice as likely to be recipients of contraceptives containing more than 50 μg of estrogen than women aged 15–19. There was an increase in the proportion of high-dose estrogen recipients among oral contraceptive recipients for each successive 5-year age group from 15–19 to 35–39 years. The authors concluded that, given the recognition of the hazard associated with higher-dose estrogen oral contraceptives, it seemed inappropriate that older premenopausal women should have the highest rates of exposure to high-dose pills. It was pointed out that this use pattern might contribute to a preventable excess of cardiovascular disease among older users of oral contraceptives. This study was based on 1980 use data, when high-dose pills constituted 17% of the market. By 1983, when the article was published, high-dose pills constituted 9% of the market.

Were the attempts of the FDA to educate physicians and patients via professional medical meetings, package inserts, patient labeling, 'Dear Doctor' letters, and *Current Drug Information* bulletins, successful? Yes, they were. The use of preparations containing more than 50 μg of estrogen decreased from 65% of the market in 1970, when the FDA first recommended use of products containing the lowest effective dose of estrogen, to 3.4% of the market in 1986. This translates to a reduction in the use of high-estrogen-dose pills from 7.5 million women in 1970 to 400 000 women in 1986.

It has been reported that a decrease in the estrogen content of oral contraceptives from 100 or 150 μg to 30 μg is accompanied by a decrease in the risk of myocardial infarction and stroke of 80%. This means that in 1986 alone, 200 deaths in the USA from myocardial infarction attributable to oral contraceptive use were prevented in women aged 30–39 years by using low-estrogen-dose pills. It also means that in 1986 alone, over 3700 cases of deep venous thrombosis in the USA attributable to oral contraceptive use were prevented by using low-estrogen-dose pills.

A pharmacy survey conducted in 1986 indicated that of the 400 000 women still using high-estrogen-dose pills, 200 000 were using pills containing 100 μg of estrogen and an additional 200 000 were using pills containing 80 μg of estrogen. Staff from FDA's Division of Drug Experience had already published an article in the *American Journal of Epidemiology* entitled 'Relationship of oral contraceptive estrogen dose to age' (Van De Carr et al, 1983), in which it was pointed out that women aged 35–39 were more than twice as likely to be recipients of high-estrogen-dose pills than women aged 15–19. The risk of myocardial infarction and stroke that is attributable to oral contraceptive use is primarily concentrated among older women. Given the hazards associated with higher-dose-estrogen oral contraceptives, it seemed inappropriate and unsafe for older, higher-risk premenopausal women to have the highest rates of exposure to high-dose pills. The 3.4% of women still taking high-dose estrogen pills represented a very significant minority of women at needless risk of thromboembolism, coronary infarction and stroke, since lower-estrogen-dose pills were just as effective in preventing pregnancy as the higher-estrogen-dose pills and were safer.

The FDA believed that the higher-estrogen-dose pills should be withdrawn quickly from the market. On January 15 1988, at a day-long public advisory committee meeting, the FDA's advisory committee also agreed that contraceptive pills containing more than 50 μg of estrogen should be withdrawn from the market.

However, the FDA lacks the legal authority to withdraw approved drugs from the market unless there is a finding of an imminent hazard to the public health or a finding that the drug is unsafe for use for the condition for which it is approved, and then only after affording the drug companies due legal process. Knowing that the legal process by the Agency of withdrawing these products from the market could take many years, the FDA was of the opinion that the Agency could be successful in persuading the three involved drug companies to quickly, voluntarily, withdraw the high-dose products from the market. Some public citizen health groups insisted that previous attempts by the Agency at voluntary withdrawals had never worked and insisted that the Agency should immediately begin the legal process that could possibly eventually ban the products. The Agency was successful, however, in persuading the three involved drug companies not only to agree to withdraw their high-dose pills from the market, but to do so in a very timely fashion. Two-and-a-half months after the January 15 meeting, two of the three companies had announced the withdrawal of these products and 2 weeks later the third drug company also complied. This was the first time in the history of the FDA that three drug companies had voluntarily withdrawn seven products from the market—and in less than 90 days. Securing the quick withdrawal of high-dose-estrogen oral contraceptives from the market was a major public health contribution that protected the health of an additional 400 000 women in the USA from the serious and potentially fatal dangers of high-estrogen-dose pills. In addition, the Agency conserved precious time and valuable resources, including manpower, money, material, equipment, and possibly even reputation, in resolving this issue, which otherwise would have been a complex, time-consuming, expensive process.

FDA regulation has resulted in the prevention of hundreds of deaths each year by reducing the incidence of thromboembolism, myocardial infarction and stroke in women using oral contraceptives.

In addition to lowering the amounts of estrogens and progestogens in oral contraceptives, three newer progestins in birth control pills have been developed in recent years. These progestins are norgestimate, desogestrel and gestodene. These third generation progestins were developed with the hope that, being less androgenic, they would reduce the incidence of weight gain, acne, hirsutism, and adverse changes in lipoprotein and carbohydrate metabolism. They are viewed as more 'selective' than other progestins in that they are less androgenic at doses that inhibit ovulation. Oral contraceptives containing norgestimate and desogestrel are marketed in the USA and Europe. Gestodene is also marketed in Europe but not, as yet, in the USA.

In December 1995, the results of three epidemiological studies on the safety of oral contraceptives in relation to venous thromboembolism were published in *The Lancet* (WHO, 1995a, b); Jick et al, 1995). Taken together, these studies provided reassurance about thromboembolic risks associated with oral contraceptives containing older progestins (levonorgestrel, norethisterone or ethynodiol). For these products, the excess risk of thromboembolism in users was around 5–10 cases per 100 000 women per year. The three new studies all indicated that combined oral contraceptives containing desogestrel and gestodene were associated with about a two-fold increase in the risk of thromboembolism, compared with those containing older progestins.

It is interesting to see how this information was handled around the world. The WHO Steering Committee of the Human Reproduction Program Task Force for Epidemiological Research in Reproductive Health advised that, until further information becomes available, low-estrogen-dose oral contraceptives containing progestogens other than desogestrel and gestodene may be preferred. The Committee on Safety of Medicines in the UK advised that combined oral contraceptives containing gestodene or desogestrel should only be used by women who are intolerant to other combined oral contraceptives and prepared to accept an increased risk of thromboembolism, and should not be used by women with risk factors for venous thromboembolism, including obesity, varicose veins or a previous history of thrombosis from any cause. Germany's Federal Drug Institute said that oral contraceptives containing desogestrel or gestodene could no longer be prescribed to women under 30 years of age who are taking oral contraceptives for the first time. The FDA did not recommend that women using the desogestrel products (gestodene is not marketed in the USA) stop using them or change to another oral contraceptive, but advised women who are taking these products to discuss them with their health care provider and make an informed choice based on benefits, risks and individual preference.

Fortunately, the risk of thromboembolism attributed to older low-dose pills and to newer low-dose pills is less than that of a woman in the year of a pregnancy, and the mortality associated with venous thromboembolic disease is 2%. Thus, the birth control pill remains a relatively safe method of contraception.

INFERTILITY DRUGS

Infertility is a condition with unique and profound psychological and emotional impacts. Advances in reproductive endocrinology have made ovulation induction one of the most successful means of treating infertility. It is estimated that at least 14% of American couples of reproductive age who desire pregnancy are infertile and unable to conceive in one year.

It is estimated that 25% of involuntary sterility in women is caused by anovulation or oligo-ovulation. Since the early 1920s, many empirical methods have been used to induce ovulation, generally with little success. The turning point in treatment of this disorder came in the late 1950s and early 1960s, with the introduction of *clomiphene citrate*, which now makes it possible to treat successfully many women whose infertility is caused by anovulation.

A furor erupted in 1967, when the FDA recommended approval of clomiphene citrate for induction of ovulation in anovulatory women who wished to become pregnant. The furor was much like that which occured in 1996 and 1997 about the topic of cloning. Congressmen demanded to know why such a potent drug was being approved that would make women pregnant who could not become pregnant naturally. Such a powerful drug could not be safe, they said. Front page articles appeared in newspapers across the country with headlines such as 'Antisterility Drug Release Questioned' and 'FDA Drug Clearance Questioned in the House'. The FDA, fortunately, was able to dispel the fears on Capitol Hill, and one of the most valuable drugs to be developed for women was approved.

Clomiphene citrate is an orally administered, non-steroidal agent, which may induce ovulation in anovulatory women in appropriately selected cases. Clomiphene is a drug of considerable pharmacologic potency. Its administration should be preceded by careful evaluation and selection of the patient, and must be accompanied by close attention to the timing of the dose. While its mechanism of action is not fully understood, it is thought to compete with endogenous estrogens in the hypothalamus and pituitary for estrogen-binding receptors and thereby disrupt the normal estrogen-controlled negative feedback release of gonadotropin-releasing hormone (GnRH).

This action augments the secretion and release of follicle-stimulating hormone (FSH) and luteinizing hormone (LH) and results in ovarian stimulation. When clomiphene is administered to anovulatory women, presumptive signs of ovulation are induced in most appropriately selected patients.

The ovulatory response to cyclic clomiphene therapy appears to be mediated through increased output of pituitary gonadotropins, which in turn stimulate the maturation and endocrine activity of the ovarian follicle and the subsequent development and function of the corpus luteum. The role of the pituitary is indicated by increased urinary excretion of gonadotropins and response of the ovary, as manifested by increased urinary estrogen excretion.

To date, clomiphene citrate is the medication of choice and mainstay of therapy for ovulation induction in suitable patients because of its relative safety, efficacy, simple mode of administration (oral) and relatively low cost. The primary indication for the use of clomiphene citrate is ovulation induction in patients with adequate levels of estrogen and normal levels of FSH and prolactin. Patients with inappropriate gonadotropin release (with an increased ratio of LH to FSH), as occurs in polycystic ovary syndrome, are also candidates for therapy. In contrast, women with abnormally low levels of FSH and estrogen generally do not respond to clomiphene.

Although a wide range of figures has been reported, approximately 80% of well-selected patients can be expected to ovulate following treatment with clomiphene citrate. However, only about 40% of these patients ultimately become pregnant.

Human menopausal gonadotropins (hMG) consist of 75 or 150 IU each of LH and FSH per ampule. Urofollitrophin consists of 75 or 150 IU of human FSH per ampule with negligible amounts (less than 1 IU per 75 IU FSH) of LH activity. Gonadotropins promote follicle growth and maturation as evidenced by increasing estradiol secretion and follicle size. They are the medications of choice for women with low levels of estrogen and gonadotropins. They may also be useful in patients who do not ovulate with clomiphene citrate therapy.

The success of gonadotropin therapy is related to the patient's diagnosis and age. Women with low levels of estrogen and gonadotropins fare better in nearly every series than those with normal levels of estrogen and gonadotropins. The cumulative pregnancy rate for the former group is up to 90% for women ages 35 and younger, with lower rates noted for older individuals. Pregnancy rates for women with normal levels of estrogen and gonadotropins are substantially lower (30–40% or less).

Purified urofollitrophin, which is a better characterized product, is now available and can be administered by the subcutaneous route as well as by the intramuscular route as used by urofollitrophin. Recombinant FSH products may be available in the near future.

Bromocriptine mesylate is a semisynthetic ergot alkaloid with dopamine receptor agonist activity. It reduces the size of prolactin-producing pituitary tumors which are associated with anovulation. Bromocriptine is the treatment of choice for ovulation induction in patients with prolactin-producing pituitary adenomas. In some amenorrheic women, an elevated level of prolactin appears to be the causative factor of anovulation. Bromocriptine inhibits the secretion of prolactin in humans, with little or no effect on other pituitary hormones, except in patients with acromegaly, where it lowers elevated blood levels of growth hormone in the majority of patients. In about 75% of cases of amenorrhea and galactorrhea, bromocriptine suppresses the galactorrhea completely, or almost completely, and reinstates normal ovulatory menstrual cycles. Menses are usually reinstated prior to complete suppression of galactorrhea, the time for this on average being 6–8 weeks. Some patients respond, however, within a few days and others may take up to 8 months. Galactorrhea may take longer to control, depending on the degree of stimulation of the mammary tissue prior to therapy. At least a 75% reduction in secretion is usually observed after 8–12 weeks. Some patients may fail to respond even after 12 months of therapy.

Every effort should be made to use the minimal effective dose of bromocriptine, as judged by the establishment of normal circulating levels of prolactin and by the resumption of normal menstrual cyclicity. The initial dose of 1.25 mg/day, orally, may be increased weekly in 1.25 mg increments. Dosages greater than 15 mg/day are seldom required.

In 1980, bromocriptine was also approved for the prevention of physiological lactation. By 1987 it was estimated that three to four million women had received bromocriptine for this indication. During this period the sponsoring drug company received 50 reports of hypertension, which sometimes occurred at the initiation of therapy, but which were often detected during the second week of therapy, 38 reports of seizures, both with and without hypertension, occurring up to 14 days after initiation of treatment, and 15 reports of stroke, mostly in post-partum patients whose prenatal and obstetrical course had been uncomplicated. Although the available evidence was insufficient to establish a causal relationship, the drug company nevertheless modified the package insert in several ways in August 1987, in an attempt to provide for safer use of the drug for the prevention of post-partum lactation. The Fertility and Maternal Health Drugs Advisory Committee to the FDA advised the Agency in 1988 that drugs should not be used routinely to suppress lactation. This indication was subsequently withdrawn by the sponsoring drug company.

Gonadotropin-releasing hormone (GnRH) is an endogenous hypothalamic peptide capable of stimulating pituitary LH and FSH release. A synthetic peptide is now available. The primary indication for pulsatile GnRH therapy is infertility associated with chronic anovulation in women with low levels of estrogen and gonadotropins. In appropriate individuals, pulsatile GnRH therapy can result in high rates of ovulation. Results in patients with chronic anovulation and normal levels of estrogen and gonadotropins, however, have been disappointing. Because both a functional pituitary and a functional ovary must be present for pulsatile GnRH therapy to be effective, patients with pituitary or ovarian failure should not be expected to respond to GnRH therapy.

THE FUTURE OF DRUG DEVELOPMENT FOR WOMEN

Drug development for women will continue to progress with the increasing complexity of science and drug technology. The continued development of valuable drugs for women will also be attributed to more women scientists, now that medical and professional schools accept a fairer percentage of women as students. Research areas will include drug development for infertility, contraception, disease control, abortion, and conditions associated with the menopause.

REFERENCES

Bottiger LE, Bowan G, Eklund G, Westerholm B. Oral contraceptives and thromboembolic disease: effects of lowering oestrogen content. *Lancet* 1980; **1**: 1097–1101.

Greenwald P. Vaginal cancer after maternal treatment with synthetic estrogen. *N Engl J Med* 1971; **285**: 390.

Herbst AL, Ulfelder H, Poskanzer DC. Adenocarcinoma of the vagina: association of maternal stilbestrol therapy with tumor appearance in young women. *N Engl J Med* 1971; **284**: 878–81.

Inman WH, Vessey MP. Investigation of death from pulmonary, coronary, and cerebral thrombosis and embolism in women of child-bearing age. *Br Med J* 1968; **2**: 193–9.

Inman WH, Vessey MP, Westerholm B, Engelund A. Thromboembolic disease and the steroidal content of oral contraceptives: a report to the Committee on Safety of Drugs. *Br Med J* 1970; **2**: 203–9.

Jick H, Jick S, Gurewich V, Myers MW, Vasilakis C. Risk of idiopathic cardiovascular death and nonfatal venous thromboembolism in women using oral contraceptives with differing progestogen components. *Lancet* 1995; **346**: 1589–93.

Kelsey FO. Thalidomide update: regulatory aspects. *Teratology* 1988; **38**: 221–6.

Lenz W. A short history of thalidomide embryopathy. *Teratology* 1988; **38**: 203–15.

Meade TW, Greenberg G, Thompson SG. Progestogens and cardiovascular reactions associated with oral contraceptives and a comparison of the safety of 50 and 35-μg oestrogen preparations. *Br Med J* 1980; **280**: 1157–61.

Nightingale SL, Morrison JC. Generic drugs and the prescribing physician. *JAMA* 1987; **258**: 1200–1204.

Rock J, Pincus G, Ramon-Garcia CR. Effects of certain 19-nor-steroids on the normal human menstrual cycle. *Science* 1956; **124**: 891.

Royal College of General Practitioners. Oral contraception and thromboembolic disease. *J Coll Gen Pract* 1967; **13**: 267–79.

Sartwell PE, Masi AT, Arthes FG, Greene GR, Smith HE. Thromboembolism and oral contraceptives: an epidemiological case-control study. *Am J Epidemiol* 1969; **5**: 365–80.

Stolley PD, Tonascia JA, Tockman MS et al. Thrombosis with low-oestrogen oral contraceptives. *Am J Epidemiol* 1975; **102**: 197–208.

Van De Carr SW, Kennedy DL, Rosa FW, Anello C, Jones JK. Relationship of oral contraceptive estrogen dose to age. *Am J Epidemiol* 1968; **117**: 153–9.

Vessey MP, Doll R. Investigation of relation between use of oral contraceptives and thromboembolic disease. *Br Med J* 1968; **2**: 199–205.

World Health Organization Collaborative Study of Cardiovascular Disease and Steroid Hormone Contraception. Effect of different progestogens in low oestrogen oral contraceptives on venous thromboembolic disease. *Lancet* 1995a; **346**: 1582–8.

World Health Organization Collaborative Study of Cardiovascular Disease and Steroid Hormone Contraception. Venous thromboembolic disease and combined oral contraceptives: results of international multicentre case-control study. *Lancet* 1995b; **346**: 1575–82.

4

Markets, Market Research and Demographic Forces

Julia M. Amadio[1] and Vanaja V. Ragavan[2]

[1]*Rhone-Poulenc Rorer, Collegeville, PA, and* [2]*FemmePharma Inc., Wayne, PA, USA*

INTRODUCTION

The pharmaceutical industry is a critical mix of science, medicine and commerce. In no other industry is there such a profound reliance on these often diametrically varying forces which, when they work in harmony, form the basis of medical and commercial success. This chapter will address the role of the commercial departments in drug development with a specific emphasis on the marketplace for women's drugs.

The global pharma market is described in Figure 4.1. From a dollar point of view, the USA, Europe and Japan dominate the markets. In many instances, marketing and market research departments will at first consider these large financial markets as the basis for generation of sales. Other markets are often added later. As can be seen in the figure, these other markets, although smaller in comparison to the expenditures of the first three, can be critical markets from a health point of view. The regulatory climate for drug development and approval will often play a vital role in determining which markets to consider commercialization at first with a new chemical entity.

When marketing departments begin to evaluate markets, demographic and disease prevalence data forms the basis for evaluating the commercial opportunity for drugs, in as much as this information is also used for scientific rationale and clinical development. These data provide both public and private sectors with the information needed to predict medical need, market size, potential use and successful commercialization of drugs. When considering a market size based on disease prevalence, an important consideration is the primary indication for the drug and its possible use in other, non-studied but related diseases. Such information can provide data on the overall use of the drug and also form the basis for further indications after initial approval. An important case in point is the fact that many drugs developed for women and men relating to their reproductive systems are non-specific and often find wider utilities than first intended.

Drug Development for Women. Edited by V.V. Ragavan. © 1998 John Wiley & Sons Ltd.

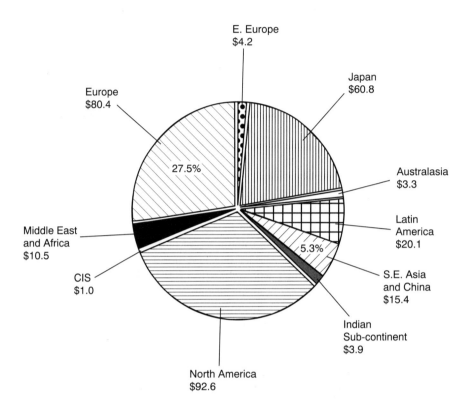

US$ 292.3 BILLION

FIGURE 4.1 Global pharma market 1996–2000: total world market by region (US$ billions). CIS = Commonwealth of Independent States (former USSR). Reproduced by permission from Pharma Strategy Group Ltd, © 1997, IMS International Inc.

Successful development of drugs should utilize a careful analysis of all the information from the very beginning of the drug development process, preferably into very early bench research, if at all possible. In the case of drugs for women, such an analysis is particularly critical, since many of the drugs discussed in this book are given to normal women for many years, and the end-user's considerations and preferences may be critical to a drug's success. Such a critical analysis encourages the marketing organization of a company to play a vital role in providing input into the development of a particular research activity. At the end of the day, it is the marketing organization that has to sell a drug and their practical knowledge of demographics, market conditions and end-user preferences could be successfully integrated into the drug development process.

In the current market condition, in both the USA and ex-US markets, the increased involvement of managed care or government-funded health delivery is beginning to profoundly affect drug development. In the USA, there are certain criteria which managed care plans dictate in drug selection for the majority of their subscribers who are covered under a given plan. For example, certain managed care plans will only cover drugs which have demonstrated cost-effective management of disease. A drug which merely delays the need for surgery for 3–5 years is less likely to be reimbursed than one which can potentially eliminate the need for surgery.

In a number of instances, the drug industry has been criticized for developing too many 'me too' type products, rather than continuing discovery into a next generation of a product line. This could be construed as a somewhat narrow view, when one realizes the cost competitiveness created by similar 'me too' products. Often, the more products entering the market in a single drug class, e.g. β-blockers for hypertension, the greater the cost competition. Also, an individual patient can react somewhat differently to a specific medication. Furthermore, women of different ages and during different times of the menstrual cycle can potentially have different pharmacokinetics and reactions to a particular drug. Each new product in a single drug class may offer a more tolerable therapeutic alternative to an added number of people. These are issues the managed care and health care companies need to consider when limiting choices for reimbursement. The 'tighter' the formularies for drugs reimbursed, the lower the incentive for companies to continue development.

Market research plays another crucial role in drug development, especially for development of drugs for chronic use, such as the products described in this book. They bring the sensitivity of the end user into drug development. Critically, a drug could be a major breakthrough scientifically, but if it has unacceptable side effects, it will not be used. Understanding the needs of the end user is thus a major contribution of market research and marketing input into drug development. This chapter will discuss the basis for conducting market research and then describe the demographics of the subjects of interest to us, namely the demographics and disease prevalence/incidence which affect women during and after their reproductive years.

COLLECTING MARKET DATA

OBTAINING DEMOGRAPHIC AND DISEASE PREVALENCE DATA

Obtaining demographic information for drug development is often both a science and an art. There is much public information on basic population demographics and these provide an important starting point. Demographic data can be obtained from a number of sources, including Census Bureau Statistics, National Health Statistics, the World Health Organization, and large-scale population-based studies which will document demographics as part of their background information. Such data are critical to create the foundation and form the denominator of interest for determining prevalence and incidence rates of disease occurrence.

Disease prevalence and incidence rates can often be culled from the medical literature, from epidemiological cohort and case control studies, and from autopsy series. Another important source of incidence rates resides in population-based databases, such as Medicaid statistics or in records of health maintenance organizations, who serve large groups of populations. Risk factors for diseases can be obtained from scientific studies and are necessary information sources which assist in determining whether the incidence of a disease will increase over time or remain stable.

Market size and growth in market size can be extrapolated using population demographics as a denominator and disease prevalence and incidence rates as the numerator. Predictions about future growth of populations, along with data about risk factors, is necessary to determine whether the market size for a particular drug will grow, remain stable or decrease.

MARKET RESEARCH METHODOLOGIES

Market research is used extensively in the drug development process to identify critical unmet needs, and determine important characteristics of the population of potential users. Market research involves both qualitative and quantitative assessments of physician and patient needs.

A qualitative study or method looks at physicians, patients, pharmacists, other health care providers and payors' perceptions of what they like or don't like about current therapeutic alternatives, or new product profiles under study. A qualitative study determines a general attitude towards a product or market. Qualitative methodologies include:

- In-depth interviews, usually one-on-one discussions.
- Telephone surveys, with select individuals to determine their general perceptions about a disease or product.
- Focus groups, a discussion group of 5–10 people, usually behind one-way mirrors. An independent discussion leader will bring out individual concepts and determine whether there is a consensus on a topic.
- Symposia to present and discuss topics with a group of thought leaders and primary researchers.

A quantitative study attempts to quantify a market or a product. By using various statistical methods, such studies can produce forecasts for a potential product or market. Quantitative methods often employ a variety of statistical single and multivariate techniques, including:

- Conjoint or trade-off analyses: a statistical multivariate method to analyze preferences and assign utility curves, or 'rankings of preference importance levels', to each parameter.
- Telephone and mail surveys of large populations for projectable data: here the key concern is gaining an adequate size and demographic representation in a sample from which to project national or regional trends.
- Mall intercept surveys: surveys administered at a mall or similar venue with a large traffic of people, subject to those population demographics.
- Multivariate forecasting: these are various statistical models used to forecast trends. They incorporate more than one or two variables from which to project influence for the outcome. Usually these are applicable only to those products with actual data from which a trend can be projected, e.g. time series analysis, step-wise regressions, etc. For new products often models of other similar products are used for projections.

For most new product or market analyses, both qualitative and quantitative methodologies are used at various stages to assist in drug development.

MARKET ANALYSIS FOR DRUG DEVELOPMENT

At the start of an assessment for the market for a particular drug or drug category, certain basic definitions and information determinations need to be established. A market may be evaluated in multiple ways.

The stage of product development helps determine the type of market research/ analysis that is needed. Very early in the development process, overall market assessment is needed to determine the size and satisfaction of a market. This will require a combination of qualitative and quantitative techniques, looking at primary and secondary information. At this stage, basic demographic trends are needed and are often ascertained by looking at potential populations. The definition of the disease or therapy area confines such an assessment, e.g. heart disease vs. hypertension vs. ACE inhibitors, etc.

Various secondary data audits (quantitative)—IMS America, Walsh America, Scott-Levin, etc.—are used to outline a current market overview. Through the various audits, journals and other secondary data sources, a number of key variables regarding a market are determined:

- The number of patients seen (patient visits) for a disorder.
- The top percentage of physician specialties seeing/treating that disorder.
- The most frequent pharmaceutical products used for treatment.
- The key reasons for using the pharmaceutical products.
- Sales volumes by certain outlets for pharmaceutical products, etc.
- Prescription volume and trends for various pharmaceutical products.

All of the above information and more is used in developing a general overview of an existing market segment from secondary sources.

Primary or qualitative information complements the quantitative database and is derived from interviewing both physicians and patients regarding the disease category, available therapeutic alternatives and desired characteristics for new alternatives. This primary research involves discussions and surveys of opinion leaders in the various specialty fields, testing of the practical approach with practicing clinicians and care givers, and acceptance testing with both care givers and patients receiving treatments. By nature, this research is more qualitative. The objective of such research is to determine the general needs of a market while defining some pragmatic boundaries for use and marketing of a drug.

Quantitative and qualitative research have their own roles in the drug development process. Quantitative research is a refining step, where relative priorities are culled out, and involves both health care providers and patients. Quantitative surveys are done with representative populations and projected statistically to the overall audience. Some examples which demonstrate the relative importance of drug features which can be modified early in the process include decisions, to, say, develop a tablet vs. a capsule; once daily vs. three-times-a-day administration; oral vs. transdermal administration; etc. Conjoint analyses, in conjunction with other multivariate statistical methods, are most commonly used to help quantify the relative importance of one feature over another.

Once a product is in later stages of development, qualitative analysis can be used to determine whether market needs and product class positioning has or has not changed over the development time of a drug. In order to determine which comparisons may be required, actual testing of a product's market positioning, and outlining its possible effects and benefits, are tested with physicians and patients. Such studies can be helpful in identifying beneficial outcomes associated with a new therapy.

In today's evolving market, the priorities of the drug payors also need to be taken into account. Pharmacoeconomic information is needed to assure product use in given managed care segments. The payors for therapy need to be presented data on the products and benefits of the drug therapy, particularly with outcome information on the benefits of the drug vs. alternative therapies such as surgery.

Role of the Marketing in R&D Activities

As has been previously mentioned, the marketing department plays a crucial role in the development of drugs. As a matter of fact, incorporating market information as early as possible in the research processes will significantly improve the marketability of a drug and ensure that the needs of the end user have been considered. One of the basic purposes of drug development is to address previously unmet needs of the market. Another purpose is to advance therapies that can have a significant effect on mortality and morbidity of disease. A classic example is that of Tagamet®, where there was no effective treatment for peptic ulcer disease other than antacids and bland diets. The anti-ulcer 'market' was developed 'overnight' with a new and innovative therapy. In fact, the need for more effective treatment had always been there but had not been adequately addressed until the discovery of H2 antagonists.

During the basic research phase of a drug's development, while highly trained and technical chemists and scientists debate the structure and function of a molecule and its potential therapeutic efficacy, market data can inform research scientists about efficacy and safety characteristics acceptable or needed in a drug in order to make it a success in the marketplace.

Additionally, assessing the value of unmet needs may also assist scientists target the 'right receptor' or 'organ system' of interest. For example, much work is being conducted today on the development of organ-specific research on steroid ligands. Knowing the marketplace for osteoporosis vs. cardiac disease can allow such designer molecules to be selected from a variety of other ligands. Market research can also provide other significant information, such as determining which side effects may be best tolerated by the target population, assuming similar product efficacy.

During the clinical development phase, marketing experts will often become closely involved in providing information about clinical parameters, safety end points and product comparators. The marketing department will also start to examine the status of the marketplace. Decisions about final packaging, dosing and pricing tend to be made towards the latter half of clinical development.

Around the time of a drug's filing, the marketing department's work will start to accelerate. Data will be collected about pricing, product positioning vis-à-vis competitors and fine-tuning of market size. Imminent product approval and product launch finally generates a frenzy of activities at the time the R&D departments have started to wind down their involvement with the drug.

Ongoing Analysis of Marketed Products

Throughout a drug's life in the marketplace, ongoing analysis of the adverse reactions and reports are monitored very closely at first and then with decreasing intensity. In some cases this information can help direct research efforts to identify unmet needs and problems. In other cases, it can also lead to synergistic combination products, for instance, development of anti-hypertensives in combination with a diuretic.

Ongoing market analyses will be carried out to determine the commercial success of products. Market analyses often collect a variety of data. For instance, compliance data can assist in identifying potential line extensions, such as sustained release versions. Acceptance within certain patient segments can also be evaluated to determine the need for other dosages and forms, e.g. a liquid or lower dose for children. Identification of issues relating to a current product can help define any remaining unmet needs, either for a drug product or a category.

The invention of new technologies in the marketplace can be evaluated for their applications to given products or diseases. The same methodologies are also used to assess the benefits and drawbacks of the new applications. Possible linking of gene therapy and biotechnology with current therapeutics to create a more targeted approach to a specific disease is one area under investigation.

PHARMACOECONOMIC CONSIDERATIONS

Economic constraints on the price of drugs and scrutiny by major payors—government and organizations—into the necessity and differences of drug therapy has spawned a new concept in drug development. Not only is it important to know what the market size for a drug will be, it is critical to analyze the pharmaco-economic climate in which the drug will be sold. These analyses were traditionally carried out towards the end of a drug's approval process at the time when pricing decisions were traditionally made. It is with considerable peril and risk that drug developers leave this aspect of a drug's future to latter phases of drug development. Many companies are presently incorporating such issues early in a drug's development and are, often at the same time, evaluating how a drug would fit into a whole disease management profile.

It must be emphasized that pharmacoeconomic considerations are even more critical for drugs used in prevention, such as drugs developed for women. Many perfectly normal women take drugs such as contraceptives and hormone replace-ment therapy for many years. The benefits of these selective therapies over the product cost and side effects need to be taken into consideration as part of an overall outcomes assessment. A comprehensive pharmacoeconomic evaluation needs to consider risk/benefit ratios, utilize careful market analysis and patient preferences and overall cost analysis to any drugs developed for these purposes. In addition, such analysis must include information from payors to understand how a woman will end up obtaining the drug.

Pharmacoeconomic evaluations may take into account the following considera-tions, which are best added to clinical trials early in Phase II and Phase III research periods:

- Simplified clinical studies evaluating health outcomes of a drug in addition to traditional efficacy and safety studies. Such studies can often be included as questionnaires tagged on to a Phase III study and/or studied independently.
- Cost-effective analysis of drug treatment and how it fits into the overall treatment of a disease, including advantages of the new drug over approved drugs or procedures.
- Quality of life issues, especially overall improvements using the new drug, not just relief of a disease entity.
- Patient surveys on drug preferences, compliance issues, satisfaction.

- Overall productivity issues, including employee absenteeism and reduction in utilization of resources; e.g. in an HMO or managed care setting, preservation of health and prevention of disease occurrence.

Pharmacoeconomic considerations could change the way traditional R&D departments operate. Often, all of the new data collection can impose a burden on clinicians conducting the studies, data management groups and writers. In addition, there continues to be general debate about whether it is still best to defer such analyses to Phase IV, when a drug is made available to the population who will use it rather than to a restricted clinical trial population. In the latter instance, typically, compliance and follow-up are often significantly better than during post-marketing periods. In some countries, regulatory agencies have required typical 'use' data prior to a drug's approval, but the reimbursement of drugs is typically determined by government agencies and not private payors.

Although this area remains one in which considerable work has begun, its utility—when best to conduct such trials, how much information to generate, how to tie it in with traditional safety and efficacy data—all remain to be determined and delineated. More information regarding the potential benefits of a drug therapy outcome on pharmacoeconomic parameters and quality and mortality issues are starting to be examined early in the drug development process. Soon-to-be-published Federal Drug Administration (FDA) guidelines indicate an approach to pharmacoeconomic evaluations with the same rigor as those in place for new drug application studies. These include assessments using two well-controlled studies for use as 'indications' or for promotion. While these evaluations may appear to be scientifically sound methods for gauging new drug effectiveness, they may not be the most practical way to evaluate true pharmacoeconomic impact or effectiveness of products, since the purpose of pharmacoeconomic trials is to assess realistic parameters for 'true therapeutic' economic influences, while the purpose of NDA trials is to evaluate efficacy and safety under idealized research conditions.

DEMOGRAPHIC ANALYSIS OF WOMEN'S HEALTH AND DISEASE

GENERAL POPULATION DEMOGRAPHICS

In 1990, there were approximately 2.6 billion women in the world. Projections show the female population reaching 3.04 billion by the year 2000, with the majority of these women found predominantly in developing nations. The population of women in the USA represents approximately 5% of the world population. The European Community accounts for almost 9% of the female population, with the other developed countries adding another 12%. Seventy-four percent of women live in developing countries. Table 4.1 provides a further breakdown of the demographic segments with historic data and projections for the year 2000.

TABLE 4.1 Population demographics by age and world segment (in millions)

Age	Developed world						Developing world			
	1990	2000	1990	2000	1990	2000	1990	2000	1990	2000
0–14	26 472	29 257	88 437	78 946	114 909	108 203	716 683	810 144	831 592	918 347
15–29	28 666	27 167	98 068	92 971	126 734	120 138	581 566	648 131	708 300	768 269
30–39	21 125	20 978	67 012	66 793	88 137	87 771	270 717	360 088	358 854	447 859
40–49	16 087	21 394	56 938	66 531	73 025	87 925	179 358	261 196	252 383	349 121
50–59	11 339	15 883	54 261	55 369	65 600	71 252	135 241	168 072	200 841	239 324
60–64	5 683	5 602	26 315	26 865	31 998	32 467	51 585	64 432	83 583	96 899
65+	18 704	20 296	70 298	81 133	89 002	101 429	98 686	134 462	187 688	235 891
Total	128 076	140 577	461 329	468 608	589 405	609 185	2 033 836	2 446 525	2 623 241	3 055 710

(From United Nations, 1994, with permission).

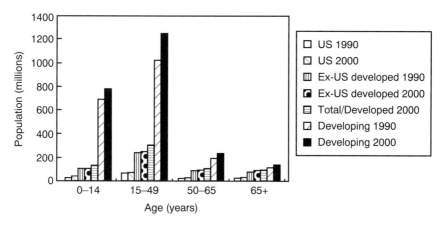

FIGURE 4.2 Population demographics by age and world segment

The world market is changing dramatically. In the USA and Europe there is an aging of the population and continued increases in longevity (Figure 4.2). As we near the end of this century, the dramatic demographic trends which started in mid-century in the post-World War era have become significantly accentuated. These trends show an increase in life expectancies for women in both developing and developed countries, but these remain at quite different rates. As a result of these trends, an increasing number of women are approaching menopause in the developed countries. In contrast, within the developing countries, the growth of populations has remained predominantly within the younger segment of women.

For pharmaceutical companies interested in developing drugs for the worldwide marketplace, these demographics pose serious challenges to global drug development. Clearly, these demographic trends result in differing needs for the different regions. Developed countries have growing needs based on an aging population. Developing countries, which still account for the majority of the world's population, have a younger and different demographics and subsequently, different product needs.

DEMOGRAPHICS AND MARKET TRENDS: DISEASE/CONDITION-SPECIFIC INFORMATION

Contraception

Demographics

In 1990, there were approximately 287.9 million women of child-bearing age in the developed countries, representing almost 30% of the world population at that time and anticipated to grow to 34% by the end of the century. The majority of women are in the under-developed countries and will also grow substantially by the year 2000 (United Nations, 1994). No doubt there will be an increasing need to provide safe and effective contraceptives to this very large population group. From a demographic and marketing point of view, there are two issues: (a) how good is the present mix of contraceptives with regard to safety and efficacy and how well are they accepted; and (b) are our distribution and educational systems performing adequately to ensure that contraceptives are used appropriately and when needed?

An examination of present use patterns of contraceptives is the first step in trying to determine present market status. Utilization of various contraceptive methods in certain major countries throughout the world is depicted in Table 4.2.

As shown in Table 4.2, contraceptive usage can vary markedly between countries/regions of the world. These differences are generally related to socio-economic status, cultural differences and governmental policies. In addition, these differences are most marked between developed and developing nations. Some of these differences are outlined in Table 4.3.

Contraceptive Market Characteristics: Market Trends/Usage Data

Since contraceptive use is often related to the very heart of social mores and government policies/philosophies, it is easy to understand why these differences very often dictate the acceptance and use of available products (and ingredients). The European market, in comparison to the USA, for example, is more tolerant of a variety of products such as the IUD and the 'abortion pill'. On the other side of the spectrum is the fact that oral contraceptives (OCs) are not yet approved for use in Japan, where there is a concern that they will encourage increased promiscuity and increase sexually transmitted diseases (STDs). Further, even within a similar geographic or demographic segment, governmental regulations dictating contraceptive drug development differ considerably from one country to another. Certain countries require extensive testing and accumulation of data for certain products or ingredients, whereas other countries are much less restrictive. In the UK, for example, an oral contraceptive product was approved as a line extension of previously existing products, based purely on pharmacokinetic data and projections. No specific clinical studies were conducted with the new combination for approval.

Contraceptive Development: Preference Data

Current preference for contraceptives can be assessed based on current usage data. When comparing use data from country to country, it is important to take into consideration the differences in the products available for the consumer in the different markets, because of the factors discussed previously. For instance, the European market, in general, has more product options available for contraception than there are in the US market. Furthermore, both these markets vary considerably

TABLE 4.2 Contraceptive usage by method, 1990

Country	Condom (%)	Pill (%)	IUD (%)	Barrier (%)	Male sterilization (%)	Female sterilization (%)	Injectables (%)	Rhythm, etc. (%)	None (%)
USA	20	25	1	2	7	17	3	7	17
Europe	10	26	11	1	3	7	0	18	24
France	4	29	26	2	0	7	0	13	19
Italy	13	14	2	2	0	1	0	46	22
Germany	6	34	15	2	2	10	0	9	22
UK	16	24	6	1	12	11	0	8	22
Canada	8	11	6	2	13	30	0	3	27
Japan	41	0	6	5	0	6	0	9	33
Latin America	2	20	4	1	1	24	1	9	38

Data from Ortho Pharmaceuticals (1996); World Health Organization (1990).

TABLE 4.3 Differences in contraceptive use between world regions

Developed countries	Developing countries
Stable child-bearing population	High growth in target population
Contraception well established	Lack of formalized contraception; usually as part of poor health care delivery
Women postponing childbirth into 30s and 40s	Younger women having children
Women using contraceptive methods longer	Condoms most frequently used method, due to cost
STDs increasing with earlier sexual activity	STDs at high level—on the rise
More women facing fertility problems	

from developing nations, where in many countries the major concern is not a product option, but a more fundamental problem of availability and distribution of products. Very often, products are not distributed to remote areas. Adequate training and education in contraception and of the various methods are often desperately needed.

To be relevant, use data must take into consideration preferences which are influenced by the local culture and religion. These cultural differences can be highlighted by an example. Significant differences can be seen in the use of oral contraceptives in the USA vs. Europe, but in some ways these are much more similar than use in developing countries. In spite of good, if not free, access and equal availability, there is a much higher percentage use of oral contraceptives in Europe compared to the USA. In addition, there has always been a higher usage of intra-uterine devices (IUDs) in Europe, which could partially be attributed to the litigious nature of the US market. Despite these differences, many similarities are also present. In both populations a similarly high percentage of women at risk of unwanted pregnancy do not use any kind of contraceptive method. There is also a significant percentage of women in these countries using sterilization on an annual basis as their primary means of contraception.

In Japan and Eastern Europe, abortion is still used extensively for contraception. This is due in part to the lack of concern about abortion and lack of access to other more effective and commonly-used methods, available in other developed countries.

Deficiencies in the Marketplace for Contraceptives

Although oral contraceptives, injectables, IUDs and implants provide safe and effective contraception, there remain unmet needs in the contraceptive market-place, as evidenced by the large numbers of women at risk for pregnancy who do not use any methods. Side effects, such as bleeding irregularities, weight gain, mood swings and other concerns, often result in discontinuations or hesitancy to start. Another significant and growing unmet need is the availability of contraceptives that also provide some degree of protection against STDs such as HIV, and which can be under a woman's control.

Effective and safe contraceptives have been available for over 30 years. Yet, research in both developed and developing sectors has consistently shown that women remain interested in new modes of contraception rather than in those widely available today, most often because of unacceptable side effects and the cost of present therapy (Population Crisis Committee, 1991). They seek, apart from protection against STDs, a variety of new contraceptive alternatives, such as long-acting contraceptives (e.g. a once-a-month pill) and products which do not cause the irregular bleeding and other side effects found in progestin-only methods, which at present account for most of the long-acting contraceptives.

Another indication of existing unmet needs in the market is the rapid response and uptake to a new product introduction. A good example of such a phenomenon in the USA is the initial success of the Norplant system. The significant and rapid adoption rate by users demonstrated clearly that there was an unmet need for a simple, long-lasting contraceptive method. But when negative publicity became associated with the product, the downfall in use was almost as rapid as the initial uptake.

A further example is the withdrawal of the Today Sponge from the market, leaving a gap in over-the-counter contraceptive availability. Depo-Provera, an old contraceptive, was well accepted when it was finally approved in the USA for contraceptive use in mid-1994. Consistent high rates of abortion (>1 million annually) also demonstrates that a large unmet segment of fertile women are not well served with existing methods.

In the European markets, availability of more products results in a more satisfied marketplace and fewer unmet needs. The IUD is one of the most frequently used methods of contraception in Europe, particularly in France. The 'abortion pill' is available in some markets and has captured an important market niche in these countries. The difficulty in producing a product with the efficacy of today's methods and acceptable side effects is significant. In developing countries, economics, distribution systems and lack of education contribute to inadequate contraception and control of reproduction.

Menopause/Climacteric

Demographics

The cessation of a woman's menstrual cycle, for at least 12 months, is known as the menopause. The average age of menopause is 51. This statistic continues to remain remarkably consistent despite demographic and cultural differences. In 1988, there were approximately 36 012 000 women over the age of 50 in the USA and approximately 434 960 000 throughout the rest of the world. By the year 2000, there will be over 700 million women over the age of 50 with a life expectancy greater than 78 years. The developed countries will face the largest growth rate in this age group over the next decade. Developing countries, in contrast, are experiencing their most significant growth in the younger, contracepting age range, with over 1 billion women in that age group. As populations grow though, developing countries will also experience growth in gross numbers in the older age group.

Menopause is also the time when women start to experience certain diseases against which they have been largely protected by their reproductive hormones. In the absence of estrogen, there is a rapid increase in the loss of bone density and, furthermore, a rapid increase in cardiovascular risk. These biological changes are reflected in a number of morbidity statistics which increase dramatically in women after the age of menopause. Cardiovascular disease, the leading cause of death in women as well as men, increases significantly after the age of 60. Osteoporosis in women, in contrast to men, increases in severity in their 50s and 60s with resultant increase in morbidity and mortality from fractures in their 70s. Many studies have demonstrated that these risks can be substantially reduced with various therapies, particularly hormonal replacement. These issues will be discussed in later chapters.

Market Trends

Women experiencing menopause today, especially educated and working women in all countries, are less likely than their mothers to 'suffer in silence'. They are information seekers and, with the onset of hot flashes, will generally visit their physicians requesting treatment of vasomotor symptoms. The additional benefits of longer-term preventive treatment with hormone replacement therapy (HRT) are often reasons for which women will initiate, but not necessarily remain on, therapy. Interestingly, market research has shown that although awareness of preventive therapies has increased amongst women, the risk/benefit of HRT has yet to be clarified within the general medical profession. Ambivalence of the treating physician often leaves the woman with ambiguous advice, and she then has to make important decisions on incomplete data. Market research has shown that these ambiguities translate into poor long-term compliance with HRT.

HRT is the most commonly used and widely tested treatment for menopausal vasomotor symptoms and osteoporosis protection. The worldwide market in 1993 was over $1.7 billion sales of HRT. The market is currently dominated by oral therapy at 76%. Transdermal products capture 14% of the total market. The remaining 10% is made up of vaginal inserts, topicals, injectables, implants/IUDs and other delivery systems. The US market is dominated by oral therapy and a single branded product—Premarin, a conjugated equine estrogen product. The international market has a larger segment of transdermal products and is much more fragmented by brands. It is also more segmented by combination products, with 17β-estradiol and several progestins. The US market share, broken down by estrogen and progestin markets, is shown in Figures 4.3 and 4.4.

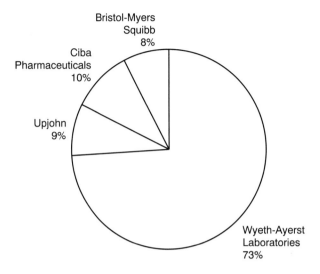

FIGURE 4.3 Non-contraceptive estrogen market: company market share by revenues (USA) 1994. All percentages given are rounded. Reproduced by permission, © 1995 Frost & Sullivan Inc. at Frost.Com

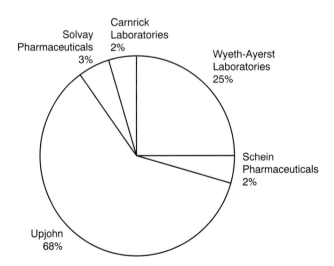

FIGURE 4.4 Non-contraceptive progestin market: company market share by revenues (USA) 1994. All percentages given are rounded. Reproduced by permission, © 1995 Frost & Sullivan Inc. at Frost.Com

While the HRT market has been growing rapidly, it is anticipated that this market could expand substantially in the next few years. It is reported that only around 20–25% of those eligible for HRT actually take it for any significant period of time. An estimated half of women with a hysterectomy and 14% of those undergoing menopause actually receive therapy (Harris, 1993). Additionally, in the USA, HRT is frequently discontinued after about a year, at the time when the majority of vasomotor symptoms have been alleviated. Thus, full benefits from long-term use, viz. decrease in cardiovascular risk and osteoporosis protection, are not gained.

There have been a number of new entries to this market recently with Wyeth-Ayerst introducing a combination estrogen/progestin in 1995 in the USA, while combination products have been available in Europe for a number of years. New components for HRT are under development, with various delivery systems making up the rest of the new products in this area.

Concerns of Women Regarding HRT

The fear of developing breast cancer is still by far the most significant concern among women preventing continued long-term usage of HRT. The inconvenience of monthly and/or irregular bleeding is also one of the top reasons women give for discontinuing therapy. Other bothersome side effects noted are breast tenderness, headache and bloating by women. The benefits of longer-term therapy are often not considered as important to women in their decisions to continue or stop hormone replacement.

Future drug development in this area must take into consideration side effects which stop women from taking or continuing HRT. Products such as those specifically developed to result in amenorrhea, or longer-term dosing regimens, are critical for development. There are a number of scientific efforts under way to produce products with activity on specific organs/tissues of interest. Furthermore, a significant group of women who cannot tolerate hormones, e.g. women with breast cancer, need non-hormonal therapy for vasomotor symptoms. There is a significant need for non-hormonal estrogen-like products which can alleviate symptoms and perhaps add protective effects for those women who can not take hormonal replacement.

Osteoporosis

Demographics

Osteoporosis is a disease where there is a loss of bone mass in areas of the skeleton made up of estrogen-dependent trabecular bone, e.g. in the vertebrae and the hip, often leading to fracture of these bones. Estrogen-dependent osteoporosis is directly correlated with increasing age. As the world population grows rapidly and ages, morbidity, hospitalizations and medical costs related to osteoporosis and osteo-porotic fractures are expected to increase exponentially. Women have two-fold greater risk than men, although some older men will also suffer the disease. The risk is clearly increased in Whites as compared to Asians, Africans or Hispanic women in the USA (Baron et al, 1994).

Approximately 1.7 million hip fractures are estimated to have occurred in 1990 worldwide. A marked increase in incidence is anticipated to occur over the next few years. Hip fractures cost about $10–20 billion annually in the USA, and these expenses continue to increase dramatically (National Osteoporosis Foundation, 1995). Hip fractures pose serious morbidity and mortality for the elderly. Of the approximately 250 000 hip fractures that occur in the USA each year, 75–80% are in women. It has also been shown that 15–25% of persons who were functionally independent before a hip fracture needed institutional care for at least a year afterward. A futher 20–25% needed at-home assistance, adding to the increasing health care costs (Cummings et al, 1985).

Some populations have been found to have a higher incidence of osteoporosis than others, although the reasons for these differences are not clear at this time. Genetic factors may play an important role in the increased incidence of osteo-porosis noted in women who come from Northern European extraction. Diet is another factor known to affect population based osteoporosis. Data from countries like China, where milk intake is often low, report a high incidence of osteoporosis after the menopause. Such demographic differences assist in targeting populations who are at particular risk.

Market Trends: Drugs for Osteoporosis

Treatment of osteoporosis is based on two prevalent trends, prevention of meno-pausal bone loss and/or treatment of fractures. Widely accepted preventive therapies include HRT, calcium supplementation and exercise. Market data have shown that approximately 14% of peri- and post-menopausal women at risk of osteoporosis receive HRT. Furthermore, there appears to be segmentation in treatment based on specialty. Primary care physicians are less likely to recommend HRT, even for treatment of fractures resulting from osteoporosis. These physicians tend to recommend only calcium supplements and exercise for prevention of osteoporosis, while specialists like obstetricians/gynecologists and endocrinologists are more likely to use HRT for osteoporosis protection. Availability of newer agents in the market for prevention and treatment may increase awareness and earlier treatment of osteoporosis. In particular, the availability of the new bisphosphonate from Merck—Fosamax®—has increased the size of the entire osteoporosis market.

Despite considerable information available to the physician and patient on the benefits of HRT for osteoporosis, the average duration of continuous use of HRT

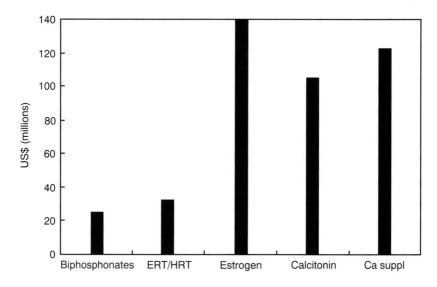

FIGURE 4.5 Market size of osteoporosis products, USA. Reproduced by permission from Point of View (PoV) Women's Health Care, *Report* (1995)

is approximately 9+ months. This figure represents all women, including those who start and stop therapy within a year. For those women who elect to take HRT for longer periods, the next average duration of use is approximately 3+ years for non-hysterectomized women and over 5 years for hysterectomized women. These data are primarily derived from the US market, but significant differences are not expected from the European market. In Europe the duration of treatment has remained relatively short. Trends extending therapy for the prevention of osteoporosis have not yet been noted in European prescribing habits (FDC Pharma, 1996).

The US market share of the various therapies is shown in Figure 4.5.

There are a number of new therapies on the market or in development for the treatment and prevention of osteoporosis. They include estrogens, bisphosphonates (e.g. Merck's Fosamax®), calcitonins, progestogens, selective (anti-) estrogens, vitamin D derivatives, slow release fluoride, parathyroid hormone and growth-related peptides, etc. In the estrogen- and steroid-related markets, a new potential product entry is a tissue-specific estrogen agonist called raloxifene, which has recently been approved in the USA for prevention of osteoporosis. This drug is part of a profile of drugs called selective estrogen receptor modulators (SERMs). Initial data demonstrates that this drug has a similar profile of bone preservation as estrogen itself.

Most therapies do not act by increasing bone mass but prevent further bone loss, thus preserving the status quo. Although etidronate, a first generation bisphos-phonate, has been on the market for a number of years for Paget's disease, it has never been approved for osteoporosis for a number of reasons. Fosamax was the first bisphosphonate to gain approval for the treatment of fractures. Studies are ongoing on the use of Fosamax in prevention of osteoporosis. Initial data from these studies appear to be encouraging, with a slight increase in bone mass seen after a couple of years of use. Although accepted and tolerated well in clinical studies, patients who take Fosamax find its gastro-intestinal intolerance to be very problematic.

Fluoride is one of the few agents known to increase bone mass when given in large doses. Fluoride-treated bone appears to be more dense, but in well-controlled studies this bone has been found to be brittle, causing an increase in bone fractures with long-term use. This may be a dose-related phenomenon, because recent data presented to the FDA showed that slow-release fluoride given in smaller doses was not found to be as toxic to the bone but was able to maintain its ability to increase bone mass strength.

Most of the agents on the market or in development work by stabilizing bone turnover and prevent further loss. Parathyroid hormone and fluoride are exceptions because they build new bone. Given the present therapeutic status, an individual with significant existing bone loss would most likely remain at risk of fracture despite interventions. But there are new data emerging in this area, such as use of bone-targeted growth factors, which hold much promise.

Market Trends: Detection of Women at Risk

Until now, detection of loss of bone mass has been a difficult task. Most physicians do not routinely perform monitoring of bone status, unless the patient has sustained fractures or has a strong familial history. A number of methods have been developed and are in use for detecting bone mass. Several technologies have been developed over the years. Dual energy X-ray absorptiometry (DEXA), single (SPA) and dual (DPA) photon absorptiometry have been applied to the lumbar spine, proximal femur, forearm and heel. The present state of the art is DEXA. These methods detect bone loss over a long-term span, about 6–12 months. A number of bone turnover chemical markers are available or are under development to provide adjunctive measures for rapid, short-term assessment of risk or therapeutic efficacy. While awareness of osteoporosis is higher among physicians and women, many people continue to believe it is an unavoidable consequence of aging.

With the availability of various forms of diagnosis/detection of bone loss and turnover, knowledge and awareness of osteoporosis becomes more tangible to the physician and patients. Recent approvals of chemical bone turnover markers can help detect changes in bone metabolism and can help the practitioner in a caregiving setting. However, their prognostic utility and population-based analysis remain unknown. Until now, physicians have not had available a simple test to determine a woman's rate of bone turnover. Densitometry is still the gold standard, but it is still not used in the majority of patients. With the approval of the bone markers and the ease of ELISA on which these are based, physicians and patients may have a means of measuring the effectiveness of therapy and evaluating trends in therapy for helping prevent further loss. Since these markers can be used to detect changes more rapidly than densitometers, they can be used to make therapeutic changes.

The importance of baseline densitometric status of bone in diagnosing true osteoporosis can not be underestimated. Bone markers provide a support structure for the identifying and treatment and monitoring therapy for those found to have rapid bone turnover rates, but to date, bone densitometry is still the only approved method for diagnosing osteoporosis.

Quality of Life Issues and Osteoporosis

The commercial environment also has had an impact on public awareness of osteoporosis. Brand name consumer goods such as orange juice and antacids are now being promoted as a source of calcium. The NIH has launched the Women's Health Initiative, the largest community-based intervention and prevention trial ever conducted, which will continue to increase awareness of this devastating illness.

Present and future market needs include effective, non-estrogenic therapy and prophylaxis with minimal side effects for long-term intervention. Continued education is also needed, because many physicians and patients are still not aware of the effective early interventions which can prevent fractures and do not realize the need for treatment. Some of the new agents under development may provide viable alternatives. The osteoporosis market is anticipated to grow substantially over the next decade. Cost of drugs and diagnosis vs. long-term outcomes of fracture will play a greater consideration for treatment and prevention therapies under the emerging health care system.

For the majority of women, market studies have found that even simple measures such as calcium/vitamin D intake appear to be problematic or unclear as to the advantage. In the Commonwealth Fund Women's Health Survey, 1993, about 61% of women over 45 lacked knowledge of osteoporosis, and again approximately 60% of women over 45 did not take calcium supplements (Harris, 1993). Educational programs aimed at coordinating the total care of women, addressing their nutritional needs, promoting preventive measures such as exercise, etc., can go a long way towards addressing the issue of osteoporosis and its impact on quality of life. Many practitioners and HMOs have put in place such programs for their patients. In addition, pharmaceutical companies have taken an active role in this process. For instance, Merck has recently formed an education institute to help increase overall knowledge and awareness of osteoporosis and its consequences, and availability of various early diagnostic methods. Information will be provided to patients and women at risk. The National Osteoporosis Foundation (NOF) is another source and contains a wealth of information for patients. The NOF is an able lobbying and educational group which serves its constituency extremely well.

Endometriosis

Demographics

Endometriosis is characterized by the presence of endometrial tissue outside the endometrial cavity and the uterus. Endometriosis can be found in the ovaries, fallopian tubes and the pelvic area and can also disseminate to remote areas such as the lung. Symptoms vary in their severity, but primarily include chronic pelvic pain, disabling periods, abnormal menstrual bleeding, dyspareunia and infertility.

In 1991, about 5 million women in the USA and 500 000 in Canada suffered from endometriosis. The prevalence of endometriosis has been reported, based on surgical series, to vary dramatically from 1% to 50%. This variability cannot be reduced in the absence of a non-invasive diagnostic procedure, which is the present state of affairs, with the definitive diagnosis dependent on a surgical laparoscopy (Wheeler, 1992). The age of onset can be any time during a woman's reproductive life, although chronic fibrosis can lead to pelvic pain in later years. Endometriosis can be found in higher socioeconomic groups, especially when women remain single longer, marry late and have few or no children. Unfortunately, infertility can be the first clinical manifestation of endometriosis.

Pelvic endometriosis has been found in approximately 1% of all women undergoing major surgery for all gynecologic indications. Approximately 20% of women who undergo laparoscopy to determine the cause of pelvic pain are found to have endometriosis. An estimated 50% of teenagers undergoing laparoscopy for evaluation of dysmenorrhea and an estimated one-third of women evaluated for infertility are found to have endometriosis.

Market Size, Cost, Trends

The total market for treatment of endometriosis is difficult to estimate and separate, since the therapies used for endometriosis are often used for many other conditions. Given the changing demographics, such as delay in childbearing and fewer children, the endometriosis market is predicted to continue to grow substantially, as shown in Figure 4.6.

In 1993, the sales of the various agents for use in treatment of endometriosis accounted for approximately $50 million ex-USA and about the same in the USA. The US market share is shown in Figure 4.7.

Treatment of endometriosis can vary depending on the severity of the disease, the size and extent of lesions and the patient's age and desire to have children. There are several treatment alternatives currently approved, including GnRH analogs (leuprolide, nafarelin, buserlin and gosarelin), progestogens, androgenic steroids such as Danocrine® danazol capsules and various surgical procedures. Gestrinone is used extensively in Europe, and is under investigation in the USA. In the USA, the GnRH analogs are the best sellers, followed by danazol. Surgery

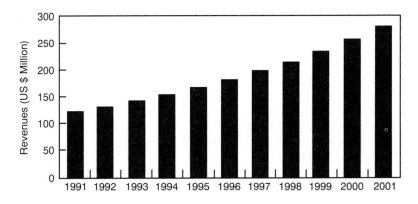

FIGURE 4.6 Endometriosis pharmaceuticals market: revenue forecasts (USA) 1991–2001. All revenues quoted are rounded. Reproduced by permission, © 1995 Frost & Sullivan Inc. at Frost.Com

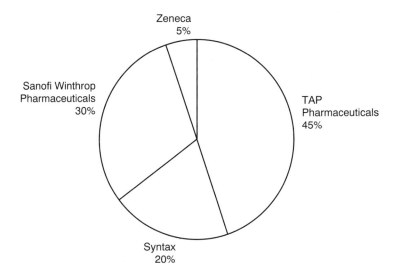

FIGURE 4.7 Endometriosis pharmaceuticals market: company market share by revenues (USA) 1994. Reproduced by permission, © 1995 Frost & Sullivan Inc. at Frost.Com

including laparoscopic removal of lesions and correction of fibrosis is used if the symptoms are severe and incapacitating.

Current therapeutic alternatives are limited and side effects can be significant. The GnRH analogs work by creating a chemical menopause and are associated with hot flashes, headache, bone loss and other symptoms associated with estrogen deprivation, and can be frequent. In the USA and Europe, surgery is an important therapeutic modality. Laser ablation has emerged as a preferred treatment for alleviating pain and eliminating fibrous clusters. GnRH therapy is often used prior to laser or surgical procedures, for three months or less, to reduce the size of endometrial nodules and ease surgical removal.

Endometriosis: Specific Concerns

Endometriosis remains a condition with unmet therapeutic needs, based on current therapeutic options. Much of the present therapy is used for short-term treatment of a chronic disease and does not cure the disease or its sequelae. In addition, current therapies work by suppressing estrogen and/or ovulation and put a woman into a chemical menopause. Once the suppression is discontinued, the symptoms and manifestation of endometriosis generally return.

Novel alternative therapies with significantly fewer side effects, and therapies which can cure disease rather than alleviate side effects, are much needed. In addition, present drugs do not address infertility. This a critical major cause of morbidity, especially in developed countries. Long-term therapy aimed at suppressing or preventing the disease in high-risk groups could significantly reduce infertility associated with chronic endometriosis. Much of the progress in this area presently has involved better detection and identification of those at risk of endometriosis but research leading to cure is still a long way off.

Ideal therapy for endometriosis would need to be targeted at the exact mechanism of growth and spread of endometrial tissue in the abdominal cavity. Recent research into the immunologic basis of endometriosis appears promising.

Cancers of the Reproductive System

Demographics

Breast cancer can occur during both pre- and post-menopausal periods and the two diseases appear to have slightly different prognosis. This is the most common cancer in women and accounts for about 350 000 deaths around the world. Breast cancer incidence has reached epidemic proportions, with a life-time risk of 1 in 8 for women in the USA. The annual incidence of this cancer is 180 000 new cases yearly in the USA, as noted by the National Cancer Institute, with an estimated mortality of 25 000 women per year. The American Cancer Society classifies the incidence by age, as shown in Figure 4.8.

Recent statistics show that although breast cancer continues to rise, lung cancer mortality is now a significant problem for women. These demographic trends, most likely due to the rise in cigarette smoking in women, are shown in Figure 4.9.

Breast cancer is detected by physical examination and mammography. Diagnosis may be confirmed by aspiration cytology, core needle biopsy or excision

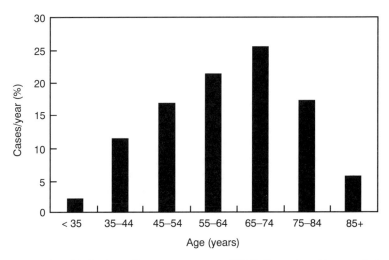

FIGURE 4.8 Age distribution of breast cancer cases (USA). Reproduced by permission from American Cancer Society, 1992

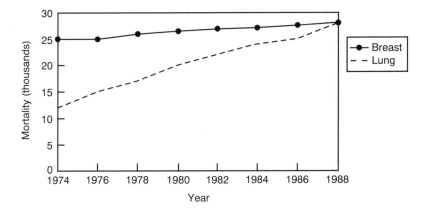

FIGURE 4.9 Breast vs. lung cancer mortality in females (USA). Adapted from Office of Research on Women's Health, 1992

biopsy. Since the increasing use of mammography to screen for breast cancer, there has been an increase in the detection of non-invasive cancer, which now comprises 15–20% of all breast cancers.

Unlike breast cancer, endometrial and cervical cancers are on the decline because of better methods of early diagnosis and aggressive surgical therapies. Endometrial cancer accounts for about 13% of cancers in women, with incidence rates of 15 per 100 000 women in the USA. Although cervical cancer remains the leading cause of cancer death among women worldwide, the number of cases and mortality rates have declined sharply in the USA, having dropped from an incidence of 44 per 100 000 women in 1947 to only 8 per 100 000 in 1982 and continuing to decline. However, the increasing incidence of human papillomavirus (HPV) infections may reverse this trend, since HPV has been associated with cervical cancer.

Ovarian cancer accounts for about 4% of all cancers in women and 6% of all cancer deaths. This cancer has a higher mortality rate than other cancers, because it is often diagnosed only after it has already spread, often into the peritoneum. Early diagnosis is the key—but only 23% of all ovarian cancers are detected while still localized. Overall, only 76% of patients survive the first year, while 5-year survival rates are about 44%. CA 125 antigen is used as a marker for ovarian cancer, especially for postmenopausal women.

The chapter will focus on breast cancer, primarily because the drugs developed for this cancer are steroid-based. The other cancers will not be covered in this book, because treatment for the other gynecologic cancers (except for early stage endometrial cancers) are typically based on oncologic drugs.

Market Trends

Treatment of breast cancer depends on the stage at diagnosis. Surgery, chemo-therapy and radiation therapy are the most common methods. Like breast cancer, a cure for uterine and cervical cancers is based on the time of diagnosis—the earlier the detection, the more favorable the outcome.

Numerous pharmacological agents have been introduced in the last 10 years to aid in the treatment and prevention of recurrence in the same or alternate breast. Treatment modalities have also changed. With increasingly earlier detection of small tumors, most women now undergo localized surgical procedures, rather than radical procedures. These are followed by chemotherapy and/or anti-estrogen therapy based on the stage at diagnosis, menopausal status and receptor status of the tumor. The chemotherapy market size for the products used in this condition worldwide, including figures for anti-estrogen, is about $800 million. Some of the products and their market share are shown in Table 4.4.

Recent interesting developments include controversy regarding high-dose chemotherapy. A controlled study evaluating high dose chemotherapy, followed by bone marrow transplant, could not be completed because initial positive results resulted in a demand that all women be treated with the same regimen and resulting in the closing of the study.

There are still many unmet needs for this disease. Unfortunately, some of the newer agents used in treatment are found to be associated with resistance. New, less toxic alternatives are needed, along with a better understanding of the epidemiology of the disease. Recent development in the isolation of the BRCA1 gene in women with high-risk breast cancer (primarily family members with breast cancer) have added another complexity to this disease. The Women's Health

TABLE 4.4 Sales of leading drugs to treat breast cancer, 1993 ($ millions)

Drug	USA	France	Germany	Italy	Spain	UK	Japan	Total
Cytotoxic agents	182.4	70.0	88.3	92.2	12.3	48.0	18.0	511.1
Cyclophosphamide	32.9	3.4	3.3	2.6	1.2	0.2	0.3	43.9
Doxorubicin	63.3	13.5	–	39.6	3.9	–	0.8	121.1
Epirubicin	–	20.6	53.5	40.1	4.7	11.2	11.8	141.9
5-Fluorouracil	4.0	4.4	17.4	4.0	0.5	13.0	4.9	48.2
Mitoxantrone	16.5	16.5	–	0.4	–	6.7	–	40.1
Taxol	37.5	–	–	–	–	–	–	37.5
Others[a]	28.2	11.6	14.1	5.5	2.0	16.9	0.2	78.4
Hormonal agents	184.1	6.4	33.7	10.9	2.7	13.0	65.8	316.6
Tamoxifen	180.3	6.4	23.9	10.1	2.7	13.0	65.8	302.2
Others[b]	3.8	–	9.8	0.8	–	–	–	14.4
Total	329.0	76.4	122.0	103.1	15.0	61.0	83.8	827.7

[a] Aminoglutethimide, carboplatin, chlorambucil, cisplatin, etoposide, methotrexate, mitomycin-C, vinblastine, vincristine, vindesine.
[b] Leuprolide acetate, medroxyprogesterone, megestrol acetate.

Reproduced from Godsey (1995) by permission of *DR Reports*, Decision Resources Inc.

Initiative, a large, NIH undertaking, has certain studies designated to understanding some of the risk factors for breast cancer.

Market Needs

The most pressing epidemiological question is to identify the reasons for the noted increase in the incidence rates of breast cancer. The NIH has plans to address this issue in its Women's Health Initiative. While therapeutic advances continue, more effective and less toxic alternatives remain to be found. A need for alternatives to anti-estrogenic therapy is needed. Preventive therapy for those with identified high risk of developing breast cancer is another substantial need for this market. Additional improvement in diagnostic measures and earlier detection are always key to successful treatment of this disease. Inadequate or non-existent health care coverage remains a barrier to many women receiving yearly mammograms, which help in earlier detection. Recent discoveries of the breast cancer gene BRCA1 raise other issues regarding detection/treatment/follow-up of women found to have the gene and the ethical issues surrounding such diagnosis.

Other Endocrine Disorders

Market data in this area are difficult to obtain, as most of the therapies are the same for these indications and often physicians do not specify which indication is the reason for treatment. Surgery also plays a very large part in treatment alternatives of these disorders.

Uterine Fibroids

Demographics

Uterine fibroids (leiomyomata) are very common benign tumors of the uterus. They occur and grow in the thick muscular uterine wall under the influence of estrogens and/or local growth factors, some of which may be stimulated by estrogens. Fibroids are frequently asymptomatic but, depending on location, symptoms, such as pain, excessive bleeding and disturbances in urination and fertility may arise. One in five women under the age of 50 develop uterine fibroids. Black women are more prone (2–3 times more frequently than in White women) and develop them at an earlier age. Fibroids remain one of the leading reasons for hysterectomy in the USA.

Uterine fibroids are primarily diagnosed by pelvic or abdominal exam, usually with ultrasonographic confirmation. Magnetic resonance imaging (MRI) is also used to diagnose and differentiate these benign tumors from ovarian tumors.

Market Trends

Typical treatments consist of drugs or surgery, depending on the size, location and symptomatology. Drug therapy includes: GnRH agonists, progesterone, gestational steroids, antiprogestins and anti-estrogens. Despite the high prevalence of this disorder, there are few therapeutic alternatives. Sales for specific treatment of fibroids accounted for just over $5.3 million in 1993 with growth in some countries and declines in others (IMS Midas, 1993). It is difficult to assess sales trends in the international markets in particular, since reimbursement, which is determined by each regulatory authority, changes annually. Surgical intervention is often the only long-term alternative for women with severe symptomatic fibroids, which can be therapeutic but can often result in loss of fertility. More research is needed to better define the causes of fibroid development.

Market Needs

As with endometriosis, treatment tends to be non-specific gonadotropin releasing hormone (GnRH) analogs prior to surgery appear to have become a primary mode of therapy. As with endometriosis, GnRH analogs are not a cure, but merely alleviate symptoms. In addition, these products are associated with sometimes unbearable side effects of estrogen deprivation. More effective therapeutic alternatives are much needed. Alternatives to surgery other than partial myomectomies or total hyster-ectomy are needed. Unfortunately, fibroids are problematic because they so often tend to be asymptomatic. In fact, they often present clinically as large masses. With growths of such size, any therapy other than surgery is usually less than successful.

Prophylactic therapeutic alternatives remain a market need. Since the exact mechanisms involved in the development of fibroids are not well defined, current pharmacologic treatments offer only immediate solutions, without significant long-term results or cure. Ongoing research into the genetic basis of fibroid growth may yield some therapeutic alternatives in the future.

Polycystic Ovarian Disease

Demographics

Polycystic ovarian disease (PCO) is characterized by abnormal gonadotropin secretion with polycystic ovaries, increased in size and functional activity of ovarian stromal tissues. These stromal cells are responsible for secretion of androgens, which can be elevated in PCO and cause many of the androgenic symptoms and signs. PCO is one of the most common endocrine disorders in women of reproductive age, with prevalence of 10–23% in this age group. Irregular menses, mild obesity and hirsutism are associated with PCO, often beginning at puberty and worsening as the woman ages.

Market Trends

There is no ideal treatment for PCO. Current therapy includes the use of combination oral contraceptives, urofollitrophin (to assist in the infertility associated with PCO) and cyproterone acetate. Spironolactone and the 5α-reductase products are in use or under study, as are GnRH analogs. These agents often assist in reduction of acne and hirsutism, while limiting the effect on ovarian size. Without a clear understanding of the etiology of PCO, treatment is often targeted at symptomatic relief.

Sales for various agents used, including progestins, oral contraceptives, etc., amounted to over $15 million in 1993 (IMS Midas, 1993). There were strong growth rates in most of the major markets, with the exception of France, where progestin use is generally quite high. This could be an anomaly of the definition of why/for what indication(s) the therapy is given.

Market Needs

Similar to the other diseases of the reproductive tract, there is a considerable need to both understand the disease and develop innovative therapies. Although there is continued effort at basic research into etiology, very little research is ongoing on the much needed therapies for this very common disease. In addition, there is still an unmet need to treat the symptoms of this disease, namely acne and hirsutism. Current alternatives are potent but some toxic side effects often limit their use. Effective alternatives which do not affect fertility are clearly needed. Effective treatment of hirsutism, which offers both cosmetic and long-term solutions, is much needed. This issue is discussed further below.

Hirsutism

Demographics

Hirsutism is defined as an increase in the density and rate of growth of typically androgen-dependent terminal hairs in women. Causes include mild to serious increase in mild androgens of ovarian or adrenal origin. No clear incidence rates of hirsutism are well established, primarily because the etiologies can be multiple. Hirsutism itself is not often considered a disease but rather a symptom of other conditions, such as PCO.

Market Trends

The use of ethinyl estradiol and medroxyprogesterone acetate is 75–85% effective in treating hirsutism. Spironolactone is approved in the USA for its anti-

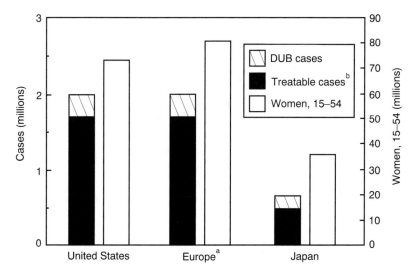

FIGURE 4.10 Potential treatment market for dysfunctional uterine bleeding (DUB), 1993. [a]'Europe' here consists of France, Germany, Italy, Spain and UK. [b]Only 85% of DUB cases are treatable. Reproduced from Godsey (1995) by permission of *DR Reports*, Decision Resources Inc.

aldosterone effect but not its anti-androgenic effect, although it can be used to treat hirsutism. It is, however, widely used as an anti-androgenic agent. Cyproterone acetate is prescribed quite readily in Europe due to its anti-androgenic characteristics. Sales of agents for the treatment of hirsutism were just over $19 million in 1993, according to IMS Midas (1993). Again, fairly strong growth was seen in most major markets. Several 5α-reductase inhibitors (finestride is such a product) are being evaluated for the treatment of hirsutism. Hirsutism can sometimes be attributed to a side effect or androgenic action of a drug.

Dysfunctional Uterine Bleeding

Demographics

Dysfunctional uterine bleeding (DUB) is defined as painless, irregular vaginal bleeding of endometrial origin which may be excessive (>80 ml), prolonged (>7 days), or unpatterned (occurring differently to the normally expected menstrual bleeding) and in which an organic or systemic disease can not be demonstrated. It is most commonly found at the extremes of a woman's reproductive life. More than 50% of cases occur in women over 45 years of age, while 20% can be seen in adolescents.

Potential market size for DUB is shown in Figure 4.10.

Market Trends

Treatment of DUB is often individualized and will depend on the severity of bleeding and the etiology. The patient's desire for cycle control, fertility, contraception or simply bleeding control are determining factors. Low-dose contraceptives, cyclic progestin, conjugated estrogens or hysterectomy procedures in extreme cases or in menopausal/perimenopausal women, may all be tried by the treating physician. The therapeutic regimen is often dependent on the underlying cause and severity of bleeding.

Fibrocystic Breast Disease

Demographics

Fibrocystic breast disease, or benign breast syndrome, refers to a range of changes in the breast observed in premenopausal women. Changes in breast stroma often seen can be due to the presence of cysts, adenosis, fibrosis, fibroadenoma and ductal hyperplasia. The condition is characterized by breast tenderness, pain, swelling and nodularity, often but not always just prior to menses.

Market Trends

Since fibrocystic breast disease can affect most women at some point in their reproductive life, pain relief is the primary intention of treatment. Apart from analgesic therapy, dietary changes are commonly recommended, such as avoidance of caffeine, theophylline and theobromine. As with most of such less well-defined conditions, further elucidation will most definitely better address targeted drug development. The market is not currently satisfied with current therapeutic alternatives and women are often obliged to continue with the presence of pain. The only other products used primarily outside the USA include chymotrypsin and acetazolamide. Sales of these agents only account for approximately $50 000 in 1993. The trends are too small to be meaningful (IMS Midas, 1993).

Urinary Incontinence

Demographics

'Incontinence' is a term used to define the physical inability to control urination. Urinary control is a complex process that is dependent on established reflexes in the spinal cord and brain. There are various causes which lead to urinary malfunction. Urinary incontinence (UI) can be caused by pathologic, anatomic or physiologic factors affecting the urinary tract, and includes psychological conditions which can also result in UI.

The types of UI are:

1. *Stress*—represents 40% of all cases and usually follows coughing, laughing, bending or lifting, i.e. some type of physical exertion.
2. *Urge*—specific urinary urge accounts for approximately 39% of incontinence cases; it may be caused by bladder infections, local tumors, bladder stones, or spinal cord damage, stroke or mental deterioration.
3. *Reflex*—loss of urine caused by the sensation of a full bladder.
4. *Overflow*—occurs when the bladder is fully distended and the urethral sphincter is malfunctioning.
5. *Functional*—can be slight, moderate or heavy; it is the involuntary emptying of the bladder, associated with chronic impairments of physical and/or cognitive function.

Prevalence of UI differs by gender. In men aged 15–64, prevalence is 1.5–5%. In women of the same age range, prevalence of UI is 10–25% (Thomas et al, 1980).

For non-institutionalized persons over the age of 60, prevalence of UI is 15–30%. The institutionalized population is estimated to have almost 50% prevalence, and incontinence is often cited as the main reason for institutionalizing patients.

Market Trends

The high prevalence of urinary incontinence has significant physiologic, social and psychological costs. Currently, there are wide variations in UI diagnosis, care and treatment. $16.4 billion is spent in the USA every year on incontinence-related care; $11.2 billion for community-based programs and at home care. Approximately $1.1 billion is spent on disposable products for adults (AHCPR, 1992). The current market for pharmaceutical products is not significant. Globally there is approximately $300 million spent annually on currently available products.

Current treatment with drug therapy can help incontinence. Banthene® and Pro-Banthene® propantheline bromide, marketed by Roberts Pharmaceutical in the USA, are approved for use in urinary incontinence. Another drug, Contigen®, is a collagen injected into the bladder, allowing the collagen to expand and close off the bladder opening. The procedure is new and costs $1,500–$2,000 for each injection plus overhead costs. This procedure is usually reserved for stress incontinence cases. Propaverine HCl, known as BUP-4, was approved for incontinence use in Japan. Farmitalia-CarloErba has introduced Cystrin® for treatment of urge and nocturnal enuresis.

Surgical procedures are also used frequently to treat the various types of incontinence. They are intended to strengthen the pelvic floor, and treat defects in the bladder, urethra or sphincter. Kegel exercises are a first line attempt at increasing muscular tone. These are geared towards strengthening the muscles, which are often weakened by childbirth. These exercises can be effective in alleviating symptoms in some cases.

The use of absorbent adult diapers or similar products has increased substantially over recent years. Women formerly would resort to using feminine protection products, shields or pads. Now there are products specifically designed for incontinence use, with less bulk and greater absorption. This over-the-counter market segment is often noted to be over $1 billion dollars annually in the USA.

Incontinence appliances are used for collecting and draining urine. Types of appliances used are external catheters, which direct urine to a bag strapped to the leg, or tubing, connectors, mechanical supports and anti-reflux valves. These products are used when surgery and alternate products are not effective.

Market Needs

There are substantial unmet needs in the UI market. The first need is to educate health care professionals in proper diagnosis and classification of this disorder. Despite the high prevalence, little has been done to acknowledge and treat the various types of UI, except when symptoms become intolerable.

Less than half the population suffering from UI consult a health care giver about the problem. Urinary incontinence is rarely fully worked up medically. Instead, many people turn to absorbent materials and supportive aids without consultation or discussions with health care providers. Dependence on caregivers is high and increases over time as the condition worsens. Increased awareness of the disorder and alternatives for treatment need to be communicated to the general population. Increased education is necessary to encourage earlier and perhaps less costly intervention. The costs associated with UI are substantial. A conservative estimate from WHO in 1990 accounted for a direct cost of $7 billion annually in the USA in the community and an additional $3.3 billion in nursing homes.

There are a number of pharmacologic alternatives available for treating UI. However, not many well-controlled studies have been conducted with these therapies that would assist in comparison of treatment benefits for the various types of UI.

Most therapies used to treat detrusor overactivity, leading to urge incontinence, are effective. Drawbacks to these drugs are their cholinergic-related side effects, viz. dry mouth, blurred vision, nausea, constipation, etc. Pharmacologic alternatives, obtained from better defined studies which target specific smooth muscle function effects and which limit cholinergic or cardiac side effects, are very much needed.

Sexually Transmitted Diseases (STDs and Vaginitides)

Demographics

Sexually transmitted diseases (STDs) are an extremely worrisome threat to women worldwide. They are the most common infectious diseases throughout the world, with substantially greater numbers being found in the developing countries. The World Health Organization (WHO), has put the incidence of bacterial and viral STDs at 125 million people worldwide. In the USA alone, the Center for Disease Control (CDC) estimates 12 million people annually contract an STD, with the majority (> 65%) under 25 years old.

In developed nations, such as the USA, Europe and Japan, the incidence of bacterial STDs has decreased since the 1970s. Viral infections, e.g. HIV, herpes simplex, human papillomavirus (HPV), in those countries have increased over the same period. The general increase of STDs worldwide is attributed to the rise in drug abuse and the resulting impact on the commercial sex industry, the decreased age of first intercourse, more lifetime sexual partners and the lack of availability of non-barrier contraceptives.

Table 4.5 shows basic incidence data on each of the main STDs in the selected countries from the developed world.

Therapeutic Options

Antibiotics remain the mainstay of therapy for all non-viral STDs. Tetracyclines, macrolides, quinolones, along with the penicillins and cephalosporins, are utilized in most of the infections. Nucleoside analogs and interferon are used in cytomegalovirus (CMV), HIV and herpes simplex virus (HSV). HIV treatment and prevention continues to take center stage in research into novel anti-viral agents. The new protease inhibitors hold promise.

Vaccine development is an important area of investigation, although no specific vaccines are available for sexually transmitted diseases.

Market Trends

From a public health point of view, prevention is by far preferable to treatment of these diseases. Safe sex behaviors and consistent use of barrier contraceptives are probably the most important messages to convey to the population at risk. Women should know about the added susceptibility they encounter to HIV.

Worldwide, the STDs marketplace was worth about $1.5 billion dollars in 1993, of which bacterial STDs accounted for about $300 million (Decision Resources, 1995). The addition of expensive HIV drugs to this portfolio will no doubt greatly increase the sales figures. Sales for HIV treatment in 1992 were currently estimated

TABLE 4.5 Incidence of STDs in selected countries

	USA	France	Germany	Italy	UK	Japan
Chlamydia	4 000 000	500 000	700 000	515 000	515 000	1 250 000
Cytomegalovirus	3 965 000	632 000	950 000	910 000	637 000	1 962 000
Trichomonas	2 500 000	560 000	775 700	570 000	460 000	1 000 000
Gonorrhea	1 500 000	225 000	310 000	230 000	230 000	500 000
HPV	878 000	164 000	296 000	201 000	210 000	310 000
Herpes simplex	1 497 800	342 700	479 350	328 440	348 550	652 150
HIV (prevalence)	940 000	146 000	96 500	97 000	43 400	10 200
Hepatitis B	290 000	62 000	109 000	630 000	51 700	1 850 000
Hepatitis C	150 500	46 000	40 000	60 100	34 500	211 000
Syphilis	130 000	17 000	23 000	17 000	17 000	37 000

Data from Decision Resources Inc., 1992.

at $392 million, according to Decision Resources, in the seven major countries throughout the world. That still leaves the majority of the $1.5 billion accounting for other treatment and non-pharmacologic treatment, i.e. surgery.

In general, almost all non-viral STDs are susceptible to antibiotics, although some resistant strains continue to emerge in some of the gonococcal infections. Complete cure of HIV remains elusive, while therapies aimed at other viral diseases often alleviate symptoms rather than eliminating the disease.

CONCLUSION

There are substantial differences in pharmaceutical availability and use during a woman's reproductive life cycle, and often these can be dependent on the developing status of the country. Those women who live in developed nations have a much greater exposure to, and alternatives to, drug therapy throughout their lifetime. Those in developing countries often suffer from little or limited drug availability, although the needs may indeed be inversely proportional.

Throughout a normal life cycle, a woman may be exposed to hundreds of pharmaceutical agents. Various antibiotics, vaccines and other prophylactic care are used predominantly in the early years of a female's life. Once she has reached puberty and becomes sexually active, a young woman must learn to use birth control options. Abstinence is common among the younger teenagers; however, there are increasing numbers of sexually active young teenagers. The choice of methods used is often the result of cultural, religious and societal peer influence.

The use and exposure to pharmaceutical agents increases generally with age. The greatest use of pharmaceutical products is with the older population of women, frequently over 60. As the body ages and, particularly with women, as the natural hormonal estrogen production ceases with menopause, there are increases in the incidence and morbidity of diseases.

This chapter has provided a quick insight into the critical importance of market data and the role of the marketing in the development of drugs. Marketing serves a unique role in being able to provide insight into the commercial success of a potential therapeutic, but also remains privileged in being able to represent the consumer in the developmental process. Marketing experts are truly a window into the world of the user for research-based companies. Wise use of these critical sources of information should provide the basis of good and socially useful drugs for women.

REFERENCES

AHCPR (Agency for Health Care Policy and Research). *Overview: Urinary Incontinence in Adults, Clinical Practice Guideline Update, Facts about Incontinence* 1992; Rockville, MD: AHCPR.
American Cancer Society. *FactBook 1992*.

Baron JA, Barrett J, Malenka D et al. Racial differences in fracture risk. *Epidemiology* 1994; **5**: 42–7.

Cummings SR, Kelsey JL, Nevitt MC, O'Dowd KJ. Epidemiology of osteoporosis and osteoporotic fractures. *Epidemiol Rev* 1985; **7**: 178–208.

Decision Resources. 1992; Waltham, MA: Decision Resources Inc.

FDM Pharma. *Hormone Replacement Therapy in Key European Markets* 1996; Valbonne, France: FDM Pharma.

Frost & Sullivan. *US Obstetrics and Gynecology Pharmaceutical Markets* 1995, pp 7–24, 7–32, 8–6, 8–12; Mountainview, CA: Frost & Sullivan, Inc.

Godsey SG. *Women's Unmet Health Needs* 1995, pp 9, 106; Waltham, MA: Decision Resources Inc.

Harris L. *The Commonwealth Fund Women's Health Survey* 1993, pp 29–31; New York: Louis Harris & Associates, Inc.

IMS International. *Total World Market by Region, 1996 Global Pharma Report* 1997; London: IMS International Inc.

IMS Midas. *IMS International Market Audits* 1993; London: IMS Midas International.

National Osteoporosis Foundation (NOF). *Report* 1997; Washington, DC: NOF.

Ortho Pharmaceutical Co. *The Ortho Annual Birth Control Survey* 1996; Raritan, NJ: Ortho Pharmaceutical Co.

Office of Research on Women's Health, Office of the Director. *Report of the National Institutes of Health: Opportunities for Research on Women's Health* 1991 Publication No. 92-3457; Hunt Valley, MD: US Department of Health and Human Services, Public Health Service, NIH.

Point of View (PoV) Women's Health Care. *Report* 1995; PO Box 238, Cedar Grove, NJ 07009: PoV.

Population Crisis Committee Report. *Access to Affordable Contraception: 1991 Report on World Progress Toward Population Stabilization.* Washington, DC: Population Crisis Committee.

Thomas TM, Phlymat KR, Blanwin J, Meade TS. Prevalence of urinary incontinence. *Br Med J* 1980; **281**: 1243–5.

United Nations, Dept. for Economic and Social Information and Policy Analysis Population Division. *The Sex and Age Distribution of the World Populations* 1994 Revision, pp 4–5, 8–9, 816–17; New York: United Nations.

Wheeler JM. Epidemiology and prevalence of endometriosis. In Diamond MP, DeCherney AH (eds) *Infertility and Reproductive Medicine Clinics of North America* 1992, vol. 3, pp 545–9; New York: Saunders.

World Health Organization. *The World Health Statistics Report* 1990; Geneva: WHO.

5

International and National Public Health Issues

Roberto Rivera[1], Karen Hardee[2] and Barbara Barnett[1]

*[1]Family Health International, Research Triangle Park, NC,
and [2]Futures Group International, Durham, NC, USA*

INTRODUCTION

The development of new drugs and medical devices is commonly driven by two factors: the evolution of scientific knowledge and perceptions of public need.

The public may perceive the need for a new drug long before the scientific base of knowledge exists to make development of the drug possible. For example, the need for a polio prophylaxis was evident long before a vaccine was developed. Similarly, the AIDS pandemic is well under way, but no curative or preventive drug is ready for distribution. To a large degree, pharmaceutical companies base decisions on the development of new drugs and medical devices on epidemiologic information (e.g. the frequency or severity of a disease or a syndrome) as well as economic issues. Development of new contraceptives, for example, may be influenced by data from demographic surveys, which document the numbers of unplanned or unwanted pregnancies among sub-groups of women in a particular region.

Increasingly, public perceptions are playing a key role in the development of new drugs, particularly contraceptives. Scientists are asking what couples want from family planning methods and seeing the importance of directing drug development to match those needs.

This chapter presents an overview of the main public health issues that should be taken into consideration in the development of drugs for women. Public health is dealt with in a broad sense, and our discussions include the needs and expectations of society at large, but particularly women. The goals of drug development should be to meet the diverse needs of women and to improve the quality of their lives. Because of the importance of reproductive health to women's overall well-being, and the authors' experience in this field, much of this chapter is devoted to discussions of contraceptive development in the context of reproductive health.

Drug Development for Women. Edited by V.V. Ragavan. © 1998 John Wiley & Sons Ltd.

THE PUBLIC HEALTH PERSPECTIVE

The ultimate goal of any public health program is to improve the quality of life of the individual and of the larger society. The Institute of Medicine's Committee for the Study of the Future of Public Health has proposed that public health be viewed as '. . . what we, as a society, do collectively to assure the conditions in which people can be healthy. This requires that continuing and emerging threats to the public are successfully encountered (National Academy of Science, 1988)'. In defining health, the World Health Organization (WHO) has concluded that health is the state of complete physical, mental and social well-being.

The declaration of Alma Ata, which resulted from the International Conference on Primary Health Care convened by WHO in 1978 (WHO/UNICEF, 1978), underscored this point. At the conference, the goal of 'Health for All by the Year 2000' was proclaimed. Based on the ideals of universal access to care, health was viewed as an integral component of economic development (Andreano, 1993).

The Alma Ata declaration recommended the need to focus health care in some basic areas, including maternal care and family planning. More recently, the World Bank has proposed a health service package that includes 11 interventions as essential components of health care for developing countries (Saxenian, 1994–95). Some reproductive health services for women are elements of this package, including family planning (both as a public health program and as a clinical service), prenatal care and obstetric delivery care. The package, affordable for most countries, gives a high priority to the development of improved methods for fertility regulation and development of drugs for the management of sexually transmitted diseases (STDs) for women in both developing and developed nations.

REPRODUCTIVE HEALTH

Reproductive health is one of the most important components of women's health; it affects numerous aspects of women's quality of life, including their emotional, social and economic well-being. Reproductive health also affects the larger public health.

In developing drugs to meet women's reproductive health needs, it is particularly important that the user's perceptions—including perceptions of risks and benefits, practicality of use, affordability, and effectiveness—be analyzed and taken into account. These perceptions may be different for women who live in developing countries and women in industrialized nations, given the large differences in health and economic climates. In developing new drugs for women, researchers must consider the realities of these women's everyday lives.

The concept of reproductive health has evolved over several decades. In the 1970s, human rights and women's health advocates began to question the rationale of traditional population policies, which focused mainly on reducing population growth rather than on individual well-being (Dixon-Mueller, 1993; Sinding & Ross, 1994). Women's advocates urged reconsideration of population policies that had encouraged fertility regulation without addressing women's needs for economic security, education and freedom from poverty and oppression. Advocates also argued that population policies that emphasized only family planning ignored other important health needs of women, such as access to basic health services, prevention of sexually transmitted diseases, screenings for cancer and treatment of infertility.

In January 1994, representatives of women's organizations and non-governmental organizations from 79 countries gathered in Rio de Janeiro, Brazil, to draft a document defining the essential components of reproductive health. The Rio Statement called for 'quality reproductive health services [as] a key right for women . . . all with the informed consent of women' (Rio Statement, 1994).

Several months later, a consensus definition of reproductive health was ratified at the 1994 International Conference on Population and Development (ICPD) in Cairo. This definition has far-reaching implications for women's reproductive health, for programs that provide reproductive health care and for the development of new drugs and therapies for women:

> Reproductive health is a state of complete physical, mental and social well-being and not merely the absence of disease or infirmity, in all matters relating to the reproductive system and to its functions and processes. Reproductive health therefore implies that people are able to have a satisfying and safe sex life and that they have the capability to reproduce and the freedom to decide if, when and how often to do so . . . It also includes sexual health, the purpose of which is the enhancement of life and personal relations, and not merely counseling and care related to reproduction and sexually transmitted diseases (ICPD, 1994).

At the Fourth World Conference on Women, held in 1995 in Beijing, this comprehensive definition of reproductive health was reaffirmed.

A public health perspective requires that the process of drug development for women be seen not only as the development of products to treat women's diseases, but as the development of interventions that enhance the quality of women's lives and provide them with improved opportunities for social, emotional and economic well-being. In other words, drug development must consider the comprehensive spectrum of women's needs. It must consider how a health intervention will affect other aspects of a woman's life—her ability to work, to care for her family, to participate in religious or community activities. With contraceptive development, there is yet another consideration: unlike drugs that are taken to cure an illness, contraceptives are generally used by healthy women. It is essential, therefore, that a contraceptive drug or device does not compromise the current health status of the user.

SOCIAL PERCEPTIONS OF GENDER AND HEALTH

Social and Cultural Perceptions of Women's Roles and Women's Health

In many developing countries, the socio-economic status of women is considerably lower than that of men; consequently, women's health status is negatively affected. For example, family preference for sons instead of daughters may mean that daughters receive less food than their brothers, leading to poor nutrition and possibly anemia. The need to produce children for economic security may mean that women undergo multiple pregnancies, putting themselves at risk of morbidities and mortality to ensure their financial survival. Women's inability to negotiate with their spouses or partners may put them at risk of sexually transmitted diseases, including AIDS. And an adolescent's desire to prove her fertility may put her at risk of teen pregnancy. In industrialized nations, where women have greater access to health care services, including family planning and abortion, maternal death rates are lower than in developed countries. However, women in industrialized nations still face some of the same risks as women in developing nations: exposure to STDs and AIDS, violence, and unwanted or unplanned pregnancy. As women in industrialized nations gain more financial equality with men, they also are facing health problems that used to affect men predominantly: lung cancer due to cigarette smoking, heart disease and alcoholism.

In her writings on gender and development, Moser presents a framework that includes the triple roles of women: reproductive roles, which include childbirth and childrearing; productive roles, which include paid and voluntary employment; and community management (Moser, 1993). In developing new drugs for women, it also is important to consider the multiple contexts in which women make decisions about their own health care and the health care of their families, and the circumstances in which women receive health care. Some of these factors are discussed below.

Marriage and Family

In many countries, women's roles are defined exclusively as wife and mother, and women's primary responsibilities are childbearing, childrearing, and care for family members. In 14 out of 42 countries in which a demographic and health survey (DHS) has been conducted, at least half of the women were married by age 18 (Carr & Way, 1994), and marriage—or a consensual union—was virtually universal. In many cultures, marriage and children are a means for women to achieve some measure of economic security. Therefore, early marriage (in adolescence) and large families are important. 'Lack of economic resources and inequality in gender relations make having children a strategy for survival', according to Sonia Corrêa of the Instituto Brasileiro de Análises Sociais e Economicas in Brazil (Barnett, 1994).

Children are often viewed as a source of labor or as a source of security for parents in old age. In Africa, women have at least five children on average, compared to three or four in Asia/Near East and Latin America/Caribbean. Women in the countries surveyed by the DHS spent an average of between 11 and 20 years in active childbearing. For example, the median age for first birth among women in Kenya was 19 and the median age of last birth was 39—a period of nearly 20 years (McCauley et al, 1994).

In addition to duties in childrearing, many women assume responsibility as the caretakers of all family members, including the elderly and the sick. These responsibilities increase where cuts in social services and economic dislocation affect access to health care.

Work

For most women in developing countries, participation in the paid work force may be temporary or part-time if it occurs at all. The home is typically the major center of work for women, and women are not paid for essential tasks such as collecting fuel, cooking, childcare or farming. Work in family enterprises or subsistence activities also may not be remunerated.

Time-use statistics, which consider all work (paid and unpaid activity and housework), reveal that women spend more of their time working than men in all developing and developed regions, except North America and Australia. Studies in Latin America and the Caribbean have found that women work an average of 3 more hours a week than men, while women in Africa, Asia and the Pacific work an average of 12–13 hours more per week than their male counterparts (United Nations, 1991).

Female heads of households are a growing phenomenon, and now comprise more than 20% of all the households in Africa, the developed regions and Latin America and the Caribbean (United Nations, 1991).

Health Status

In much of the developing world, the health status of adults and children is poor. Lack of adequate food and safe water, poor sanitation, and poor health-care infrastructures contribute. For boys and girls alike, poor health begins before birth; mothers who are anemic, who suffer from infectious and parasitic diseases and who lack access to antenatal care are likely to give birth to unhealthy babies. Infant mortality rates are highest in developing countries, with an average of 90 deaths per 1000 live births in Africa, 44 per 1000 in Latin American and the Caribbean and 62 per 1000 in Asia (World Population Data Sheet, 1995). Thirteen percent of children born in developing countries die before their third birthdays (National Research Council, 1989).

Children who survive infancy face uncertain health prospects. Lack of safe water and sanitation contribute to children's health problems; in Africa, 33% of the population still lacks safe drinking water, and in the 1980s approximately 80% of people living in rural areas and 50% living in urban areas lacked adequate sanitation facilities (United Nations, 1991). Malnutrition continues to be a devastating health problem. In 21 of 42 developing countries surveyed by the DHS, at least one-quarter of children under the age of 3 are undernourished to the point that their growth is stunted (Carr & Way, 1994).

For girls, often considered an economic burden by their families and of less value than sons, the prospects for a healthy future are particularly bleak. Social and cultural discrimination against girls takes many forms, and these can have an impact on the physical well-being of the girl child. In countries where there is a strong preference for sons, girl children tend to receive less food and less medical care. A study in Bangladesh found that boys were seen 66% more often than girls at a treatment center for diarrhea (Chen, Huq & D'Souza, 1981). Selective abortion of female fetuses are practices in some countries, and infanticide or abandonment of females soon after birth occurs as well.

Starrs observes that:

The root causes of a woman's death can begin before her birth and are perpetuated during childhood and adolescence and continue later in her life. She generally has less access to food and education. Her childhood days were taken up by the endless search for water, food and fuel (Starrs, 1987, cited in Kwast, 1993, p. 105).

Anemia, one indicator of malnourishment, is prevalent among women in developing countries and increases women's vulnerability to illness, complications during pregnancy and maternal death.

Worldwide over 500 000 women die each year from causes related to childbearing. According to Koblinsky (1995, p. 830), 'Pregnant women and newborns have had no advocates; if they die it is often attributed to fate'. In 30 of 42 countries surveyed by the DHS, at least one-quarter of the women had experienced the death of at least one child (Carr & Way, 1994).

Adolescent pregnancy is a problem of growing concern in both developed and developing nations. Pregnancy before age 20 places both mother and infant at higher risk of mortality and morbidity. Pregnant teens may suffer from anemia, miscarriage, toxemia or eclampsia. Because their bodies have not fully matured, prolonged or obstructed labor may occur, which can lead to a ruptured uterus or vesicovaginal fistula. Infants born to teen mothers may suffer complications due to low birth-weight and prematurity. The incidence of stillbirths is higher among teens, who are less likely to seek prenatal care due to economic and social barriers.

Sexually transmitted diseases, including AIDS, are health problems drawing increased attention from researchers and women's health advocates. Women are, by virtue of culture and biology, more vulnerable to STDs than men. Some researchers have suggested that anatomical differences make reproductive tract infections more easily transmissible to women but more difficult to diagnose. STDs are more frequently asymptomatic in women than in men, and when symptoms do occur in women, they are more subtle and often more difficult to diagnose. Because of their lower social status and their economic dependence on men, women may not be able to negotiate the use of condoms as an STD prevention measure (Cates & Stone, 1994).

According to the World Health Organization, AIDS is now the leading cause of death for women ages 20–40 in some major cities in western Europe, Sub-Saharan Africa and the Americas. Other types of STDs can lead to infertility—a drastic consequence in countries that place a high value on women's role as mothers and on large family size—and STDs are responsible for 0.5–1.0% of maternal deaths in Sub-Saharan Africa and 20% of the maternal deaths in the USA (United Nations, 1991).

In addition to these health concerns, women also are vulnerable to rape, sexual assault and domestic violence.

WOMEN'S ACCESS TO HEALTH CARE

Within the world's medical community, women's health has been viewed primarily in terms of obstetrical and gynecological services. Within the field of public health, women's needs have been addressed primarily through the provision of maternal and child health programs (Francisco, 1989; Krieger & Fee, 1994). This perception ignores large groups of women in need of reproductive health services—specifically, those who are not pregnant, often including adolescents, unmarried women and menopausal women. In many parts of Africa, for example, the medical community ignores women who are not mothers (McFadden, 1994). McFadden (1994) states her point emphatically: few health programs in developing countries target non-pregnant and non-lactating women. Because they are neglected at health centers unless they are pregnant or are already mothers, women often seek care only for conditions linked to childbearing; for other conditions they tend to depend on self-care or tolerate the pain and associated discomfort.

An example of this tolerance for pain can be found in the preliminary results of a five-country study coordinated by Family Health International (FHI). Researchers found that approximately three-quarters of the 16 000 women interviewed in household surveys reported a morbidity related to their last pregnancy, delivery or post-partum period, or a chronic condition stemming from pregnancy or childbirth. Morbidities included a wide range of conditions, such as obstructed labor, complications from unsafe abortions, bacterial infections, anemia, eclampsia and hemorrhage. From preliminary results, researchers speculated that in Egypt, Ghana and Indonesia there were some 240–330 maternal morbidities for each maternal mortality. In spite of the apparent prevalence of morbidities, women often do not view less serious conditions as anything extraordinary; this perception of morbidities as 'normal' has hampered research in this area (Finger, 1994).

Although the emphasis in women's health care has been on maternal care, antenatal services nonetheless remain limited in developing countries. In 10 of 41 countries surveyed by the DHS, women received prenatal care for 90% of their pregnancies, while in 18 of 42 countries surveyed by the DHS, fewer than half of deliveries received professional medical assistance (Carr & Way, 1994).

Emergency obstetrical care, including treatment of hemorrhage, infection, hypertension and obstructed labor, is often severely limited in the developing world. Life-saving interventions, such as referral to medical centers, antibiotics and surgery are unavailable to many women, especially those in rural areas who may lack the money for health care or the transportation to a health center.

In the developed world, where maternal and infant mortality rates are typically lower due to broad access to antenatal services, fragmentation of health care services is a concern. During her reproductive years a woman might receive care from several physicians, not just one; she might receive care from a family physician, an internist and an obstetrician/gynecologist, all in different clinics (Commentary, 1992).

THE DRUG DEVELOPMENT PROCESS

Principles Guiding Research

Several principles must guide drug development for women around the world, particularly for reproductive health. The 1994 ICPD called for reproductive health research—including applied biomedical and social science research—to strengthen reproductive health services. These measures include:

- The need for a life-cycle approach to reproductive health.
- Inclusion of men, adolescents and the unmarried.
- The importance of reproductive choice.
- The need for safe childbearing and freedom from unwanted pregnancy and coercion.
- The right to full information and services to regulate fertility.
- The right to complete well-being, freedom from disease and a focus on positive health outcomes including infant and child survival.
- Linkages to reproductive rights and women's rights (see Hardee & Yount, 1995).

In particular, the conference emphasized the need to strengthen research in the areas of new methods of contraception that meet users' needs and are acceptable, easy to use, safe, free of side effects, effective and affordable. The ICPD called for research on contraception for men, STDs, infertility and various aspects of abortion. International declarations very clearly indicate the high priority given by the public health sector to women's health.

When developing new drugs for women, the unique needs of women in less-developed countries must be taken into consideration. Differences in mortality or morbidity rates should be a factor, but there are other considerations as well. For example, culture can dictate which drugs a woman will or will not use. Routes of administration (e.g. an injection, a patch, vaginal administration) are perceived differently by women in various cultures. Which side effects are tolerable and which are not also varies. Preliminary results of a multi-country study on women's perspectives of contraception, conducted by Harvard University's School of Public Health, found that women in Phnom Penh, Cambodia, said they might be willing to tolerate some disturbances in menstrual bleeding; however, women in Udaipur, India, said they would not tolerate side effects well because of fears that amenorrhea would be viewed as a symptom of pregnancy and that family members would become suspicious (Snow, 1995).

The resources within the health structure necessary to deliver a new drug appropriately may not be present in a developing country situation, or even within certain social sectors of a developed country. The problems that the field is now facing with Norplant$^®$ (lack of access to trained providers who can perform removals) illustrate these points very well. However, since developing countries account for relatively little of the total world's health spending—10% in 1990 (Saxenian, 1994–95)—their influence on drug development is minor. Consequently, the needs of women living in developing countries exert limited influence in a market-driven economy of drug development.

The impression that drugs to be used in developing countries under primary health care conditions are economically unattractive for the pharmaceutical industry is misplaced, however. The need and potential use of these drugs is enormous, and reasonable economic benefits may be expected. Also, the need for 'new technologies' for fertility regulation and for the management of reproductive tract infections, including STDs, is universal. Furthermore, policy-makers with a primary interest in reproductive health agree that reproductive health services should extend beyond the childbearing years, and that these services should be integrated to the basic health services provided (Progress in Human Reproductive Research, 1994). This approach is an important medical and economic justification for the development of new drugs for women.

Life-cycle Approach

An important consideration in the development of new drugs, particularly contraceptives, is that women's health needs change over time.

One of the principles underlying the ICPD is the need to take a life-cycle approach to women's health (Sai & Nassim, 1989; OWL, 1994), rather than to view women in their more narrowly defined reproductive role.

The stages of a woman's life could include birth, childhood, menarche, marriage, childbearing, childrearing, menopause and old age. At each of these stages a woman's health needs will be different. For example, in their study in Gamileya, Egypt, Lane & Meleis (1991) found that the health risks for young girls are infectious diseases and accidents; for married women, pregnancy-related morbidity and burns; and for older women, respiratory infection, trachoma, and other age-related chronic conditions.

Forrest, who has studied women's reproductive health in developed countries, has observed five stages of reproductive life and notes that women's health needs vary considerably at each stage: menarche to first intercourse; first intercourse to marriage; marriage to first birth; first birth to attainment of desired family size; and attainment of desired family size to menopause. Women in the USA have a potential reproductive life (between menarche and menopause) of 35.9 years; spacing of children accounts for only 11% of a woman's reproductive life, and women spend about 75% of their reproductive lives trying to avoid unintended pregnancy and STDs (Forrest, 1993). Women's contraceptive needs (as well as larger reproductive health needs) change over time, depending upon fertility goals, sexual behavior and perceived exposures to STDs.

While quality of life research has long been used in association with drug trials in the West, notions of what constitutes quality of life are likely to be culturally bound. Nevertheless, the methodology for studying quality of life is rigorous (Spilker, 1990; Schipper, Clinch & Powell, 1990; Fletcher et al, 1992) and could be adapted to cultures outside of the West (Keller, 1987; Leelakulthanit & Day, 1992).

RESEARCH PRIORITIES AND GENDER ISSUES

In examining the development of drugs for women, it appears that women often have not been consulted or included in the research and development process. There has been concern in the USA and around the world that the practice of medicine was based on a male model (Council on Ethical and Judicial Affairs, 1991). Krieger & Fee (1994, p. 270) wrote that:

> In fact, by the time that researchers began to standardize methods for clinical and epidemiological research, notions of difference were so firmly embedded that whites and non-whites, men and women, were rarely studied together. Moreover, most researchers and physicians were interested only in the health status of whites and, in the case of women, only in their reproductive health.

Krieger and Fee argued for studies based on gender, race and class.

Gender also appears to be a factor in the delivery of health services. The doctor–patient relationship is often viewed as hierarchical, and this is complicated by gender roles that discourage women from questioning or challenging a traditional authority figure. While a US survey found that 82% of women did not feel that gender affected the way they were treated by their doctors, 25% of women, compared to 12% of men, said that doctors 'talked down' to them (Associated Press, 1993). Complicating this scenario is evidence that women, in fact, receive more health care services than men, including more physician visits per year and more services per visit—even when they visit the doctor for the same complaint (Council on Ethical and Judicial Affairs, 1991).

Until recently, women have had little influence in the development of health care technologies (Stauning, 1993). That appears to be changing.

The scientific and medical communities have been asked, in collaboration with women's health advocates, to develop a research agenda to study diseases and conditions affecting women. One approach is to integrate basic science, clinical trials and new technologies in six areas, including reproductive biology, early development biology, cardiovascular diseases, malignancies, immune and infectious diseases, and the aging process (Pinn, 1992).

Another effort began in 1988 with the establishment of the first World Health Organization Collaborating Center for Women's Health, located at the Key Centre for Women's Health in Society at the University of Melbourne in Australia (Morrow, 1995). The objectives of the Centre are to identify factors that constrain the health and well-being of women, to conduct research on those factors, to encourage changes in policies and service practices, and to encourage women in the mainstream of the development process. Most importantly, the Centre 'serves to strengthen links between health professionals and women's groups throughout the region, facilitate research, and elicit views on crucial issues in each country' (Morrow, 1995, p. 180). Thus far, the Centre has worked with groups from nine countries in the region.

The National Institutes of Health (NIH) Women's Health Initiative, based in the USA, has undertaken a comprehensive study of heart disease, stroke, cancer and osteoporosis. These diseases and conditions represent the major causes of death, disability and frailty in women of all races and socio-economic strata in the USA. The study will also look at the effects of menopause in older women, and diet modification, smoking cessation, use of hormones and physical exercise (Editorial, 1991). The study will eventually include 140 000 women who will be followed-up for 9 years in 50 clinics. The estimated cost of the study is $600 million (Marwick, 1992).

A major concern with drug development in the USA has been the limited inclusion of women as subjects in drug clinical trials. Many have argued that studies conducted on men have been generalized to women, even though women might react differently to drugs or treatments (Council on Ethical and Judicial Affairs, 1991). Critics argue that the assumption that a drug's effects on men will be the same for women is erroneous and ignores biological as well as socio-cultural factors. In addition, women's advocacy groups have pointed out that drug trials tend to exclude groups such as adolescent, anemic and breastfeeding women.

To address the issue of women's representation in drug trials, the National Institutes of Health established the Office of Research on Women's Health in 1990.

The role of the Office is to strengthen efforts to improve the prevention, diagnosis and treatment of illnesses that affect women. The Office is also charged with promoting research to understand diseases and conditions related to women. Included in its research function is the assurance that women are adequately represented in clinical research, including clinical trials.

Among pharmaceutical companies, a 1991 survey of 33 companies found that 94% routinely tested medicines in women and monitored data for differences between women and men (Gershon, 1992). A little more than three-quarters (76%) said that they recruit representative numbers of women for clinical trials. Still, issues remain regarding the inclusion of pregnant women (or even women with childbearing potential) in drug trials. According to Kessler, Merkatz & Temple (1993), 'There has been an understandable reluctance on the part of investigators and manufacturers to do so, for both ethical and medico-legal reasons'. The FDA has been working on guidelines for inclusion of women, including pregnant women, in clinical trials. The FDA's Working Group on Women in Clinical Trials will review new drug applications for compliance with the policy that a reasonable number of women are included in the study, including, as appropriate, pregnant women (Hall, 1995; LaRosa et al, 1995).

As evidence that drug development is meeting women's broad health needs, a survey by the Pharmaceutical Manufacturers Association identified 236 drugs that were being developed for use by women. The drugs being developed are mostly for cancer, obstetric and gynecological diseases and cardiovascular/cerebrovascular diseases, the three leading causes of death for women (Gershon, 1992).

WORKING WITH WOMEN'S HEALTH ADVOCACY GROUPS FOR CONTRACEPTIVE DEVELOPMENT

Nowhere is the need to include women's perspectives in drug development more critical than in the area of contraceptive technology. Women are the primary users of contraception; therefore, understanding their needs is essential if pharmaceutical companies are to develop drugs whose use is not only safe and effective but practical (e.g. can fit into a woman's daily routine) and drugs that enhance, not diminish, a woman's quality of life (WHO/IWHC, 1991).

In observing the traditional path of contraceptive development, Faúndes has noted:

> I don't know of a time that the development of a new contraceptive was started by saying, what women need is this, so let's try to study a method that responds to this need. What really happens is that there is an opportunity of developing a new contraceptive method because of a new discovery in the biological sciences (WHO and IWHC, 1991).

In 1991 a landmark meeting, bringing together scientists and women's health advocates, was convened by the World Health Organization's Special Programme of Research, Development and Research Training in Human Reproduction and by the International Women's Health Coalition. The goal of the meeting was to provide a forum in which members of the scientific community and women's advocates could share concerns, discuss common goals, and develop strategies in which scientists and women could work collaboratively in the selection and introduction of contraceptive methods.

At the meeting, women's advocates and scientists uncovered differences in perspective. For example, scientists defined contraceptive safety in terms of a drug that causes no dangerous or permanent side effects, using toxicological and clinical studies to determine whether a method might be carcinogenic or might affect major physiological functions, such as heart, kidneys or reproductive organs. Women's health advocates suggested that safety also includes the method's affect on overall health, including sexual interest, physical stamina and emotional well-being. In other words, women were concerned about side effects such as decreased libido, fatigue, depression. While not life-threatening, these side effects can tremendously alter a woman's quality of life. Women also suggested that safety should take into account the use of methods in regions where disease and malnutrition are prevalent and there is a high incidence of STDs, including AIDS.

Another area of differing perspectives was efficacy. While scientists defined effectiveness in terms of how well a method did or did not prevent pregnancy (method failure or user failure), women's measures of efficacy also included satisfaction. For example, women asked, 'is the method easy and convenient to use', 'does the woman have control over method use', 'how does method use affect sexual relationships'.

Acceptability also is an important area of difference. Scientific measurements typically include acceptance rates (agreement to start a method) and continuation or discontinuation rates. Women's advocates recommended that acceptability include a woman's ability to select a method in a climate of informed choice and her satisfaction or dissatisfaction with a particular method.

Women's perceptions about family planning—its benefits and side effects—can be crucial to their continued use of contraceptive methods. To better understand women's perceptions of family planning, the Women's Studies Project at Family Health International is exploring how women feel they have benefited or not benefited from use of contraceptive methods. A conceptual framework examines the relationships between (a) women's experiences with family planning methods and services, their pregnancy and childbearing experiences and their use of other reproductive health services, and (b) various domains of women's lives, including family roles, psychological and physical factors and societal/economic roles. The framework takes into account the effects of social, political and economic factors, gender norms and life cycle (Hardee et al, 1996).

Women's health advocates have suggested that the development of new contraceptive technologies does little to improve women's spectrum of choice or quality of life if methods are not introduced to consumers in a setting where health personnel are well-trained, where the health infrastructure is strong enough to support the new method, and where clients can be assured they will be able to make informed choices about method use and not be subjected to coercion or abuse.

Claro noted that:

> It is our [women's advocates'] task . . . to assist scientists in the . . . challenge of creating fertility regulation methods that take into account the welfare, sexuality, mental and physical health of women . . . Male researchers can themselves become more receptive (WHO/IWHC, 1991, p. 12).

Another key meeting on inclusion of women's perspectives in contraceptive development occurred in 1993 in Mexico City. The message of the international symposium 'Contraceptive Research and Development for the Year 2000 and Beyond' was that priority should be given to methods that meet women's perceived needs (particularly those under the user's control and that offer protection from STDs), postovulatory methods, and those that involve the shared responsibility of men for both birth control and disease prevention (Van Look & Perez-Palacios, 1994; Marcelo & Germain, 1994).

At a 1995 meeting on contraceptive research and development, sponsored by the Rockefeller Foundation and held in Bellagio, Italy, participants called for contraceptive development that accommodates 'the woman-centered agenda'. In a report from the conference, participants observed:

> The first contraceptive revolution was needs-driven, with emphasis on methods that can have a demographic impact . . . In the second contraceptive technology revolution, the field must again be needs-driven, with the emphasis this time on the needs and perspectives of women (Fathalla, Diczfalsy & Spieler, 1995).

The women-centered agenda includes the development of a broader array of contraceptives, to expand women's options. However, it also identifies three unmet needs in contraceptive development: the need for menses-inducers; the need for barrier methods that are controlled by women and can protect against both pregnancy and sexually transmitted diseases; and the need for new methods for men, who are now limited to the use of withdrawal, periodic abstinence, condoms or vasectomy.

With the advent of the global AIDS pandemic and the increase in rates of various STDs, there is an urgent need for the development of microbicides that can function as both an STD prophylaxis and a contraceptive (Wasserheit, 1989; Norsigian, 1992; Elias & Heise, 1993; Lange, 1993). The Population Council, which is working on development of a vaginal microbicide, is involving women's health advocates in all facets of product development, including design, clinical trials and, eventually, introduction of the product into the worldwide market. Studies also have examined women's preferences for microbicide delivery systems, including films, gels and suppositories. The collaboration between researchers and women's health advocates will be mutually beneficial, Claro suggests:

> When researchers become allied with women's health advocates in the health centers when clinical trials are conducted, information about the product being tested is dispersed through local networks . . . If involved in this process women's health advocates would establish open and meaningful communication with the study participants, which would provide, for the scientists, more accurate and complete reactions to the product (Population Council, 1994).

The National Institute of Allergy and Infectious Diseases (NIAID) is supporting research that includes a group often left out of clinical trials—adolescents. NIAID, in collaboration with the University of Pittsburgh, is studying the safety and efficacy of microbicides containing lactobacilli. These bacteria occur naturally in the vagina and they produce hydrogen peroxide, which scientists believe may prevent infection. Researchers are studying the use of lactobacilli suppositories among 900 adolescent women attending an urban health clinic. Scientists will try to determine the effects, if any, of suppositories on micro-organisms normally occurring in the vagina and whether suppositories decrease the incidence of bacterial vaginosis and gonorrhea. Equally as important as the effects of suppositories, researchers also will study whether teens will use this method and how they use it.

Researchers also are considering refinements and improvements in existing barrier methods, to satisfy women's needs for a female-controlled method that protects against STDs and pregnancy. The female polyurethane condom, which protects against pregnancy and some STDs, is being studied by Family Health International to determine whether it can be used more than once, as is now recommended. Studies have been conducted by the Centro de Pesquisas e Controle das Doenças Materno-Infantis de Campinas (CEMICAMP) in Brazil to examine the acceptability of a diaphragm used with and without spermicide. Family Health International, WHO and the Population Council are conducting a study on diaphragm use to determine women's views of acceptability and effectiveness. Lea's Shield, a cup-shaped barrier device that covers the cervix and can be worn for up to 48 hours, has been studied by the USA-based Contraceptive Development and Research Program (CONRAD) and may eventually be marketed for distribution without a prescription.

At the same time that scientists are working on microbicides and the development of female-controlled barrier contraceptives, the development of 'vaccines' for controlling fertility and the use of quinacrine as a method of non-surgical female sterilization are causing outcries among women's groups, who are concerned about safety, efficacy and acceptability factors associated with their use (Claro, 1995). In the case of the vaccine, women's groups worry about the potential for abuse of the method, which would offer non-reversible protection from pregnancy for 1 year.

From the client's perspective, not enough is known about women's preferences for windows of non-reversibility (Snow, 1994).

Another area of research is the development of emergency contraceptives—those that can be used by women after unprotected sexual intercourse but before pregnancy occurs. Currently, oral contraceptive pills, given in higher-than-usual doses within 48–72 hours after unprotected intercourse, can be used as emergency contraceptive methods. Copper intrauterine devices also can be used, if inserted within 5 days after unprotected intercourse. However, researchers are studying new formulations that might produce fewer side effects (nausea and vomiting may occur with current regimens), and they are examining new service delivery methods, such as the automatic provision of emergency contraceptive pills as a back-up method of contraception for couples who use barrier methods or over-the-counter emergency pills.

The makers of drugs for women's health will increasingly need to include women in the design, testing and evaluation of the products. This is particularly crucial in the development of new barrier contraceptives, said Dr Barbara Brummer of the USA-based pharmaceutical company, Advanced Care Products. Marketing studies have shown that women want a contraceptive method that is, first and foremost, safe. They also want a method that is effective in preventing pregnancy, effective in preventing STDs, and acceptable to their partners. 'We need to make sure that whatever we develop, we can satisfy the needs of women,' she said. 'Women want multiple formulations. They want options. If we develop one formulation, it won't satisfy all women' (Barnett, 1997).

Involving women in all phases of the drug development process may facilitate use of products when developed. Some researchers suggest a technology assessment approach to drug development, which would encourage health care policy-makers, drug companies, providers and researchers to take into account the user context before marketing a new drug (Hardon, 1992). The Pan American Health Organization (PAHO) suggests a risk approach to women's health (Chelala & Gorgas, 1991), including biological factors (e.g. age, parity), medical factors (e.g. chronic illness, personal habits, family system and support system), environmental factors and access to health services. Developers of drugs could also use such an approach to assess the feasibility of use of drugs in different settings. The Harvard University School of Public Health study is using a market research approach to determine which attributes of methods women like or dislike (Snow, 1995).

The Women and Pharmaceutical Project, established by one group of women's health advocates, reviews standard medical practices for contraceptive development and evaluation (Hardon, 1991). Similar groups could be constituted to review other drug trial protocols. For example, developers of drugs for women will have to be clear on the side effects of the drugs and the synergy between the drugs and underlying health conditions affecting women in different social, cultural and economic conditions (Snow, 1994). They will need to consider how a drug may affect women with differing nutritional statuses. Drug trials offer an opportunity to collect additional data on women's health, including their reproductive health.

Individual countries may prefer to collect their own data from drug trials, often stating that local residents have different perspectives, living conditions and cultural values to women in other countries.

Involvement of women's health advocates in the regulatory process, which governs approval and marketing of new drugs, is also important. The National Women's Health Network, founded in the USA in 1976, has conducted several campaigns to influence FDA guidelines and policies (Pearson, 1995). In the 1970s, the Network worked for inclusion of package inserts for users of oral contraceptives containing estrogen. The effort, supported by the FDA, was done to inform women of the risks and benefits of estrogen use. In 1977, the FDA implemented a new regulation that required all manufacturers of estrogen drugs to include patient package inserts in their products. The Network also was successful in its attempts to modify package labeling, to clarify that many of the drugs used during pregnancy had not been approved by the FDA specifically for obstetrical use. During the FDA approval process for the injectable contraceptive, Depo Provera, Network members created a registry for women who had used Depo Provera, to answer questions about their experiences with the drug, and members developed a user consent form, which has been included by some drug manufacturers. The Network also has worked to expedite approval of barrier contraceptives, which could protect against STDs and pregnancy; to improve protection for participants in trials of tamoxifen, a drug to prevent breast cancer; and to increase women's access to information about the long-term safety of silicone breast implants.

The challenge for developers of contraceptives is to accommodate the diverse needs of women—needs that vary from woman to woman and that may change over the course of one woman's lifetime. While many women see efficacy as the main concern when choosing a contraceptive method, others would cite user-control as the most important feature. For some women, secrecy of use is paramount, while for others, having a non-coitally-dependent method is important. All women want a safe method, but definitions of safety may vary. For example, some women disapprove of hormonal contraceptives because they can produce systemic changes; these women believe hormonal methods are not safe for long-term use. Some would argue that there will never be an 'ideal' hormonal method; consequently, dosages should be tailored to a particular woman's needs (Elstein & Furniss, 1996).

THE NEEDS AND PARTICIPATION OF THE PUBLIC SECTOR

The public sector and non-governmental organizations (NGOs) have played an important advocacy role in the development of new drugs for women. The precursors of the now existing organizations, such as the American Birth Control League, established in the USA in 1921 and the National Birth Control Council, founded in the UK in 1930, called the attention to the need of fertility regulation and initiated the social and political process of legitimization of contraception. More recently, international organizations such as the Contraceptive Research and Development Program (CONRAD), Family Health International (FHI), the International Planned Parenthood Federation (IPPF), the Program for Applied Technology in Health (PATH), the Population Council and the World Health Organization (WHO), among others, have played important roles in advancing and directly participating in the process of research and development of new drugs for women, particularly those needed for the management of reproductive health problems.

These organizations were concerned with consideration of women's perspectives and of involvement of women groups' representatives in the process of research, development and introduction of new drugs for women. Senanayake & Turner (1994) state that NGOs 'should be encouraged to play a more leading role in the development of contraceptive products that address priority needs of the public health sector, especially in developing countries'. However, to date, the communication and collaboration between these organizations and the pharmaceutical industry has been limited, given the magnitude of the need.

Mechanisms that insure a mutually satisfactory and complementary collaboration between the public sector and the pharmaceutical industry must be established. The International Conference on Population and Development in Cairo noted that 'to expedite the availability of improved and new methods for regulation of fertility, efforts must be made to increase the involvement of industry, including industries in developing countries and countries with economies in transition. A new type of partnership between the public and private sectors, including women and consumer groups, is needed that would mobilize the experience and resources of industry while protecting the public interest' (ICPD, 1994).

In recent years there has been a renewed interest in collaboration between the public and private sector in contraceptive research and development. The Rockefeller Foundation has played a leading role in reviving the interest of the industry in the area of contraceptives development and in establishing links between public sector organizations and industry. The Consortium for Industrial Collaboration in Contraceptive Research (CICCR)/CONRAD works to encourage private industry to expand its contraceptive research and development work. Established in 1995 by CONRAD, CICCR's goal is to foster the development of new contraceptive methods—particularly vaginal methods and postcoital methods—by awarding grants to not-for-profit research institutions working with for-profit industries. This effort is supported by the Rockefeller Foundation and the Andrew W. Mellon Foundation. The Institute of Medicine recently released a study on the need for new contraceptive research; among its priorities were continued research to meet the priorities of the 'woman-centered agenda' and public sector support for basic research in reproductive biology and applied research that would transform promising leads into reality. FHI and CICCR/CONRAD recently organized a conference to identify areas of collaboration for not-for-profit and for-profit entities. Participants recommended the establishment of a database on microbicide research; a future symposium that brings together researchers and consumers; and additional work between researchers and women's groups to better determine women's needs and perspectives.

CONCLUSION

Public perspectives and expectations must be a guiding force in the development of new drugs for women. Relying solely on epidemiological information on mortality and morbidity provides an incomplete picture of what women want and need. The development and marketing of any new drug, particularly contraceptive technologies, must consider women's sociocultural and health status, and may be more successful if done with the aim of enhancing women's well-being and empowerment. Improving the quality of women's lives should be the ultimate goal of any drug development program.

REFERENCES

Andreano R. Reflections on the economist and health economics in an international setting. *Soc Sci Med* 1993; **36**(2): 137–41.

Associated Press. High cost, insurance keep many from care. *Herald–Sun* July 1993; p 15.

Barnett B. Family planning and development. *Network* 1994; 15(1).

Barnett B. *Opportunities for Industrial Collaboration in Contraceptive Research* 1997. Proceedings from a meeting held by Family Health International and The Consortium for Industrial Collaboration in Contraceptive Research, November 7–8, 1996; Durham, NC: Family Health International.

Carr D, Way A. *Women's Lives and Experiences. A Decade of Research Findings from the Demographic and Health Surveys Program* 1994; Calverton, MD: Macro International Inc.

Cates W, Stone K. Family planning: the responsibility to prevent both pregnancy and reproductive tract infections. In C Wayne Bardin, DR Mishell Jr (eds) *Proceedings from the Fourth International Conference on IUDs* 1994, pp 93–129; Newton, MA: Butterworth-Heinemann.

Chelala CA, Gorgas MR. Maternal health: the perennial challenge. In *Communicating for Health Services, No. 1* 1991; Washington, DC: Pan American Health Organization.

Chen LC, Huq E, D'Souza S. Sex bias in the family allocation of food and health care in rural Bangladesh. *Population and Development Review* 1981; **7**(1): 55–70.

Claro A. Some views from developing countries about the pros and cons of male contraception. Paper presented at a Mellon Foundation and Family Health International seminar on male contraception March, 1995; Durham, NC.

Commentary. American women's health care. A patchwork quilt with gaps. *J Am Med Assoc* 1992; **268**(14): 1918–20.

Council on Ethical and Judicial Affairs, American Medical Association. Gender disparities in clinical decision-making. *J Am Med Assoc* 1991; **266**(4): 559–62.

Dixon-Mueller R. *Population Policy and Women's Rights: Transforming Reproductive Choice* 1993; Westport, CN: Praeger.

Editorial. Women's health, public welfare. *J Am Med Assoc* 1991; **266**(4): 566–8.

Elias CJ, Heise L. The development of microbicides: a new method of HIV prevention for women. In *Programs Division Working Papers* 1993, No. 6; New York: The Population Council.

Elstein M, Furniss H. The fiction of an ideal hormonal contraceptive. *Adv Contraception* 1996; **12**: 129–38.

Fathalla MF, Diczfalsy E, Spieler J. Public/private sector collaboration in contraceptive research and development: a call for a new partnership. Report from a Rockefeller Foundation Bellagio Conference, April 10–14, 1995.

Finger WR. Maternal morbidities affect tens of millions. *Network* 1994; **14**(3): 8–11.

Fletcher A, Gore S, Jones D et al. Quality of life measures in health care II: design, analysis, and interpretation. *Br Med J* 1992; **305**: 1145–8.

Forrest JD. Timing of reproductive life stages. *Obstet Gynecol* 1993; **82**(1): 105–11.

Francisco JS. Women's reproductive health care: research notes. *Women and Health Booklet Series* 1989, No. 5; Manila, The Philippines: Institute for Social Studies and Action.

Gershon D. Drugs tested for women. *Nature* 1992; **355** (January): 287.

Hall JK. Exclusion of pregnant women from research protocols: unethical and illegal. *IRB* 1995; **17**(2): 1–3.

Hardee K, Yount K. Delivering reproductive health promises through integrated services. *Women's Studies Project Working Paper* 1995, No. 2; Durham, NC: Family Health International.

Hardee K, Ulin P, Pfannenschmidt S, Visness C. *The Impact of Family Planning and Reproductive Health on Women's Lives: A Conceptual Framework* 1996; Durham, NC: Family Health International.

Hardon A. Development of contraceptives: general concerns. Contraceptive research: women's perspectives. In B Mintzes (ed.) *A Question of Control. Women's Perspectives on the Development and Use of Contraceptives* 1992, pp 7–16; Report on an international conference held in Woudschoten, The Netherlands, April, 1991. Women and Pharmaceuticals Project (WEMOS).

Hardon A. The needs of women versus the interests of family planning personnel, policy-makers and researchers: conflicting views on safety and acceptability of contraceptives. *Soc Sci Med* 1992; **35**(6): 753–66.

ICPD (International Conference on Population and Development). *Programme of Action of the International Conference on Population and Development* 1994; New York: United Nations.

Keller RT. Cross-cultural influences of work and nonwork contributions to quality of life. *Group Organiz Studies* 1987; **12**(3): 304–18.

Kessler DA, Merkatz RB, Temple R. FDA policy on women in drug trials. *N Engl J Med* 1993; **329**(24): 1815–16.

Koblinsky MA. Beyond maternal mortality—magnitude, interrelationships, and conse-quences of women's health, pregnancy-related complications and nutritional status on pregnancy outcomes. *Int J Obstet Gynecol* 1995; **48** (suppl): S21–32.

Krieger N, Fee E. Man-made medicine and women's health: the biopolitics of sex/gender and race/ethnicity. *Int J Health Services* 1994; **24**(2): 265–83.

Kwast BE. Safe motherhood—the first decade. *Midwifery* 1993; **9**: 105–23.

Lane SD, Meleis AI. Roles, work, health perceptions and health resources of women: a study in an Egyptian Delta hamlet. *Soc Sci Med* 1991; **33**(10): 19–208.

Lange J. Experts call for urgent development of microbicides. *Global Aidsnews* 1993; **4**: 9–10.

LaRosa JH, Seto B, Caban CE, Hayunga EG. Including women and minorities in clinical research. *Appl Clin Trials* 1995; **4**(5).

Leelakulthanit O, Day RL. Quality of life in Thailand. *Soc Indicators Res* 1992; **27**: 41–57.

McFadden P. Health is a gender issue. *S Africa Polit Econ Monthly* 1994; **7**(3–4): 59–61.

Marcelo AG, Germain A. Women's perspectives on fertility regulation methods and services. In *Contraceptive Research and Development 1984–1994. The Road from Mexico City to Cairo and Beyond* 1994, pp 325–42. Delhi: Oxford University Press.

Marwick C. Women's health initiative. *J Am Med Assoc* 1992; **268**(14): 1824.

McCauley AP, Robery R, Blanc AK, Geller JS. *Opportunities for Women Through Reproductive Choice* 1994, Population Reports, Series M, No. 12; Baltimore: Center for Communications, Johns Hopkins School of Public Health.

Moser CON. *Gender Planning and Development: Theory, Practice and Training* 1993; London: Routledge.

Morrow M. First WHO collaborating centre for women's health. *World Health Forum* 1995; **16**: 179–80.

National Academy of Science. *The Future of Public Health* 1988; Institute of Medicine, Washington, DC: National Academy Press.

National Research Council. *Contraception and Reproduction: Health Consequences for Women and Children in the Developing World* 1989; Washington, DC: National Academy Press.

Norsigian J. Women's perspectives on contraceptive development. Paper presented at the Annual Meeting of the Society for the Advancement of Contraception, Barcelona, November, 1992.

Older Women's League (OWL). *Campaign for Women's Health: A Model Benefits Package for Women in Health Care Reform* 1994, Washington, DC: OWL.

Pearson CA. National Women's Health Network and the US FDA: two decades of activism. *Reprod Health Matters* 1995; **6**: 132–40.

Pinn VW. Women's health research. *J Am Med Assoc* 1992; **268**(14): 1921.

Population Council. *Partnership for Prevention: A Report of a Meeting Between Women's Health Advocates, Program Planners, and Scientists, 3–12 May, 1994*, New York and Washington, DC.

Progress in Human Reproduction Research. *Reproductive Health and Reproductive Choice: The WHO Perspective* 1994; **30**: 1–5. Geneva: WHO.

Rio Statement: Reproductive Health and Justice International Women's Health Conference for Cairo 1994; Rio de Janeiro: International Women's Health Coalition.

Sai FT, Nassim J. The need for a reproductive health approach. *Int J Gynecol Obstet* 1989; Suppl 3: 103–13.

Saxenian H. Optimizing health care in developing countries. *Issues Sci Technol* 1994–5; **XI**(2): 42–8.

Schipper H, Clinch J, Powell V. Definitions and conceptual issues. In B Spilker (ed.) *Quality of Life Assessments in Clinical Trials* 1990; New York: Raven.

Senanayake P and Turner J. Fertility regulation: history and current situation—an NGO perspective. In *Contraceptive Research and Development 1984–1994. The Road from Mexico City to Cairo and Beyond* 1994, pp 249–62; Delhi: Oxford University Press.

Sinding SW, Ross JR. Seeking common ground: unmet need and demographic goals. *Int Family Planning Perspect* 1994; **20**: 23–32.

Snow R. Each to her own: investigating women's responses to contraception. In G Sen and RC Snow (eds) *Power and Decision. The Social Control of Reproduction* 1994; Boston, MA: Harvard Series on Population and International Health.

Snow R. Presentation to staff at Family Health International, Durham, NC, 16 June 1995.

Spilker B. Introduction. In B Spilker (ed.) *Quality of Life Assessments in Clinical Trials* 1990; New York: Raven.

Stauning I. Women, health and technology. *Health Care Women Int* 1993; **14**(4): 355–63.

Van Look PFA, Perez-Palacios G. Declaration of the International Symposium: contraceptive research and development for the year 2000 and beyond. In *Contraceptive Research and Development 1984–1994: The Road from Mexico to Cairo and Beyond* 1994; New Delhi: Oxford University Press.

United Nations. *The World's Women 1970–1990: Trends and Statistics* 1991; New York: United Nations.

Wasserheit J. The significance and scope of reproductive tract infections among third world women. *Int J Gynecol Obstet* 1989; Suppl 3: 145–68.

WHO/IWHC (World Health Organization and International Women's Health Coalition). *Creating Common Ground* 1991; Geneva: WHO/HRP/ITT/91.

WHO/UNICEF (World Health Organization and United Nations Children's Fund). *Primary Health Care* 1978; A joint report by The Director-General of the World Health Organization and The Executive Director of the United Nations Children's Fund; Geneva/New York: WHO.

World Population Data Sheet 1995. Wall chart. Washington, DC: Population Reference Bureau.

6

Legal Issues

Marlene J. Tandy

Health Industries Manufacturing Association, Washington, DC, USA

INTRODUCTION

Drug development in modern times is not only an art and a science, but also a major business investment. In the pervasive litigation atmosphere within the USA, a business activity such as pharmaceutical research and development must be pursued with an awareness of legal issues that can have an adverse impact on the success of the product.

The end result of successful pharmaceutical research and development is the advancement of public health through the availability of drug therapies. Legal issues, particularly product liability exposure, can (and do) have an adverse impact on drug development for the treatment of disease and life cycle management in women.

This chapter will explore these legal issues. First, an overview of the drug development process and the law of personal injury will be presented. Next, there will be a brief review of some of the more prominent personal injury litigation cases involving medical products (both pharmaceuticals and medical devices) used primarily by women. The following section will focus on the impact of these legal issues on drug development for women, including the effects on research choices for new products as well as the participation of women in clinical trials. The chapter will then conclude by offering some potential solutions for the problems these legal issues raise.

OVERVIEW OF DRUG DEVELOPMENT PROCESS

Phases of Drug Research

The phases of drug research can be divided into pre-clinical and clinical. The pre-clinical phase is the work that is accomplished prior to introduction into human beings, such as discovery of the compound, basic molecular design, biochemical

Drug Development for Women. Edited by V.V. Ragavan. © 1998 John Wiley & Sons Ltd.

research, as well as short-term and long-term animal studies.[1] Clinical research, meaning studies undertaken in human beings, is generally divided into phases 1, 2 and 3.

Phase 1 studies involve a small number of subjects, in whom the basic metabolic and pharmacologic actions, as well as side effects, of the drug will be determined. Phase 2 studies are larger than those in phase 1, are controlled studies, and are performed to evaluate effectiveness of the drug in the target patient population, as well as to determine shorter-term side effects. In phase 3, large controlled (and uncontrolled) trials are conducted to gather additional effectiveness data and to evaluate the overall risk/benefit of the study drug.[2]

FDA Review

Prior to starting clinical research with a new investigational drug, a study sponsor must obtain approval from the Food and Drug Administration (FDA) of an investigational new drug application (IND). The IND contains the results of pre-clinical testing and the protocol (study design) for the upcoming clinical study, as well as other pertinent information. Once FDA approves the IND, or if no negative response from FDA is received after 30 days from the date of the IND submission, the sponsor may start the clinical research study contained in the IND.[3]

When the clinical research through phase 3 is completed, the new drug sponsor submits a new drug application (NDA) to FDA for permission to make the drug commercially available in the USA. The NDA contains, among other items, the results of the pre-clinical and clinical research, manufacturing information, and proposed labeling. The new drug is not to be marketed in the USA until FDA has reviewed and approved the NDA.[4]

Development Time and Cost

In a January 1988 article, Dr Frank Young, then Commissioner of Food and Drugs, provided the following time-line for drug development: pre-clinical research, 1–3 years (average time 18 months); research for NDA, 2–10 years (average time 5 years); NDA review, 2 months–7 years (average time 24 months). From these figures, the average time for new drug development from research through to marketing is 8.5 years (Young, 1988).

---

[1] For a general description of this process, as well as the clinical research process, see FDA (1988).
[2] The three phases of clinical drug research are described in 21 CFR, Part 312.21.
[3] The IND process is described in Section 505(i) of the Federal Food, Drug, and Cosmetic Act (FFDCA) (21 USC, Part 355(i)) and its implementing regulations in 21 CFR, Part 312.
[4] The NDA process is described in Section 505(b) of the FFDCA (21 USC, Part 355(b)).

Other information suggests that the time period may be even longer. The Pharmaceutical Research and Manufacturers of America (PhRMA) (formerly PMA) noted in a report in 1993 that the average time for a new drug product to go from pre-clinical research through to marketing is 12 years. PhRMA also stated that only 1 in 5000 compounds tested in the pre-clinical stage makes it to marketing. In addition, the average cost to develop a new drug is approximately $359 million (Wierenga & Eaton, 1993).

Post-marketing

Once a new drug has been approved by the FDA, the drug sponsor must continue to submit reports to the FDA on a regular basis, including information about adverse effects as well as other pertinent manufacturing information. For some new drug products, the FDA may require post-marketing clinical studies (often called phase 4 studies) to gather information about long-term effects or additional data from certain sub-populations who are taking the drug. While these post-marketing requirements are not technically a part of the new drug development research time and cost, they figure into the overall investment time and cost for a pharmaceutical company becoming involved with a particular line of drug products.

OVERVIEW OF PERSONAL INJURY LITIGATION

If a person believes that he/she has been injured by a product (or by another person), the law gives the injured person an opportunity to bring a lawsuit in an attempt to remedy the injury. This field of law is referred to as 'tort' law (for a detailed explanation of tort law principle, see Lee & Lindahl, 1988, 1995; Prosser, Wade & Schwartz, 1988).

The doctrines of tort law, meaning the various types of injuries that are appropriate subjects for lawsuits, are established by state law. The relevant state law can be found in state statutes (enacted by state legislatures and signed by the governor of the state) as well as in cases (i.e. lawsuits) that have been decided by the state courts and federal courts in each state.[5]

One of the types of injuries recognized in tort law as a basis for litigation is an injury alleged to be related to a product, such as a pharmaceutical product. This area of law is referred to as product liability.

---

[5] Every state in the USA has within its territory a number of state courts as well as federal courts. For tort law purposes, the federal court will be applying the law of the state in which it hears the lawsuit. Whether a tort law case is brought in state court or federal court depends on various rules of civil procedure, such as where the parties to the lawsuit reside and the amount of money in controversy.

Product Liability Litigation

A manufacturer of a product is the most likely party to be sued in a product
liability lawsuit. The plaintiff is the injured person who files the lawsuit; the
defendant is the entity being sued. According to the doctrines of tort law, there are
two basic legal theories for product liability lawsuits—negligence and strict liability
(for additional information on product liability lawsuits in the area of pharmaceutical products, see Dixon & Woodside, 1995).

Negligence

To support a product liability lawsuit involving negligence, the plaintiff must prove
four basic elements: (a) the defendant owed the plaintiff a legal duty; (b) the
defendant breached that duty; (c) the plaintiff suffered an injury from the product
as a result of the breached duty; and (d) the plaintiff incurred damages as a result
of the injury.

Legal duties owed by a manufacturer to a person who used the manufacturer's
product include: a duty to manufacture the product properly (i.e. in a safe and
effective fashion); a duty to design the product properly; and a duty to warn the
person (generally through the health care professional) about known or reasonably
foreseeable side effects. In addition, a manufacturer (as well as a clinical investigator and a research institution) owe various legal duties to a person who is
participating in a clinical trial of a product, such as a duty to carry out the research
properly and a duty to inform the potential participant of the known or reasonably
foreseeable risks of being a part of the research. This duty to inform of risks may
include, if appropriate, the duty to inform of the possibility of damage to a person's
reproductive potential and/or damage to a fetus.

One of the most common claims in product liability lawsuits about pharmaceutical and medical device products is that the manufacturer breached the duty to
warn about the product through appropriate labeling. During the product approval
process prior to marketing, the FDA reviews proposed labeling and ultimately must
approve the labeling that appears with the product once it is commercially available.
Compliance with FDA requirements does not generally insulate a manufacturer
from litigation or provide an absolute defense to the lawsuit. Instead, the FDA
requirements are usually viewed as a minimum standard to be met.[6] However,
manufacturers can introduce evidence that compliance with the FDA requirements
shows the product is properly labeled and it will be up to the decision-maker (judge

---

[6] For certain types of medical devices, complying with FDA requirements can pre-empt lawsuits that
involve state tort law claims, such as failure to warn labeling claims. However, after the recent US
Supreme Court case, *Medtronic vs. Lohr*, 116 S. Ct. 2240 (1996), this pre-emption doctrine has been
narrowed significantly.

or jury, depending on the case) to evaluate the merits of that evidence. On the other hand, non-compliance with FDA requirements can be used as significant evidence of a manufacturer's negligence.

State law may also establish a duty of a manufacturer to an unborn child, exposed in utero either to an investigational drug or a marketed drug product, allowing the child (once born) to bring a product liability case against the manufacturer for injuries such as birth defects or other injuries related to drug exposure. In a research setting, this duty to an unborn child may also extend to clinical researchers and research institutions involved with investigational drug research.

A plaintiff in a negligence case must also show that the defendant failed to perform the required duty, hence that the defendant was somehow at fault. This is where the difference between the theories of negligence and strict liability lies.

Strict Liability

In this type of product liability action, the plaintiff must prove the following elements: (a) the product is defective and unreasonably dangerous; (b) the plaintiff suffered an injury as a result of the defective product; and (c) the plaintiff incurred damages as a result of the injury. The plaintiff does not have to prove that the defendant (the manufacturer) failed to do something properly, i.e. the plaintiff does not have to prove fault on the part of the manufacturer.

Strict liability is a relatively recent theory in the development of tort law, dating from the early 1960s. In addition to state statutory law and case law, which define the elements of a strict liability case, there is also a general commentary on tort law which sheds light on the basic principles of strict liability theory, referred to as the Restatement (Second) of Torts, Section 402(A).[7]

Two of the most commonly alleged product defects by plaintiffs are defect in manufacturing and defect in design. According to comment (k) of Section 402(A) of the Restatement, if a product can be considered 'unavoidably unsafe', such as a pharmaceutical product might be considered, the product will not be subject to a strict liability claim if the manufacturer has properly prepared the product and has provided appropriate warnings about the product.

Often the most difficult and complex parts of a product liability lawsuit, whether using negligence or strict liability theory, is the battle over whether the product caused the injury (i.e. that the plaintiff suffered an injury as a result of the product). Much evidence in litigation will be produced to the judge and jury on the topic of

---

[7] The Restatement (Third) of Torts has recently become available in 1995. Although the most basic principles of strict liability as discussed in this chapter are still intact in the Restatement (Third), there have been some modifications that at least one author characterizes as pro-defendant (see Schwartz, 1995).

causation. This evidence can include research studies, epidemiological data and testimony from expert witnesses.

Monetary damages sought in product liability lawsuits can be for various items, such as out-of-pocket costs (like medical expenses), lost earnings, pain and suffering and emotional distress, as well as punitive damages to punish the defendant for wrongdoing and deter additional misconduct. The damages awarded in a product liability lawsuit can reach into the millions of dollars.

Wrongful Death/Wrongful Life/Wrongful Birth

These three types of torts may also serve as the basis for litigation in a context that could involve a manufacturer, a clinical researcher, and/or a research institution.

In a wrongful death lawsuit, the death of a human being is claimed to have occurred in a wrongful (i.e. negligent) way on the part of another person and the family of the decedent is seeking to recover compensation. The law in some states has also recognized a legal right for parents to obtain recovery for the wrongful death of an unborn child.

In a wrongful life lawsuit, a child born with an injury claims that if it were not for the defendant's negligence, the child would not have been born to suffer the pain of the injury. In essence, the injured child is claiming that the defendant failed to prevent the plaintiff's birth and that action was negligent.

In a wrongful birth action, the parents of an injured child are claiming that the negligence of the defendant prevented the parents from exercising their right to decide, in an informed manner, whether to have a child that would be born with an injury (i.e. a birth defect).

These tort actions are less commonly brought against a manufacturer than product liability lawsuits. Nevertheless, it is possible to see how including women of childbearing age (and pregnant women) in clinical trials of investigational drugs— without due care on the part of the manufacturer, clinical researcher and research center—could expose the fetus to risks that may result in injury and form the basis of a wrongful life and/or wrongful birth lawsuit.

To be involved in any type of lawsuit is an arduous process, involving lengthy contacts with attorneys and the court process. This represents a significant psychological burden for the defendant, as well as a major expense. For a company, defending a lawsuit also means that there will be substantial lost time of company personnel who will be participating in the defense process, rather than the research and development duties, for example, that they were hired to perform. Moreover, if a judge or jury awards a monetary amount to a plaintiff, it can represent a major financial loss for the defendant manufacturer. It is thus no surprise that manufacturers seek to avoid litigation risks in the conduct of their business activities.

PROMINENT MEDICAL PRODUCT LIABILITY CASES INVOLVING PRODUCTS USED BY WOMEN

One of the reasons that a pharmaceutical (or medical device) manufacturer might be wary of developing drugs (and devices) used particularly by women is a litigation track record where many of the most famous (and costly) product liability cases involve this type of product. The following examples should be considered.

Thalidomide

Thalidomide was a pharmaceutical product developed outside the USA, beginning in the 1950s, for a number of uses related to sedation (e.g. local anesthesia, anti-seizure properties, and inducing sleep). It was marketed extensively outside the USA, beginning in the late 1950s, as a sleeping pill and also for morning sickness.

A short time after marketing, the drug began to be linked to the development of serious birth defects in babies whose mothers took the drug while pregnant. The birth defects included babies born with extensive limb deformities, such as phocomelia (flipper limb).

In the USA, thalidomide never received marketing approval by the FDA, although some amounts of the drug had been domestically distributed for research. Worldwide, an estimated 10 000 babies were born with birth defects associated with thalidomide (for more information about the thalidomide incident, see Leuz, 1988; Teff & Munro, 1976).

Intra-uterine Devices (IUDs)

In the 1980s, there were a large number of product liability suits brought against manufacturers of these products, which were introduced to the US market in the 1970s for use as contraceptive devices. Some of the injuries claimed in these lawsuits were pelvic infections, ectopic pregnancies and uterine perforations. In 1985, the A.H. Robbins company (manufacturer of the Dalkon Shield device) filed for bankruptcy after the costs of litigation, including settlements and some awards for punitive damages, ranged in the several hundred million dollars. In addition, in the 1980s, the G.D. Searle company expended many milllions of dollars in product liability litigation involving the Copper 7 product, and ultimately this product was no longer marketed.

A newer generation of IUDs are currently marketed in the USA. These products have design features different from the earlier IUDs. In addition, the newer IUDs have extensive labeling, including a patient package insert to provide information directly to the user. The labeling pays particular attention to selecting the appropriate patient population for using the device and emphasizes precautions and warnings regarding the potential side effects of using the device. Even though IUDs are commercially available, only a small number of women are estimated to be using them (2%) and physicians often do not present them to their patients as a contraception option, likely because of the lingering memory of the previous litigation and concern over malpractice risk (see, e.g., Dixon & Woodside, 1995, §15.42; Randall, 1992; Glamour, 1996).

Diethylstilbestrol (DES)

This drug was used originally in the 1940s and 1950s for the prevention of miscarriage. In the 1970s, there was an increased incidence observed of a type of unusual vaginal cancer in the daughters of women who had taken the drug.

There have been many product liability cases involving DES, probably numbering in the thousands of cases. Some of these cases were combined into a single proceeding, known as a class action lawsuit. In addition to the cases brought by the so-called 'DES daughters', in the 1990s, product liability lawsuits have also been filed by the 'third generation'—granddaughters of the women who originally took DES.

Revised labeling for the drug has contraindicated its use in pregnant women. It is being used currently as a 'morning after' contraceptive (see Dixon & Woodside, 1995, §15.26).

Bendectin

Bendectin was a drug used for the treatment of morning sickness, first marketed in the USA in the late 1950s. There have been an enormous number of product liability lawsuits involving Bendectin, claiming various types of birth defects related to the drug. These lawsuits began in the 1980s and continue to the present day. The expense of the overall litigation effort led the manufacturer of the drug to discontinue its marketing in June 1983 (see Dixon & Woodside, 1995, §15.64).

Breast Implants

Silicone gel breast implants have been available in the USA since the 1960s. In the early 1990s, questions arose about the possibility of long-term side effects relating to implanted silicone, such as leakage or rupture of the implant, leading to reactions such as hardening of tissue in the breast and other tissue diseases. At that time, there were a few product liability lawsuits brought involving breast implants which resulted in awards of large monetary amounts (in the millions of dollars).

In April 1992, FDA instituted a policy that silicone gel breast implants would be available only for women with indications relating to reconstruction after cancer surgery or severe deformity or in clinical studies to evaluate safety issues. Since

1992, there has been massive product liability litigation against breast implant manufacturers. Thousands of individual cases have been filed and the manufacturers of the product decided that it would be best to try to achieve a global settlement of these claims in one class action lawsuit. Hundreds of thousands of women have registered to participate in this settlement and the cost of the settlement is expected to reach billions of dollars. Also since 1992, several studies on the safety of breast implants have been published in the medical literature, casting doubt on any association between breast implants and connective tissue diseases (see Daniel & Weiss, 1995; Dixon & Woodside, 1995, §15.71; Kolata & Meier, 1995).

Norplant

Norplant is a product whose indicated use is contraception. It contains an active ingredient, levonorgesterel, a hormone, which is contained in capsules (made of a material called Silastic) that are implanted under the skin of the arm. Gradual release of the active drug into the bloodstream is designed to provide effective contraception for up to five years. Norplant had been available outside the USA for a number of years prior to its approval by FDA in 1990. Norplant was marketed in the USA in 1991 and since that time several hundred product liability suits have been filed against its US manufacturer. These lawsuits allege various side effects from the drug, such as scarring, vaginal bleeding, headaches and nausea (see Norplant Study, 1995).

IMPACT ON DEVELOPMENT OF DRUGS

Research Choices for New Products

Several important concepts emerge from the previous sections of this chapter. First, drug development is a long and expensive process, in which many compounds are evaluated but comparatively few are commercially viable. Second, the risk of legal liability is real, because there are so many different legal theories under which to sue a manufacturer (or clinical researcher or research center) and so many incentives in our society to pursue litigation against a 'deep pocket'. And third, many of the most costly product liability actions historically have arisen from drugs and devices intended primarily for women. They have been costly, in part, because of the potentially large numbers of women exposed to these products. In addition, damage awards can be larger (as can lawsuit settlements) when the person injured is otherwise young and healthy, with the potential for more years ahead of living with the injury and its aftermath.

It is easy to see why a manufacturer engaged in research and development of new products needs to try to minimize business risks, including the risk of product liability exposure. Accordingly, a company might understandably choose to pursue research and development in any number of exciting and important therapeutic areas that have nothing to do with indications focused primarily on women, such as contraception.

For example, in 1992, one of the speakers at the Annual Meeting of the American College of Gynecology emphasized the problem that advances in contraceptive choices are not emerging from research in the USA. This speaker referenced a study, published in 1990 by the National Research Council and the Institute of Medicine, which linked existing product liability law with obstacles in developing new contraceptives in the USA. That study noted that in the previous three decades, only one new contraceptive method (Norplant) had been made available in the USA. The study concluded that tort liability may be the single most important barrier to contraceptive development (see Randall, 1992, note 12; Mastroianni et al, 1990).

The problem of fear of legal liability creating disincentives to develop new drugs has not disappeared since 1990. In fact, the following statement by PhARMA appeared in the May 1 1995 edition of *The Washington Post*:

> Why don't women in the US have more choices in contraceptives? The risk of liability. Lawsuits against American drug companies have caused the US to fall decades behind Europe and other countries in the contraceptive choices offered women. In fact, since 1970, the number of major US drug companies involved in contraceptive R&D has dropped from 20 to just two. Product liability has also slowed other areas of research like vaccines, AIDS and cancer. Prudent limits on liability for drugs that meet the FDA's high standards are essential to stimulate research for new medicines to help women—and all Americans.

Participation of Women in Clinical Trials

In July 1993, FDA modified its policy guidelines about the appropriateness of including women of childbearing potential in clinical trials for drugs (FDA, 1993). An earlier FDA (1977) policy had recommended excluding women of childbearing potential from most early drug trials. FDA identified the reason behind the 1977 policy as a concern over birth defects (Merkatz et al, 1993). Another author has offered these reasons for excluding such women from drug research: (a) protection for the fetus and childbearing potential of women; (b) concern over legal liability for the fetus; (c) the need by researchers for easy recruitment of large, identifiable cohorts of subjects, like military recruits; and (d) the potential for hormonal interference with blood tests that are a part of the research (Bennett, 1993).

The new FDA policy establishes expectations that reasonable numbers of women of childbearing potential will be included, as appropriate, in clinical studies, that clinical data will be analyzed by gender, that potential pharmacokinetic differences between genders will be evaluated, and that women of childbearing age will be considered for inclusion in clinical studies in the early phase 2 and even phase 1 stages of research. FDA emphasizes several safety factors that should be included in phase 1 and 2 trials so that serious risk of reproductive toxicity is lessened: careful protocol design with respect to dosing and dose escalation; availability of extensive animal toxicological testing; ensuring that women enrolling in these studies are not pregnant; requiring that the women in these trials take appropriate measures not to become pregnant while exposed to the investigational drug; and the continuing requirement for informed consent (including, where appropriate, the notification that the investigational drug has not been fully characterized with respect to its potential effects on conception and fetal development).[8]

Including women of childbearing potential in early phase clinical studies makes sense from a scientific point of view. Nevertheless, what makes good sense for science does not necessarily translate into the absence of legal liability.

Manufacturers, clinical researchers, and research institutions (including Institutional Review Boards) could all be subject to tort lawsuits for injuries to a woman (and potentially to a fetus) for injuries that are claimed to result from an investigational drug. The earlier the phase of research that includes women of childbearing age, the greater is the risk of potential tort liability because so much less is known about the effects of the investigational drug. While a woman's informed consent may be a good defense to a failure-to-warn claim, whether a woman can consent on behalf of her fetus is an open legal question. And, as the earlier examples of medical product liability cases show, merely having to participate in litigation can be such an expensive process that a company may choose to stop its research work in a certain area or may even be forced to declare bankruptcy.

It is too early to tell whether including women of childbearing potential in early phase clinical research will result in the legal liability nightmares that many people are concerned about. Serious thought needs to be given to preventing this type of result, both by prudent clinical practice and tort reform.

POTENTIAL SOLUTIONS

The two adverse impacts identified in this chapter of tort liability on the development of drugs for women—choices not to develop certain types of new drugs (like contraceptives) and a backlash on including women of childbearing age in early phase clinical research—could be minimized by some type of reasonable tort reform.

Proposals for tort reform have been considered off and on by Congress in recent years, but to date no meaningful reform has occurred. Some options for reform include setting a cap on damages (particularly punitive damages); a 'government standards' defense, whereby compliance with federal requirements (like FDA

---

[8] See Merkatz et al, 1993, note 20; October 27 1994 FDA Response to Citizen Petition, Docket No. 92P-0494; September 16 1994 'Dear Colleague' letter from FDA (Suydam L) re: July 22 1993, *Guideline for the Study and Evaluation of Gender Differences in the Clinical Evaluation of Drugs.*

policies) would be a defense to product liability actions; and limitations on the legal theories that can be used to support claims.

Another creative solution could be some type of federal legislation similar to the National Childhood Vaccine Injury Act, which was enacted in 1986 to create an alternative to the existing tort law system for resolution of product liability claims against childhood vaccine manufacturers. One of the purposes of this legislation was to prevent a crisis in the availability of childhood vaccines due to manufacturers leaving the market as a result of excessive product liability expenses.

The system of compensation under the NCVIA is funded through a tax on every dose of childhood vaccine. Claims for compensation are heard by a special master (not a jury) appointed by a federal court, with the government (not the manufacturer) serving as the defendant. The elements of a claim for compensation (and the defenses available) are established by the statute, as are the type and amount of damages available.[9] This type of system for pharmaceutical products with indications exclusively for women, or more generally for all new drug products, could make a difference in encouraging research and development of these products.

Everyone benefits from the continued availability of safe and effective pharmaceutical products. A strong federal regulatory system and a more rational tort liability system work together to ensure that goal.

REFERENCES

Bennett JC. Inclusion of women in clinical trials—policies for population subgroups. *N Engl J Med* 1993; **329**(4): 288–91.

Daniel BD, Weiss M. FDA on the loose—implanting fear. *National Review* 1995; **October 9**.

Dixon MG, Woodside FC. *Drug Product Liability* 1995; New York: Matthew Bender.

FDA. *From Test Tube to Patient: New Drug Development in the United States—An FDA Consumer Special Report*, January 1988, HHS Publication No (FDA) 88–3168; Rockville, MD: FDA.

FDA. Notice of availability of FDA 'Guideline for the Study and Evaluation of Gender Differences in the Clinical Evaluation of Drugs'. 58 *Fed. Reg.* 39406 (July 22 1993).

FDA. *General Considerations for the Clinical Evaluation of Drugs* 1977; FDA Publication No. 77-3040. Rockville, MD: FDA.

Glamour. Editorial: American women are missing out on a birth control method they shouldn't be ignoring. *Glamour* 1996; **May**: 91.

Kolata G, Meier B. Implant lawsuits create a medical rush to cash in. *New York Times* 1995; **September 18**: A1.

Lee JD, Lindahl BA. *Modern Tort Law: Liability and Litigation*, revised edn, 1988; New York: Clark, Boardman & Callaghan.

Lee JD, Lindahl BA. *Modern Tort Law: Liability and Litigation (Cumulative Supplement)* 1995; New York: Clark, Boardman & Callaghan.

Leuz W. A short history of thalidomide embryopathy. *Teratology* 1988; **38**: 203–15.

Mastroianni L, Donaldson PJ, Kane TT. *Developing New Contraceptives: Obstacles and Opportunities*

---

[9] The NCVIA, Pub. L. No. 99–660, 100 Stat. 3755, is codified at 42 USC §§300aa-1 through 300aa-34. For its legislative history, see H.R. REP. No. 908, 99th Cong., 2d Sess., 3–7 (1986), reprinted in USCCAN 6287, 6344–48.

1990; Washington, DC: National Research Council and Institute of Medicine (cited in Randall, 1992).

Merkatz R, Temple R et al. Women in clinical trials of new drugs—a change in Food and Drug Administration policy. *N Engl J Med* 1993; **329**(4): 292–6.

Norplant Study. *USA Today* 1995; **September 18**: 1.

Prosser WL, Wade JW, Schwartz VE. *Cases and Materials or Torts*, 8th edn, 1988; Westbury, NY: Foundation Press.

Randall T. United States loses lead in contraceptive choices, research and development, changes in tort liability: FDA review urged. *JAMA* 1992; **268**(2): 176–9.

Schwartz TM. The impact of the New Products Liability Restatement on prescription products. *Food Drug Law J* 1995; **50**(7).

Teff H, Munro C. *Thalidomide—The Legal Aftermath* 1976; Farnborough: Saxon House.

Wierenga DE, Eaton CR. The drug development and approval process. In *In Development—AIDS Medicines—Drugs and Vaccines*, November 1993; Washington, DC: Pharmaceutical Manufacturers' Association.

Young FE. The reality behind the headlines. In *From Test Tube to Patient: New Drug Development in the United States—An FDA Consumer Special Report*, January 1988, HHS Publication No (FDA) 88–3168; Rockville, MD: FDA.

B

Reproductive Years

7

Contraception

Christine Mauck
CONRAD Program, Arlington, VA, USA

THE ROLE OF CONTRACEPTION

A woman's reproductive years represent the time in her life when she is generally in good health and balancing education, work, marriage, and children. In order to maximize the health and quality of life of herself and her family and to manage daily activities, women are faced with the need to time or space births. In the past, control of reproduction was accomplished largely by behavioral means: delaying marriage, limiting coital frequency within marriage, avoidance of mid-cycle coitus, and coitus interruptus. Some attempts at contraceptive technology go back thousands of years, such as condoms and vaginal barriers, but the development of most methods has been quite recent.

While this chapter will focus on contraceptive development, it must be noted that the availability of contraceptive technology is not sufficient to optimize use. 'Modern contraceptives' are used by about 80% and 50% of women at risk for pregnancy in developed and developing countries, respectively, with wide variation between individual countries and socio-economic groups. The desire and availability to use contraception is affected not only by its availability but also by a woman's status in society, opportunities for education and employment, family influence and religious norms.

THE 'IDEAL' CONTRACEPTIVE METHOD

There is no 'perfect' contraceptive because women have different needs at different times in their lives. The risks and benefits of any method should be weighed against alternative methods as well as against the risks associated with unprotected intercourse and subsequent delivery or abortion. With very few exceptions (primarily the use of oral contraceptives by smoking women over age 35), the use of contraceptives is safer than undergoing an abortion or a delivery. This is particularly true in developing countries, where the lifetime risk of dying from pregnancy or childbirth-related causes is estimated by the World Health Organization (WHO) to

Drug Development for Women. Edited by V.V. Ragavan. © 1998 John Wiley & Sons Ltd.

be 1 in 20, compared with 1 in 10 000 in developed countries. The use of effective contraception by women who wish to delay or prevent births would reduce maternal mortality by an estimated 17–35% (Ashford, 1995).

Although there is no perfect contraceptive that meets the needs of all women at all times, some desirable attributes of contraceptives may include:

- High efficacy (including postcoital and postovulatory use).
- Safety and few side effects.
- Convenience (coitus-independent, non-detectable).
- Accessibility and low cost.
- Minimal provider intervention.
- Easy reversibility by the user (or predictable onset of complete irreversibility if a method of sterilization).
- Easy storage and disposal.
- Predictable bleeding patterns.
- Non-contraceptive health benefits, including protection against sexually transmitted diseases (STDs).

Prevention of STDs as a non-contraceptive benefit of contraceptives deserves special attention. Pregnancy has been likened to a sexually transmitted disease that can only be transmitted during a brief part of the menstrual cycle. Interventions which prevent STDs also prevent pregnancy. However, when used to prevent STDs, they require diligent, coitus-dependent use throughout the entire menstrual cycle. This need for a high level of user compliance makes these methods generally less effective at preventing pregnancy than other contraceptives. There is clearly room for a coitus-independent, long-acting means of preventing both STDs and pregnancy.

PRESENTLY AVAILABLE PRODUCTS: AN HISTORICAL PERSPECTIVE

Until the middle of this century, the means to limit family size included behavioral modifications including delayed marriage, infrequent coitus in marriage, coitus interruptus, and avoidance of intercourse during fertile periods. Available contraceptive technologies consisted of condoms, spermicidal douches, sponges, cervical caps and vaginal diaphragms. In 1846, the development of cold-vulcanized rubber improved the quality and availability of some of these.

Despite this limited choice, the desire to control child-bearing resulted in a demographic transition in the USA between 1800 and 1940, during which the average number of children borne by a woman declined from 7.0 to 3.6 (Reed, 1978).

In the late 1930s and early 1940s, efforts were made to increase research in female physiology and new methods of contraception. These early initiatives did not yield significant progress until the mid-1960s with development of the oral contraceptive (OC) pill.

Hormonal Methods—Oral

Scientists began investigating the use of exogenous hormones to suppress ovulation in the 1920s. Estrogen was isolated in 1923 and synthesized in 1936. Progesterone was synthesized in 1943. It was later found that synthetic progestins were more potent, caused fewer side effects, and were less costly to produce. Gregory Pincus and Carl Djerassi, in collaboration with the G.D. Searle Company, successfully synthesized the first progestin for use as an oral contraceptive in 1956. Synthetic estrogen was added to control bleeding. In 1960, the Food and Drug Administration (FDA) approved the first combined oral contraceptive, Enovid, which had a theoretical failure rate of 0.1 pregnancy per woman per year. By 1965, 'the pill' became the leading reversible method of contraception in the USA. In 1969, studies reported that contraceptive effectiveness could be maintained despite reduced levels of estrogen, leading in 1975 to the introduction of the first low-dose pill (Modicon 21). The product contained a fraction of the original pill's estrogen and progestin content, but had a safety and efficacy profile equivalent to its predecessor's.

Oral contraceptives contain either ethinyl estradiol or mestranol, which inhibits follicle stimulating hormone (FSH) and luteinizing hormone (LH) secretion and therefore ovulation. Progestin inhibits LH secretion and ovulation and impedes implantation of the fertilized egg. In addition, progestin interferes with both ovum and sperm transport by thickening cervical mucus and altering secretion in the fallopian tubes. These mechanisms of action provide a 'perfect use' first-year failure rate of 0.1% and a 'typical use' failure rate of 3%.

Because progestins are derived from testosterone, they can cause side effects such as acne, hirsutism, weight gain and changes in lipid and carbohydrate metabolism. These latter changes do not appear to translate into higher risk of myocardial infarction or stroke, due perhaps to the mitigating effects of estrogen on lipoprotein and the arterial wall. Nevertheless, recent efforts have been directed towards developing progestins with high progestational–androgenic activity ratios (or high 'selectivity index'). Norgestimate, desogestrel and gestodene have high selectivity indices; that of norgestimate is the highest. These new progestins may have some beneficial effects on serum lipoproteins (Collins, 1994; Darney, 1995). Norgestimate and desogestrel are available in OCs in the USA.

The combined OC pill offers non-contraceptive health benefits which were recognized by the FDA in 1988. OC users have a risk of endometrial and ovarian cancer that is only 60% that of non-users; this reduction in risk lasts 15 years. No other drug offers such a reduction in cancer risk. In addition, OCs reduce the risk of benign breast disease and anemia (Grimes & Economy, 1995).

Numerous epidemiological studies have been performed on the incidence of breast and cervical cancer among women using oral contraceptives. While there are conflicting reports, most studies suggest that use of oral contraceptives is not associated with an overall increase in the risk of developing breast cancer. Some studies have reported an increased relative risk of developing breast cancer, particularly in younger women. OC use also appears to increase the risk of cervical cancer, possibly by increasing transmission and expression of human papillomavirus (HPV). In areas of the world where HPV screening is readily available, the protective effect of OCs against ovarian and endometrial cancer outweighs the increased risk of cervical cancer. The situation may not be as clear in areas where access to cytological screening is poor (Grimes & Economy, 1995).

OCs have been associated with an increased risk of chlamydia, due to increased cervical ectropion. The risk of chlamydial pelvic inflammatory disease (PID), however, appears to be lower in women using OCs. Evidence regarding the risk of gonorrhea among OC users is conflicting. Studies on the risk of acquiring HIV among OC users have also shown conflicting results (Rowe, 1994). For women who are sexually active and not in a mutually monogamous relationship with an uninfected partner, use of a barrier method, such as a condom, is essential.

Hormonal Methods—Implants

The first steroid implant, Norplant®, was approved by the FDA in 1990 after development and testing by the Population Council. The implant is approved for use in 27 countries with estimated use by approximately three million women worldwide. This device consists of six silicone capsules containing levonorgestrel. The contraceptive steroid slowly diffuses through the capsules, initially releasing 85 μg/day of levonorgestrel and declining to 30 μg/day after 18 months of use.

Although the mechanism of action is not fully understood, this progestin-only contraceptive may prevent pregnancy through ovulation inhibition, changes in cervical mucus, and interference with cyclic maturation of the endometrium.

The cumulative 5-year probability of pregnancy among Norplant® users is 1% (Sivin 1994; Thomas & LeMelle, 1995). While pregnancies among Norplant® users are rare, those that occur are more likely to be ectopic than pregnancies among women not using contraception.

Norplant® offers a variety of non-contraceptive health benefits, including decreased overall menstrual bleeding and decreased dysmenorrhea. Since Norplant® is a progestin-only method, the potential risk of thrombophlebitis may be reduced compared with combined estrogen–progestin methods. Although unfavorable metabolic changes in lipids and carbohydrates are seen, the overall effect on the risk of cardiovascular disease is felt to be small (Sivin, 1994; Thomas & LeMelle, 1995).

One of the most frequent reasons for discontinuation of Norplant® is irregular bleeding, ranging from an increased number of days of light or heavy bleeding to amenorrhea. Implant use has also been associated with headache, weight change, mood changes and acne bothersome enough to result in discontinuation. Lack of an estrogenic component may be associated with decreased bone density.

Recently, removal of Norplant® has become an issue. Removal should be a relatively simple, short procedure without complications. Among 3416 users in 11 countries, complications were reported in only 4.5% of removals, and were most commonly associated with deeply placed or broken implants (Dunson, Amatya & Krueger, 1995). However, in the USA, stories of difficult removals have been covered in the press and have led to class action suits against the marketing company. A number of new removal techniques have been devised to overcome these problems, including the 'pop-out', 'Emory', 'U', and 'modified U' techniques.

Hormonal Methods—Injectables

Depo-Provera® and norethindrone enanthate have been available in more than 90 countries for decades and are used by about nine million and one million women, respectively. Depo-Provera® was approved in the USA in 1992.

Depo-Provera® is injected intramuscularly every 3 months in 150 mg doses. It suppresses FSH and LH levels and eliminates the LH surge which inhibits ovulation. In addition, the injectable causes the development of a shallow and atrophic endometrium and, as with oral contraceptives and Norplant®, promotes the development of a thick cervical mucus which inhibits sperm penetration. The injectable has a first-year probability of failure in typical use of 0.3% (Trussel et al, 1995).

Depo-Provera® shares many of the same advantages and non-contraceptive benefits of other progestin-only contraceptives. Its influence on menses differs from that of Norplant® in that users are more likely to experience amenorrhea than irregular or heavy bleeding. Depo-Provera® reduces the risk of endometriosis as well as endometrial cancer.

Depo-Provera® is associated with relatively minor side effects, such as weight gain, headache, mood changes and acne. Return to fertility may be delayed 9–10 months after the last injection and small unfavorable changes in lipids have been seen. Depo-Provera® users have also been found to have lower bone density than non-users; this is the subject of Phase IV clinical trials (Kaunitz, 1994).

Depo-Provera® was not approved in the USA for 25 years due to concern over breast tumors in dogs exposed to it. However, it was later determined that dogs are an inappropriate model for progestin-related breast cancer and WHO studies did not find any overall increased risk of breast cancer in women using the method. However, women who started use of Depo-Provera® within the 5 years of the study were estimated to have a relative risk of breast cancer of 2.0 (95% CI 1.5–2.8), suggesting that Depo-Provera® enhances the late stages of tumor promotion or accelerates the growth of pre-existing tumors (Skegg et al, 1995). Selection, surveillance and recall bias may have affected study results. Research is needed to fully understand the relationship, if, any between Depo-Provera® and breast cancer (Chilvers, 1994).

Depo-Provera® did not appear to decrease ovarian cancer in WHO trials, but the women studied were parous and thus already at reduced risk for ovarian cancer. Ever-use of Depo-Provera® was shown in one case-control study to be associated with a relative risk of cervical cancer of 1.43 (95% CI 1.22–1.67) in long-term users. However, the risk appeared to decrease with time, suggesting that the effect was reversible or the result of an unidentified bias (Thomas, Ye & Ray, 1995).

Intra-uterine Devices

The first intra-uterine device (IUD) was developed by Ernst Gräfenberg in 1909 and consisted of a ring of silk gut and silver wire. Lack of antibiotics and the resulting high incidence of infection caused IUD contraception to fall into disrepute. Nevertheless, a few clinicians continued to develop and test the efficacy and safety of IUDs, and in 1948 the results of a study of women using the silk suture ring were reported. There were 0.9 pregnancies per 100 years' exposure, the lowest rate ever recorded for a contraceptive.

More modern versions of the IUD were developed by various pharmaceutical companies. These devices were made of plastic and included Lippes Loop® and the Safe-T-Coil®. In 1969, it was discovered that attaching copper wire and sleeves to the plastic device increased the contraceptive effect, and modern IUDs were introduced. In 1988, the TCu 380A was developed by the Population Council and first marketed in the USA under the trade name ParaGard®. It is approved for 10-year use.

IUDs which release hormones have also been developed. The Progestasert®, introduced in 1976, is the only hormone-releasing IUD marketed in the USA. It releases progesterone over the course of 1 year. The progesterone reduces uterine contractility and therefore pain and bleeding, the two most common side effects seen in users of any inert or copper IUD. The drawback to the Progestasert® is that it must be replaced every year, exposing the user to the postinsertion risk of infection.

The levonorgestrel-releasing IUD is approved in several European countries for 7 years of use. Its efficacy is similar to or better than that of the TCu 380A. It is associated with more removals for amenorrhea but fewer for pain and bleeding.

While the exact mechanism of action is not fully understood, all IUDs appear to inhibit the capacity of gametes to fertilize, alter the transport of both ovum and sperm, and cause other enzymatic and biochemical effects on the endometrium. Hormonal IUDs also thicken cervical mucus. Since the IUD acts primarily before the egg reaches the uterus, it does not abort established pregnancies. The average annual failure rates for the TCu 380A and the Progestasert® are 0.42% and 2%, respectively (Trussel et al, 1995). The 7-year cumulative failure rate of the levonorgestrel IUD and the TCu 380A are 1.1% and 1.7%, respectively. The 10-year cumulative pregnancy rate for the TCu 380A is 2.6 per 100 women.

In the mid-1970s, studies showed that users of the Dalkon Shield IUD had higher rates of pelvic inflammatory disease (PID) than women not using IUDs and women using other IUDs. The problem was felt to be due to the multifilament tail, which allowed bacteria to migrate from the lower reproductive tract to the endometrium. The device was withdrawn from the market and was the subject of thousands of lawsuits. It has since been established that the risk of PID among monogamous IUD users is not significantly greater than the risk of PID among monogamous users of no contraception, and that most of the risk that does exist is confined to the month immediately following insertion. As with other STDs, the IUD does not protect a woman from the HIV virus. Whether the device increases the risk of acquiring the virus is unknown.

Some of the most common reasons for IUD removal are pain and bleeding. Counselling often helps to alleviate the concern associated with these side effects. In addition, between 2% and 10% of women using the IUD experience spontaneous expulsion during the first year. Risk factors for expulsion are young maternal age, heavy menstrual flow, and severe dysmenorrhea prior to IUD insertion.

IUDs are as safe and effective in monogamous nulliparous women as in monogamous parous women. However, many practitioners are hesitant to prescribe the IUD to women of unproven fertility for fear of litigation should infertility become evident after removal of the IUD.

Barrier Methods—Mechanical and Chemical

Barrier methods are the oldest form of contraceptive technology. Penile sheaths were first described in Egypt in 1350 BC. In the eighteenth century, the name 'condom' was given to penile sheaths made from animal intestines and used to protect from STDs and unwanted pregnancy. The first diaphragms were pessaries, which varied in form and were used to support the uterus. Edward Bliss Foote is credited with inventing the 'womb veil' in the early 1800s, the first diaphragm used expressly for contraception. Friedrich Wilde described the first cervical cap in Germany in 1836.

The contraceptive sponge called 'Today' was approved in 1983 and was used by 1.5 million couples by 1985. However, in 1994, the FDA revealed problems with sanitization, microbiological test methods and bacterial contamination of the water supply used to make the sponge, which resulted in the manufacturer's voluntary withdrawal of the product from the market.

The female condom, called Reality® was approved in 1993. Unlike male condoms, the female condom covers the perineum and should offer protection of that area against herpes, human papillomavirus, syphilis and chancroid.

Chemical barriers have been used for centuries and include salt solutions, astringents and many other compounds thought to kill sperm. Nonoxynol-9 and octoxynol are available in the USA, although benzalkonium chloride is available in other countries. Recent concerns about these products center around the risk of epithelial disruption with frequent use which is felt to predispose to infection with STD-causing organisms, including HIV. Mechanical barriers are often used in conjunction with spermicides.

The efficacy of barrier contraceptives varies dramatically from method to method and differs for parous and nulliparous women. The first year failure rates for 'perfect' use are as follows: cap-parous, 26–27%; cap-nulliparous, 8–10%; sponge-parous, 19–21%; sponge-nulliparous, 9–10%. Parity does not appear to affect the efficacy of the diaphragm (Trussel, Strickler & Vaughan, 1993).

Barrier methods do not cause systemic side effects and do offer protection from STDs and invasive cervical cancer (Grimes & Economy, 1995).

The main disadvantages associated with barriers, depending on the specific method, are reduced sensitivity, interruption of intercourse, breakage, allergy to latex, and difficulties with fit and placement.

SPECIAL POPULATIONS WITH UNMET NEEDS FOR CONTRACEPTION

Despite the availability of numerous and effective methods of contraception, half of all pregnancies in the USA are unintended. This results from: failure to use contraception at all, inconsistent or incorrect use of contraception, or failure of a method correctly used. Clearly some needs are not being met by available methods.

No method has all the characteristics of an 'ideal' contraceptive and none ever will. But it is useful to look at groups of potential contraceptive users who may have specific needs which can be addressed by methods incorporating some 'ideal' characteristics.

Spacers vs. Preventers

The terms 'spacing births' and 'preventing births' may at first sound synonymous. But the terms differentiate between women who desire children at some point in the future (birth spacing) and women who consider their families complete (birth prevention). The characteristics and needs of these two groups differ considerably. Spacers tend to be younger, have fewer children, and to be concerned with effects on future fertility. Preventers tend to be older, with more children, and to desire a highly effective contraceptive for use during the rest of their childbearing years.

Adolescents

In the USA, half of teenagers have had intercourse by age 17, but only 40% used contraception at first intercourse. The average time between initiation of intercourse and seeking of contraception is 1 year. About half of adolescent pregnancies occur in the first 6 months after initiation of intercourse.

US teens have the highest pregnancy rates in the world, not due to higher rates of sexual activity but rather to poor use of contraceptives. Adolescents report that inadequate knowledge of contraceptive methods and lack of access, due to cost and confidentiality concerns, are major barriers to contraceptive use. Studies show that adolescents have misperceptions about the efficacy and side effects of various methods and are easily deterred from obtaining methods by requirements such as pelvic exams (Braverman & Strasburger, 1993).

Sexually active adolescents have higher rates of STDs than older women, even when corrected for sexual activity, suggesting that adolescents are physiologically more susceptible to STDs. Teens who become pregnant and deliver have higher rates of low birth weight, prematurity and intra-uterine growth retardation than older women, even when education, prenatal care and marital status are taken into account (Fraser, 1993).

Thus, adolescents need highly effective, accessible methods that require minimal user compliance and professional intervention. In addition, protection against STDs, predictable cycle control and reduction of dysmenorrhea and androgenic side effects are desirable. While the combination of condoms and hormonal methods comes close to meeting these requirements, the intensive counseling required to convince teens to use two methods makes further development essential (Sulak & Haney, 1993).

Post-partum and Breastfeeding Women

Women who do not breastfeed become pregnant, on average, 8 months after delivery in the absence of contraception. Women who fully breastfeed, on the other hand, do not become pregnant until 20 months after delivery. Breastfeeding women are more likely to bleed first and then ovulate, thereby receiving a signal of returning fertility, than women who do not breastfeed.

Thus breastfeeding exerts a significant contraceptive effect and prevents more pregnancies worldwide than any other form of contraception. The 'Lactational Amenorrhea Method' of contraception calls for a woman to fully breastfeed until either she begins to supplement, or menses return, or the baby is 6 months old. This method is 98% effective.

A need for post-partum contraception still exists, however, for women who do not wish to fully breastfeed and for those who, for any of the three reasons given above, can no longer count on the contraceptive effect of the Lactational Amenorrhea Method.

Combined OCs are not recommended for use in breastfeeding women due to reduced milk volume, although no detrimental effects have been documented in babies. Progestin-only pills are highly effective in the post-partum period and may be used by lactating and non-lactating women alike. The incidence of irregular bleeding among post-partum women using this and other progestin-only methods may be lower than that among non-post-partum users.

The labeling for Norplant® states that it may be inserted 6 weeks after delivery with no documented harmful effects. However, Depo-Provera® is used immediately post-partum and, despite higher serum progestin levels, does not affect milk production. Thus, Norplant® is probably safe for immediate post-partum use as well.

Periodic abstinence may be used in the post-partum period, but users may have difficulty recognizing the signs of ovulation. Mechanical barriers may also be used, although the cervical cap and diaphragm may not fit reliably until 6 weeks after delivery.

IUDs may be inserted immediately post-partum or 6 weeks later. Immediate insertion may be associated with somewhat higher expulsion rates and resulting higher pregnancy rates.

The ideal post-partum contraception would be one that would incorporate prediction of the first post-partum ovulation, thereby assuring that the method would be used soon enough, but not so early as to unnecessarily expose mother and infant to potential side effects.

Perimenopausal Women

Most women in this age group consider their families complete. Some women assume they are no longer fertile and become careless about contraception; the ratio of abortions to live births for women over 40 is second only to that of teenagers. An effective, easy-to-use method is needed for this group, whose contraceptive needs are affected by the natural decline in fertility with age, the greater risk associated with pregnancy, and the increase in health problems in general seen with advancing age.

The method used by two-thirds of older women is voluntary surgical contraception. However, there are reversible alternatives that may be less costly and offer additional non-contraceptive health benefits.

Low-dose OCs offer benefits to non-smoking women over 35, such as protection against ovarian and endometrial cancer, control of bleeding problems, and protection from osteoporosis. The revised labelling states that for these women, the benefits of OCs may outweigh the risks. A woman may continue to use OCs until she reaches menopause, when she may choose to use hormone replacement therapy. While Norplant®, Depo-Provera® and IUDs are also good choices for older women, they do not provide the bone-sparing effects of estrogen. A progestin-releasing IUD may provide contraception followed by endometrial protection when hormone replacement therapy is begun. Barrier methods are appropriate for older women, especially those not in mutually monogamous relationships.

The ideal contraceptive for perimenopausal women would bridge the gap—providing contraception until menopause and non-contraceptive benefits both before and after menopause.

Women with Clinical Problems

The ideal contraceptive for these women would provide highly effective pregnancy prevention without exacerbation of the clinical condition, and possibly with amelioration of it.

Women Who Cannot Take Estrogen

Such women include those with a history of clotting problems, lipid disorders or hypertension, and smokers over 35 years old. A progestin-only pill, implant, or injectable is a safe alternative to combined OCs. Each has the common but manageable drawback of irregular cycles. A barrier method or an IUD may also be a good choice. Women whose only risk factor is a family history of thrombo-embolism may be prescribed low-dose OCs. Those on oral anticoagulants can also use low-dose OCs to reduce bleeding and to avoid conception while taking teratogenic drugs (Comp & Zacur, 1993).

Diabetes

High-dose OCs (≥ 50 μg estrogen) have a detrimental effect on carbohydrate metabolism which causes a form of insulin resistance and could increase the risk of coronary heart disease. Low-dose OCs (30–35 μg estrogen) do not, however, and may be prescribed to diabetic women. Norplant® does not cause changes in basal glucose or insulin levels, but may cause insulin resistance under hyperglycemic, hyperinsulinemic conditions, thus putting a long-term user at possible risk of cardiovascular disease (Shamma et al, 1995). Depo-Provera® may impair glucose metabolism, but not in a clinically significant way. The IUD is a good choice for appropriately selected diabetic women.

Cardiovascular Disease

Young non-smoking women with controlled hypertension can safely take low-dose OCs, provided that blood pressure is monitored. Some may develop a significant increase in blood pressure. Women who are older, smoke, or whose hypertension is uncontrolled would do better on a progestin-only method or an IUD (Sullivan & Lobo, 1993).

Women with angina and atherosclerosis are at high risk of experiencing a myocardial infarction (MI) should pregnancy occur. Low-dose OCs and long-acting progestin-only methods may be used by women with angina who do not have a history of MI. If a history of MI exists, a non-steroidal method should be chosen (Sullivan & Lobo, 1993).

Epilepsy

Most anti-epileptic drugs induce metabolism of estrogens; OCs may not be appropriate for women taking such drugs. Norplant® is also affected by the use of certain anti-epileptic medications, increasing the risk of pregnancy. Depo-Provera®, on the other hand, does not appear to be affected by antiseizure medication and its use may actually decrease seizure frequency.

Benign Breast Disease

Combined OCs reduce the incidence and severity of benign breast disease.

Anemia

OCs, Depo-Provera®, Norplant®, and the levonorgestrel IUD reduce overall menstrual blood loss and are beneficial for women with or at risk for anemia.

Women with History of Ectopic Pregnancy

OCs, Depo-Provera®, Norplant® and the TCu 380A IUD reduce the likelihood of an ectopic pregnancy.

Women with HIV

Barriers are especially important for these women to reduce the likelihood of transmission of the infection, but steroidal methods are not contraindicated to prevent conception. IUDs may be used with caution: the severity of PID, should it occur, may be increased in women with HIV. In addition, the increase in menstrual blood may facilitate transmission.

Women with Hyperandrogenic Disorders

These may include acne, hirsutism, obesity and polycystic ovaries. Most OCs have positive effects on androgenic complications. The more selective progestins such as norgestimate appear to be more effective in ameliorating these side effects.

Women with Few Resources

Poor women have less access to contraception than women of higher income. Less than half have access to Medicaid (which does pay for the full range of contraceptives, including Norplant®), and approximately a third have no form of insurance at all. For these women, Title X clinics offer contraceptive services on a sliding scale, but these fees have increased in recent years.

Nevertheless, over 80% of poor women in the USA do use contraception, mostly OCs and tubal ligation. However, they use contraception less successfully than women of higher incomes. About 20% of poor women will have an unplanned pregnancy during their first year of use compared with only 10% of higher-income women.

The reasons for these difficulties are not clear, but are likely related to lower levels of education, accessibility difficulties, and societal and cultural influences. Contraceptives that are easy to use, inexpensive, and do not require frequent resupply will provide the most useful options for disadvantaged women (Donovan, 1995).

In a recent analysis, the Paragard® IUD proved to be the most cost-effective of any method of contraception, reversible or irreversible, after two years of use, including the cost of managing side effects and unwanted pregnancies. First year costs were lowest for injectables, OCs and then IUDs (Progestasert® followed by Paragard®) (Trussell et al, 1995). It should be noted, however, that these methods do not adequately address the need for STD protection, and counseling regarding concomitant use of barrier methods is required.

Other Groups

Other groups of potential users may also have special needs. Women who are poor compliers with methods requiring daily attention do better on long-acting methods. Women having infrequent intercourse may prefer a coitus-dependent method with few side effects. Certain cultural aspects of a woman's environment (e.g. implications of vaginal bleeding) may play a role in her choice of methods. For some couples, use of a contraceptive by the male may be medically necessary or simply preferred.

ISSUES IN CONTRACEPTIVE DEVELOPMENT

Drug Development Steps in a Nutshell

Drug development includes non-clinical and clinical testing. Non-clinical testing refers to laboratory and animal studies aimed at demonstrating effectiveness and lack of drug toxicity. Clinical testing is generally divided into three, sometimes four, phases. Phase I is the first exposure of humans to the test product and generally involves less than 50 volunteers who are usually not at risk for pregnancy and are observed for side effects and other aspects of drug safety. Phase II involves a few hundred volunteers, continues to monitor safety, and may look at efficacy to determine a sample size estimate for Phase III. Phase III studies are large, involving hundreds or thousands of volunteers, and usually compare a test product with a marketed one in a prospective, randomized, double-blind design which evaluates efficacy, safety and acceptability. If the results are favorable, the product is then submitted for FDA approval. Phase IV (post-marketing) studies may follow, which could be used for pharmacoepidemiology surveillance, determining new indications, and collection of additional safety data. Development of a new contraceptive takes about 10 years and costs about $200 million.

Who Should Develop New Contraceptives?

Only a few pharmaceutical firms remain involved in the basic research that could result in new methods and in licensing new products developed by public sector agencies. The potential market for contraceptives is not large compared with the market for other products, the public willingness to pay high prices for a drug or device that will be needed for many years is not great, and the potential liability incurred by a drug manufacturer should there be a contraceptive failure and fetal abnormality is enormous. Finally, the threat of boycott by groups opposed to abortion and equating contraception with abortion is looming ever larger.

Thus, most contraceptive development in the USA is being carried out by two public sector agencies: the National Institutes of Health, through the Institute for Child Health and Human Development, and the United States Agency for International Development (USAID), which funds the Population Council, Family Health International (FHI), and the Contraceptive Research and Development (CONRAD) Program. When a product reaches the latter stages of testing, a commercial partner is sought to assist with final manufacturing and distribution, in exchange for royalties and a public sector price. These agencies have a good track record, with the Population Council developing the TCu 380A IUD and Norplant®, and CONRAD and FHI supporting clinical evaluation of the Reality® female condom.

It is unlikely that this situation will change any time soon, and indeed it is a system that functions fairly well. The greatest risk in the development of any new product is in its early stages, when many leads are found not to be promising and are weeded out. A lead that proves successful enough to make it to Phase III trials often requires resources greater than those available to public sector agencies in order to move into those trials and/or general distribution. Thus, public sector agencies assume the initial risk of investigating a new product, and commercial companies invest the large amount of capital required to move a promising lead into actual approval and marketing.

One criticism of contraceptive development is that women's perspectives have not received adequate attention. Development has been driven largely by scientific discoveries rather than by establishing what potential users want. Greater emphasis on market research is needed and should be channeled back to improve drug development.

Issues in Study Design

Contraceptive trials should be prospective, comparative, randomized, and masked whenever possible. The optimal study design should lend itself to providing results that are generalizable to the typical contraceptive user. The study population must be large enough to provide adequate statistical power to differentiate between outcome measures. Information on every act of coitus should be collected, rather than relying on patient recall at follow-up visits which can bias 'perfect use' pregnancy rates upward (Dominik et al, in preparation). Enrolling women without prior experience with the method being tested is preferred. The underlying fecundity of the participants should be known, or at least estimated, by other parameters such as age and gravidity. Pregnancies should be diagnosed using sensitive urine pregnancy tests which capture early miscarriage, possibly accounting for 22% of all pregnancies seen in a study (Trussell et al, 1990). Follow-up must be rigorous in order to maintain an adequate representation of study outcomes.

CONTRACEPTIVE EFFICACY

Contraceptive efficacy may be expressed in a variety of ways. Efficacy is most commonly represented by Pearl indices or cumulative life-table rates. The Pearl Index is a measure of the pregnancy rate relative to the total cumulative duration of exposure, regardless of whether this was accumulated by a few subjects exposed for a long period of time or many subjects for a short period of time. This index is independent of how many subjects were in the study at the time of each conception. Traditionally, the 12-month formula (number of pregnancies × 1200/ total number of months of exposure) has been used. However, since a calendar year contains 13 menstrual cycles, a formula with 1300 rather than 1200 in the numerator has also been used.

The cumulative annual life-table pregnancy rate reflects the proportion of subjects who conceived at a particular moment relative to the number of subjects at risk at that time. This contrasts with the Pearl Index analysis, which determines the pregnancy rate relative to the cumulative duration of exposure of all subjects and is independent of the number of subjects in the study at the time of a conception. For example, in a 12-cycle study, if 1000 subjects participated for 10 cycles, and 900 discontinued after cycle 10, the life-table pregnancy rate would be 10-fold higher if pregnancies were limited to cycles 11 and 12, than if an identical number of pregnancies had occurred in cycles 1 to 10. The Pearl Index would be identical for the two situations. The life-table method of analysis was designed for use with long-acting methods, such as implants or IUDs, where it provides an accurate pregnancy risk assessment and characterizes the contraceptive effect in relation to duration of use.

Two particularly important expressions of efficacy are 'user failure' and 'method failure' rates. 'Method failure' rates are often incorrectly calculated. The correct way to calculate such a rate is to use pregnancies occurring during periods of 'perfect use' as the numerator and the number of periods (months or cycles) of 'perfect use' as the denominator. Often, however, all periods of use, whether perfect or typical, have been included in the denominator, which biased method failure rates downward (Trussell et al, 1990).

Calculation of bleeding episodes has been done in many different ways. The reference period method, developed by WHO, is currently preferred. In this, bleeding days are recorded whenever they occur within a certain time period, usually 90 days, without regard to when menses was expected. Bleeding is distinguished from spotting by the need for sanitary protection, although this should probably be re-evaluated for studies done in developed countries in which 'panty-liners' have become available and may be used when no protection would have been used in the past. The number of bleeding and spotting days and bleeding episodes (consecutive days of bleeding) can be recorded and compared among studies.

Methods of Determining Patient Compliance

OCs have a theoretical efficacy of 99.9% but first year failure rates average around 3% due to less-than-perfect compliance. Failure rates among users outside of clinical trials may be much higher. Thus, there is interest in studying non-compliance and the patient and product characteristics that lead to it. These data should support the design of contraceptive methods to facilitate compliance.

Older methods of estimating compliance include pill counts, interviews, diaries, and blood and urine levels of steroids or other markers. A more modern and precise method is electronic compliance monitoring. The Medical Events Monitoring System (MEMS), developed by the Aprex Corporation for Ortho Pharmaceuticals, is a battery-powered optical sensor that fits into a slightly modified oral contraceptive pill pack and records the date and time at which a pill is removed from the pack. A recent study (Potter et al, in preparation) followed 101 women for 3 months and compared pill-taking patterns as recorded on diary cards and by the MEMS packs. Between 51% and 66% of women reported missing no pills each month; only 23–37% of MEMS recordings corroborated these findings. Pills were most often missed on weekends. The women who, by MEMS recording, missed the most pills were those who reported forgetting the fewest pills in their diaries. These women may have also been most likely to forget to fill out their diaries until the end of the month. The poorest compliers were women who had been pregnant in the past. These data are difficult to analyze, but are valuable in obtaining estimates of compliance patterns.

Determining STD Protection

Clinical trials of STD-preventing measures present significant challenges. While 80% of a non-contracepting population may be expected to achieve pregnancy in the course of a year, most non-STD-preventing populations would become infected at a much lower rate. To see the effect of an intervention in an STD trial would therefore require a much larger sample size than in a contraceptive trial. In addition, it is unethical not to advise participants at risk of STDs to use condoms. Participants who comply with this instruction provide no useful data on the efficacy of the means of STD protection being tested. It is only those participants who fail to heed the instruction to use condoms but who do use the test product who provide useful information about it. The investigator is caught in the bind of having to advise participants to do something that is in their best interest but, if followed by everyone, would severely limit the usefulness of the study.

CONTRACEPTIVE METHODS IN DEVELOPMENT

New Steroids

Computer-assisted design dramatically improves the synthesis of new steroids. This allows known compounds and their nomenclature to be examined for structure–activity relationships and new compounds designed to incorporate the structures associated with desired activities.

As mentioned earlier, three progestins have been recently developed: norgestimate, desogestrel and gestodene. Others are in development, most notably nesterone (formerly called ST 1435), which is readily absorbed from transdermal gels, microspheres, implants and vaginal rings. The drug's poor oral bioavailability makes it a promising contraceptive option for breastfeeding women; any drug appearing in breast milk is unlikely to be absorbed by the infant.

New estrogens may be on the way as well. All oral contraceptives in the USA contain ethinyl estradiol or its 3-methyl ether, mestranol. Estrogenic components under consideration include natural estrogen and highly potent synthetic compounds in an effort to improve the safety profile.

New Applications of Existing Steroids and Related Compounds

Methods Which Extend Lactational Amenorrhea

Natural progesterone in vaginal rings and suppositories is being studied in clinical trials as a means to prolong lactational amenorrhea. Rings releasing nesterone alone or in combination with ethinyl estradiol, and rings releasing norethindrone acetate and ethinyl estradiol are being studied in humans by the Population Council. In addition, gonadotropin releasing hormone (GnRH) agonists appear to delay return to ovulation in breastfeeding women. These compounds are probably safe for the infant, since they are poorly orally absorbed. The possibility of maternal hypo-estrogenism and bone loss must be evaluated (Fraser, 1993).

Over-the-counter Oral Contraceptives

Changing the status of oral contraceptives to that of an over-the-counter medication has been considered by the FDA. The advantages include convenience and privacy for the user, elimination of a clinic visit and pelvic exam, and greater user control. Significant disadvantages are higher cost and lack of the clinician counseling which could enhance compliance and improve STD prevention practices. In addition, physician intervention is required to insure appropriate patient selection in the case of women with contra-indications to the pill. Furthermore, essential preventive health services for women, such as screening for cervical neoplasia, are currently linked to physician-prescribing of pills (Reproductive Health Technologies Project, 1995).

Antiprogestins

Antiprogestins have been approved in France and other European countries for use as abortifacients. Antiprogestins act by binding to the progesterone receptor and preventing progesterone from exerting its normal effects. Hundreds of antiprogestins have been synthesized, but only mifepristone (sometimes called the 'French Abortion Pill') has been marketed. It is currently in clinical trials sponsored by the Population Council and submission to FDA for approval as an abortifacient is expected in the next few years. It is given in a 600 mg oral dose, followed by one of several prostaglandins, and is approximately 95% successful in inducing complete abortion. Issues requiring further research include determination of the minimum effective dose, the maximum gestation at which it remains efficacious, the best prostaglandin to use, and the acceptability of non-surgical abortion.

Methotrexate used with misoprostol appears to be an alternative to mifepristone used with misoprostol. In a randomized study of 61 women with pregnancies of 56 days or less, methotrexate combined with misoprostol resulted in abortions in 90% of women, compared with only 47% of those given misoprostol alone (Creinin & Vittinghoff, 1994). In a larger, non-randomized study of 178 women who received the combination, 96% had successful abortions. Side effects were minimal and the participants preferred the medical approach to the surgical one (Hausknecht, 1995).

Other potential uses for antiprogestins include contraception as a daily, weekly or monthly pill, and as emergency contraception. Use as a daily 'minipill' is directed at altering the endometrium without affecting ovulation. Antiprogestins may also be used as 'menses inducers' or compounds taken when a period is late or at the end of each cycle in which intercourse has taken place before there is any evidence of pregnancy.

'Emergency Contraception'

Contrary to popular belief, 'emergency' or 'morning-after' contraception is currently available in the USA. It consists of taking two oral contraceptive pills followed by another two pills 12 hours later. This method is 75% effective in preventing pregnancy if the pills are taken within 3 days of unprotected intercourse. If fully utilized, emergency contraception could prevent half of the unintended pregnancies and abortions occurring each year in the USA (Hatcher et al, 1995).

Despite the fact that emergency contraception has been well studied, its use has been limited. Currently no oral contraceptive is labeled for this purpose, although it is legal for clinicians to prescribe them for it. The FDA recently published requirements for approval of such labeling; no clinical studies would be required for certain regimens. However, as emergency contraception is widely perceived as an abortifacient, the threat of boycott or more violent measures against the manufacturer may deter efforts to change labeling.

A common source of confusion is the distinction between emergency contraception and mifepristone. Mifepristone, available in other countries as an abortifacient, also acts as an emergency contraceptive that prevents implantation when 600 mg are taken within three days of unprotected intercourse. The World Health Organization is studying the use of mifepristone during the first five days after unprotected intercourse.

An additional emergency contraceptive is the copper IUD, which may be inserted up to 1 week after unprotected intercourse. This method is particularly effective for women who have failed to use the emergency contraceptive pill within 3 days of unprotected intercourse, would like to continue using the IUD for contraception, or have contra-indications to oral contraceptives. Fertilization may not be prevented by either hormonal measures or the IUD but implantation, which defines the beginning of pregnancy, is prevented. An established pregnancy is not disrupted by the use of emergency contraception.

New Delivery Systems for Steroids

New delivery systems for steroids are being sought in an effort to simplify compliance and avoid the first-pass effect of oral administration. Implants and injectables are available but can be improved. Vaginal products are under investigation and are fairly close to being marketed. Transdermal, buccal and nasal administration have been studied, with varying results.

Implants

There is a demand for an implant which would provide less than 5 years' contraception for women who want fewer years of protection or who would like to try out an implant without the lengthy initial commitment of Norplant®. Norplant 2® is a two-rod implant system approved by the FDA for 3-year use. The rods are stiffer than Norplant® rods and fewer in number and therefore removal should pose fewer problems.

In addition, there is a need for more potent and less androgenic progestins in implants which would permit development of smaller and/or longer-acting systems with fewer androgenic side effects. Single implant systems under development include a 3-keto-desogestrel implant which is less androgenic than the levonorgestrel in Norplant 2®. An implant containing nesterone and one containing nomegestrel acetate are also in development (Darney, 1994).

Implant technology would be greatly enhanced if removal were not required. Capronor® is a single implant system which releases levonorgestrel and breaks down into CO_2 and water over time. Animal studies suggest that it may be effective for 2 years. Removal is not necessary but is easily done because the adherent fibrous tissue build-up seen with Norplant® does not occur. A system of biodegradable cholesterol pellets containing norethindrone is also being studied.

The risk of ectopic pregnancy in women with implants releasing sub-contraceptive levels of progestin has been an issue. Such a situation would happen after the implant has delivered its usable contraceptive effect but before all steroid is exhausted. Concern stems from the fact that women who discontinue Depo-Provera® have an increased risk of ectopic pregnancy during the time between the end of the efficacy afforded by their last injection and the decline of progestin to undetectable levels. There are insufficient data from Norplant® users who fail to have their implant removed after 5 years to draw similar conclusions about the product.

A potential solution is to release the remaining steroid in a burst once release levels go below a certain point that would occur at a predictable time after insertion. Such a burst would be unlikely to cause blood levels of steroid that would be harmful.

Injectables

New monthly injectables for women are being developed in an effort to overcome the irregular bleeding associated with longer-acting, progestin-only injectables. These new injectables contain a progestin and an estrogen, and bleeding results from falling levels of these hormones at the end of the month, similar to the pill-free week among OC users. WHO has developed two such injectables, Cyclofem (25 mg depo-medroxyprogesterone acetate and 5 mg estradiol cypionate), and Mesigyna (50 mg norethindrone enanthate and 5 mg estradiol valerate). Both have been found to be very effective and allow a faster return to fertility than Depo-Provera® or norethindrone enanthate alone. Both were registered in several countries in 1993. In the future, combined injectables with a duration of action of greater than one month may be developed.

Another development in injectables is the use of preparations with a more steady release profile than current preparations. This would avoid the burst in hormone levels that usually occurs immediately after injection and would permit longer delivery at steady levels. Microcapsules and modified crystal sizes are two approaches. The latter is less expensive and is being testing by WHO using levonorgestrel butanoate.

Vaginal Preparations

Vaginal rings releasing constant small amounts of steroid are the only long-acting method under a woman's control. Rings may contain either progestin alone or a combination of estrogen and progestin. WHO developed a levonorgestrel-releasing ring appropriate for 3 months of continuous use. Efficacy was acceptable and the main side effects were menstrual irregularity in half the women and expulsion, particularly among parous women. Red patches on the vaginal wall were also seen and are being investigated.

Rings that release the natural hormone progesterone are also being studied for use in breastfeeding women to prolong the period of lactational amenorrhea. Efficacy, safety and acceptability look promising in early trials. Rings releasing nesterone alone or in combination with ethinyl estradiol, and rings releasing norethindrone acetate and ethinyl estradiol, are being studied in humans by the Population Council.

Other

Gels, creams and patches, including iontophoretic ones, are being studied as contraceptive delivery systems. Patches delivering estrogens are currently marketed for use in hormonal replacement therapy. Patches need application only once a week, but require constant vigilance to ensure that the patch remains secure.

Buccal and nasal approaches have also been studied; maintenance of a constant dose is one of the major obstacles to be overcome.

Reversible Male Methods

Although this volume concerns itself with drug development for women, the development of contraceptives for men is included since their availability would have an impact on the need to take contraceptive drugs for many women.

Condoms, vasectomy, and coitus interruptus are the only current options for men who wish to participate in family planning. These require that the man either permanently compromise his fertility or temporarily compromise his pleasure. A number of new methods are in development that may impact on the need to take contraceptive drugs for many women.

Hormonal methods suppress spermatogenesis via suppression of LH and/or FSH. Testosterone enanthate (TE) injections, which cause superphysiological levels of testosterone, have been studied in multicenter trials in which men who achieved azoospermia were infertile for at least 12 months (with continued TE administration). Men who achieved oligospermia (less than three million sperm per ml of semen) rather than azoospermia had reduced fertility, but not to the extent of azoospermic men.

A limitation of this approach is that TE must be injected weekly. Efforts are currently directed at identifying longer-acting preparations, including microspheres, pellets, and esters such as testosterone bucyclate. Other limitations are the time required for onset and offset of the contraceptive effect, the need for superphysiological levels of testosterone, and occurrence of systemic side effects. Testosterone undecanoate and bucyclate are longer-acting than testosterone enanthate and allow testosterone to remain within the physiological range. The addition of a progestin to suppress spermatogenesis could permit use of a physiological range of testosterone. Depo-medroxyprogesterone acetate looks promising, as do levonorgestrel and desogestrel. The effect of these hormonal methods on men's lipoprotein levels and prostate size, and clinical side effects such as acne, must be studied. The synthetic androgen 7-α-methyl-19-nortestosterone (MENT) is more potent than testosterone and is being studied in humans as an implant. It is not subject to 5-α reduction and is thus not expected to stimulate prostate growth (Sundaram, Kumar & Bardin, 1993). In addition, differences in bioavailability of parenterally administered testosterone have been seen in different ethnic groups and need to be explored further.

Additional approaches to a male method are 'testicular' and 'post-testicular' methods. These would have a faster rate of onset and offset than hormonal methods and would avoid endocrine effects. Testicular methods are targeted at spermatocytes or spermatids and structures that first appear in them, such as the acrosome. Post-testicular methods are aimed at sperm stored in the epididymis and proteins secreted by the epididymal epithelium. WHO is working with Chinese researchers on an extract of the plant *Triptergynium wilfordii*, used to treat psoriasis and noted to cause decreased sperm concentration and motility. One problem with antispermatogenic compounds is that many are alkylating agents and have adverse side effects on other rapidly dividing cells. Indenopyridines and ketoconazole derivatives are non-alkylating agents with antispermatogenic properties in animals.

Calcium channel blockers have been proposed as a systemic contraceptive method for men. These compounds appear to interfere with sperm capacitation by interfering with binding to mannose of ZP3 (a protein from the zona pellucida). A patch that delivers testosterone is also being studied.

Other new male methods, discussed below, include peptides, sterilization and immunization.

Peptides

GnRH analogs have been proposed for use as contraceptives for both men and women. Both agonists and antagonists reduce gonadotropin secretion through different mechanisms. In women, they would probably be combined with low-dose estrogen and progestin replacement to avoid hypoestrogenism and irregular bleeding. The effects on cardiovascular disease and the risk of breast, ovarian and endometrial cancer will need evaluation; it is possible that the risk of these conditions will be reduced. In men, testosterone replacement will be required. The cost and route of administration of GnRH analogs present potential challenges (Fraser, 1993).

Gonadal peptides such as inhibin, activin and follistatin regulate FSH. They are not orally active and would probably be used in vaccines.

Other leads include certain intregins and cytokines which may play a role in implantation, angiogenesis-inhibiting factors which may prevent ovulation, and oocyte maturation factor (OMF).

IUDs

Cu-Fix

The most common reasons for discontinuation of an IUD are pain and/or bleeding. The Cu-Fix or Flexigard is a frameless IUD designed to reduce pain and bleeding and also expulsion that may result from the disproportion between the size of the IUD and the uterine cavity. It consists of a monofilament suture strung with six copper sheaths and topped by a knot for anchoring. The device is embedded into the fundal myometrium with a specially designed inserter. WHO has carried out trials in 10 countries to evaluate this IUD. Unexpectedly high expulsion rates have resulted in design changes and studies are continuing.

Post-partum IUDs

Immediate (within 10 minutes of delivery of the placenta) post-partum placement of copper IUDs is associated with an expulsion rate somewhat greater than insertion done 6 or more weeks post-partum, but may offer advantages in areas where the likelihood of the patient's returning for an interval insertion is low (Xu, Reuschê & Burdan, 1994).

The Cu-Fix, modified by the addition of a biodegradable cone near the knot, is being tested in post-partum use by WHO. Results, including expulsion rates, are promising.

Barriers—Mechanical

Condoms

Male condoms are the only method proven to reduce the risk of both pregnancy and STDs, yet relatively few people opt to use them. Improvement in condom technology includes the use of new, synthetic materials, such as Tactylon® and polyurethane, which should provide lower breakage rates, better resistance to petroleum-based products, improved sensitivity and longer shelf life. In addition, these materials should lack odor and not cause allergic reactions in persons sensitive to latex. New designs include baggy condoms and condoms with a pouch over the glans (Pleasure Plus®) designed to improve friction between the condom and the skin.

Diaphragms and Cervical Caps

Improvements in diaphragms and cervical caps include use of synthetic materials for the same reasons as above, and development of one-size-fits-all devices which could be sold over the counter. Phase III trials are currently being planned for Lea's Shield®, a new one-size-fits-all diaphragm. The Femcap® is a new cervical cap that still requires fitting; a Phase III trial was recently completed.

Barriers—Chemical

There is a demand for topical preparations that can be applied well before coitus and thus not interfere with spontaneity. Compounds that are not cytotoxic but interfere with sperm or micro-organism function would be less likely to cause epithelial disruption. Compounds that do not cause ulcerations or that reduce the risk of diseases that cause ulceration would be beneficial. New spermicides that penetrate cervical mucus better than nonoxynol-9 (N-9) are being studied.

There is a need for vaginal gel or cream formulations that coat the vaginal walls and provide contraception and protection against STDs. Advantage 24® is a new spermicidal preparation that claims to adhere to the vagina for 24 hours, via the negative charges on the organic polymer polycarbophil contained in its base. While the product does not make claims about STDs, and data on its efficacy as a contraceptive have not been published, it may be the first in a line of new products which could have application as microbicides (Contraceptive Technology Update, 1995).

The National Institute of Allergy and Infectious Disease recently awarded grants for the study of vaginal microbicides, to include investigation of polysulfated carbohydrates, bile-acid derivatives, pulmonary surfactants, N-9, benzalkonium chloride, chlorhexidine, methyl esters of short-chain fatty acids, lactobacillus, myeloperoxidase and protegrins (Rowe, 1995).

Ovulation Prediction

'Natural family planning' involves recording changes in cervical mucus, body temperature and ovulatory symptoms and prospectively predicting the timing of 'unsafe' periods. Current efforts at refining this technique involve the development of home urine tests that measure estrone glucuronide, which rises several days before ovulation, and pregnanediol glucuronide, which rises afterwards. So far, such tests have run into problems with reproducibility and high costs, but efforts continue.

Sterilization—Male

A 'no-scalpel' vasectomy technique that uses dissecting forceps to make a small hole in the scrotum has been well-received in China. The lack of an incision increases acceptability. Other advantages include fewer complications, especially bleeding, and the requirement for fewer instruments and less time for completion.

Percutaneous chemical vas occlusion has also been studied in China, using a mixture of carbolic acid and n-butyl-α-cyanoacrylate, with 95.6% of men achieving azoospermia.

Intravasal polyurethane and silicone plugs have been studied as potentially reversible methods of male sterilization. External clips have also been studied, but present problems in terms of movement along the vas, slippage, formation of adhesions and painful nodules, and irreversible crush injury. None of these methods is ready for clinical use (Xiaozhang & Shunqiang, 1993).

In addition, since copper is known to have toxic effects on sperm, intravasal placement of copper is being studied in animal models in the hope of developing a method for men.

Sterilization—Female

The Filshie clip, recently approved by the FDA for tubal occlusion, may have advantages in terms of reversibility since it does not occlude as large a segment of the fallopian tube as some other devices, such as the tubal ring and Wolff clip. To date there are no data on reversibility. Hysteroscopically placed in situ wired silicone plugs have been studied and appear feasible, but would not be useful in resource-poor areas.

The antimalarial drug quinacrine has been studied as a non-surgical means of permanent female sterilization. It involves two insertions, one month apart, of seven quinacrine pellets, which cause inflammation and occlusion of the tubes a few millimeters into the isthmus. Field studies have been done in Chile, India, Vietnam and other countries, and pre-hysterectomy studies have been conducted in the USA. The risk of ectopic pregnancy, should occlusion be incomplete, is a concern. In addition, since quinacrine is teratogenic and embryocidal, method failure could have unacceptable consequences should an intra-uterine pregnancy occur. Moreover, Ames testing suggests that quinacrine may be carcinogenic. Vietnamese trials involving 31 781 women who received at least one insertion demonstrated a pregnancy rate of 2.6 per 100 users at 12 months and 4.3 at 24 months. While no deaths occurred, because of the potential risk of carcinogenesis the method will not be available unless and until long-term follow-up can be done to resolve the issue of carcinogenicity (Pies, Potts & Young, 1994).

Immunocontraception

Immunocontraception offers potential advantages, including suitability for both men and women, long-acting but reversible efficacy, low cost, and ease of distribution and administration within most health care infrastructures. Difficulties encountered in animal models and in limited clinical trials include unacceptable efficacy profiles and unpredictable duration of infertility. Efforts are ongoing to ensure that any immunologically-based method of fertility regulation is well-characterized, safe, and will be utilized only with informed consent.

The objective of vaccine development is to find a preparation that provides reliable contraception for 6 months or longer. The target antigen may be a peptide hormone or part of the egg or sperm. Reversibility could occur either by natural waning of immunity or on demand by administration of a neutralizing agent. Although most efforts so far have been directed at developing injectable vaccines, the administration of oral vaccines may prove simpler and more effective, since mucosal immunity within the reproductive tract could be stimulated.

Numerous antigens have been assessed in animal trials. The most advanced antigen tested is human chorionic gonadotropin (hCG), the hormone produced by the early embryo and required for maintenance of progesterone production. One form of an hCG vaccine has undergone a Phase II efficacy trial in India. Some but not all women developed titers sufficient to prevent pregnancy. Importantly, this induced infertility has been shown to be reversible. WHO began Phase II trials in Sweden in 1994 with a slightly different prototype hCG vaccine. WHO has also worked on a vaccine derived from the trophectoderm (WHO, 1992–93).

A GnRH vaccine for men has been studied in men with prostate cancer as an alternative to orchiectomy. Testosterone levels decreased and no adverse effects were seen. Such a vaccine would also have contraceptive application (Ladd, 1993).

A vaccine directed against FSH appears to be immunogenic in animal models and humans and significantly inhibits fertility in male primates. Safety studies are under way in humans in India.

ZP3, a protein from the zona pellucida, is the primary oocyte-derived antigen currently under study. Efforts have been complicated by autoimmune reactions in the ovary, leading to ovarian failure. Current approaches focus on using epitopes that stimulate B cells rather than a T-cell response. It is possible that multiple B-cell epitopes will be required for an adequate antifertility response.

Numerous sperm-derived antigens are actively under investigation, including PH-20 and PH-30, LDH-C_4, SP-10, FA-1 and SP-17. Many others have been tested to varying degrees in the past. PH-20 and PH-30 proteins are involved in penetration of the cumulus oophorus, binding of sperm to the zona, and fusion with the egg. Immunization induces reversible infertility in guinea pigs and primate studies have begun with PH-20. Another sperm antigen, LDH-C_4, has shown promise in primate efficacy trials; human safety studies are planned. Other candidate antigens have achieved varying degrees of success in primate studies. One problem observed in animal studies of several vaccines is the production of high serum titers of antibodies against the target antigen without accompanying antifertility effects.

A reversible vaccine that combines antifertility effects with protection against STDs would come very close to being an 'ideal' contraceptive. Efforts are being directed at the development of passive immunization, using monoclonal antibodies directed at reproductive targets and/or STD-causing organisms. Protection would be immediate, unlike active immunization which may require several vaccine doses.

Although development of a safe and highly effective immunocontraceptive has proved to be problematic, the potential advantages of its unique characteristics have led to continued interest in this approach. The moderate effectiveness observed in primate trials for single antigens may be overcome by the use of multiple antigens or improved adjuvants, delivery systems and vaccine technology. Indeed, the recent finding that administration of 'naked' DNA can lead to a significant immune response in animal models, including primates, may open a new avenue for immunocontraception (Wolff et al, 1990).

SUMMARY

Contraception has benefits for women and men as individuals and for society as a whole. No one method will be ideal for all users at all times; the existence of special user populations makes this particularly true. The need for protection against STDs is critical as well.

More research is needed into mechanisms that control endometrial bleeding and the functions of vaccine antigens. Development of a longer-acting male hormonal method without side effects, and reversible 'sterilization', is also necessary. More work also needs to be done in the area of public/private sector cooperation and collaboration between developing countries, where the greatest demand for contraception exists, and developed ones, in which the most resources exist.

Providing a wider choice of acceptable methods to couples worldwide, combined with societal changes and greater opportunities for women, will improve health and quality of life and reduce the threat of unchecked population growth.

ACKNOWLEDGEMENTS

The author is indebted to Henry Gabelnick, Michael Kafrissen, Haya Taitel, Susan Allen, Doug Colvard, Linda Potter and Doris Thompson for their help in writing, reviewing and preparing this manuscript.

REFERENCES

Ashford L. New perspectives on population: lessons from Cairo. *Population Bulletin* 1995; **50**(5): 2–44.

Braverman PK, Strasburger VC. Contraception. *Clin Pediat* 1993; **32**(12): 725–34.

Creinin MD, Vittinghoff E. *JAMA* 1994; **272**: 1190–5.

Chilvers C. Breast cancer and depot-medroxyprogesterone acetate: a review. *Contraception* 1994; **49**: 211–22.

Collins DC. Sex hormone receptor binding, progestin selectivity, and the new oral contraceptives. *Am J Obstet Gynecol* 1994; **170**: 1508–13.

Comp PC, Zacur HA. Contraceptive choices in women with coagulation disorders. *Am J Obstet Gynecol* 1994; **168**: 1990–93.

Contraceptive Technology Update. New Advantage 24 contraceptive gel claims 24-hour effectiveness. *Contraceptive Technol* 1995; 45–51.

Darney PD. Hormonal implants: contraception for a new century. *Am J Obstet Gynecol* 1994; **170**: 1536–43.

Darney PD. The androgenicity of progestins. *Am J Med* 1995; **98** (suppl 1A): 104–10S.

Dominik R, Trussell J, Walsh T. Failure rates among perfect users and during perfect use: a distinction that matters. *Family Health Int*, in preparation.

Donovan, P. *The Politics of Blame* 1995; New York: Alan Guttmacher Institute.

Dunson TR, Amatya RN, Krueger SL. Complications and risk factors associated with removal of Norplant implants. *Obstet Gynecol* 1995; **85**(4): 543–8.

Fraser HM. GnRH analogues for contraception. *Br Med J* 1993; **49**(1): 62–72.

Grimes DA, Economy KE. Primary prevention of gynecological cancers. *Am J Obstet Gynecol* 1995; **172**: 227–35.

Hatcher RA, Trussell J, Stewart F et al. *Emergency Contraception, the Nation's Best-Kept Secret* 1995; Atlanta, GA: Bridging the Gap Communications, Inc.

Hausknecht RU. Methotrexate and misoprostol to terminate early pregnancy. *N Engl J Med* 1995; **333**(9): 357–40.

Kaunitz AM. Long-acting injectable contraception with depot progesterone acetate. *Am J Obstet Gynecol* 1994; **170**(5): 1543–9.

Ladd A. Progress in the development of anti-LHRH vaccine. *Am J Reprod Immunol* 1993; **29**: 189–94.

Pies C, Potts M, Young B. Quinacrine pellets: an examination of nonsurgical sterilization. *Internat Family Planning Perspect* 1994; **20**: 137–41.

Potter L, Oakley D, Wong E, Cañamar R. Measuring oral contraceptive pill use: comparison of diary and electronic data. In preparation.

Reed, J. *From Private Vice to Public Virtue* 1978; New York: Basic Books.

Reproductive Health Technologies Project. *Oral Contraceptives: Over-the-counter: What If?* 1995; Washington, DC: Reproductive Health Technologies Project.

Rowe PJ. You win some and you lose some—contraception and infection. *Aust NZ Obstet Gynaecol* 1994; **34**(3): 299–305.

Rowe PM. Research into topical microbicides against STDs. *Lancet* 1995; **345**: 1231.

Shamma FN, Rossi G, HajHassan L, Penzias A. The effect of Norplant on glucose metabolism under hyperglycemic hyperinsulinemic conditions. *Fertil Steril* 1995; **63**(4): 767–72.

Sivin I. Contraception with Norplant® implants. *Human Reprod* 1994; **9**(10): 1818–26.

Skegg DCG, Noonan EA, Paul C et al. Depot medroxyprogesterone acetate and breast cancer. *JAMA* 1995; **273**(10): 799–804.

Sulak PJ, Haney AF. Unwanted pregnancies: understanding contraceptive use and benefits in adolescents and older women. *Am J Obstet Gynecol* 1993; **168**: 2042–8.

Sullivan JM, Lobo RA. Considerations for contraception in women with cardiovascular disorders. *Am J Obstet Gynecol* 1993; **168**: 2006–11.

Sundaram K, Kumar N, Bardin CW. 7-α-methyl-nortestosterone (MENT): the optimal androgen for male contraception. *Ann Med* 1993; **25**: 199–205.

Thomas AG, LeMelle SM. The Norplant system: where are we in 1995? *J Family Pract* 1995; **40**(2): 125–8.

Thomas DB, Ye Z, Ray RM. Cervical carcinoma *in situ* and use of depot-medroxyprogesterone acetate (Depo-Provera®). *Contraception* 1995; **51**: 25–31.

Trussell J, Hatcher RA, Cates W et al. A guide to interpreting contraceptive efficacy studies. *Obstet Gynecol* 1990; **76**(3): 558–67.

Trussell J, Leveque JA, Koenig JD et al. The economic value of contraception: a comparison of 15 methods. *Am J Publ Health* 1995; **85**(4): 494–502.

Trussell J, Strickler J, Vaughan B. Contraceptive efficacy of the diaphragm, the sponge and the cervical cap. *Family Planning Perspect* 1993; **25**(3): 100–5, 135.

WHO (World Health Organization). *Biennial Report* 1992–93. Geneva: WHO.

Wolff JA, Malone RW, Williams P et al. Direct gene transfer into mouse muscle *in vivo*. *Science* 1990; **247**(4949, Pt 1): 1465–8.

Xu JX, Reuschê C, Burdan A. Immediate postplacental insertion of the intra-uterine device: a review of Chinese and the world's experience. *Adv Contraception* 1994; **10**: 71–82.

Xiaozhang L, Shunqiang L. Vasal sterilization in China. *Contraception* 1993; **48**: 255–65.

8

Reproductive Diseases

Vanaja V. Ragavan[1] and Michael Gast[2]

[1]FemmePharma, Inc., Wayne, PA, and [2]Wyeth-Ayerst Research, Philadelphia, PA, USA

BACKGROUND

Several diseases are intimately linked to the reproductive cycle. Together, these diseases account for a significant proportion of the morbidity among young, active women. A common denominator amongst these diseases is their dependence, in one form or another, on steroids secreted during the reproductive cycle. However, it must be pointed out that although most of the diseases described in this chapter are, in general, closely linked to some aspect of reproduction, many others may only bear a peripheral relationship. For instance, the clinical manifestations of endometriosis or premenstrual syndrome are often closely linked to the reproductive cycle but the underlying etiology of endometriosis may not be directly linked to the reproductive cycle. The endometrial tissue and/or its reactions to its foreign environment may play a more critical role.

Because of the dependence on sex hormones for either etiology or clinical manifestation and maintenance, most present therapies for diseases of the reproductive tract are restricted to inhibition or elimination of ovarian function. Such systemic therapies may result in multiple side effects as a significant part of their mechanism of action. For instance, the gonadotropin-releasing hormone (GnRH) analogs are used to treat endometriosis. Complete suppression of ovarian function can result in accelerated symptoms of menopause.

In addition, since present therapies often do not address the underlying disease process, they remain, at best, temporary measures, often non-specific 'shot in the dark' treatment modalities, restricted to a few months at most because of acute and chronic side effects. Since many of the diseases are chronic in nature, the woman is left with a rather difficult choice: bear the side effects of potent therapies or suffer from the disease itself.

In this chapter, we will examine available therapies, and discuss the clinical end points which have led to therapeutic success in the past, bearing in mind that the therapies used are not specific to the disease process. We will also discuss the basis of research which could identify therapies directed at underlying pathophysiologies which are clearly targeted to either cure the disease or alleviate a specific symptom.

Drug Development for Women. Edited by V.V. Ragavan. © 1998 John Wiley & Sons Ltd.

ENDOMETRIOSIS

Prevalence and Epidemiology

Endometriosis is a disorder characterized by clinical symptoms associated with the presence of ectopic endometrial tissue in non-uterine locations in women aged 15–45, although it can affect women at any time after menarche, and has been sporadically reported in postmenopausal women on estrogen replacement. The most common sites of ectopic endometrial implants are the posterior cul-de-sac, ovaries, uterosacral ligaments and bladder or bowel serosa. Less frequently involved sites include the fallopian tubes, vagina and cervix. Rarely, endometriotic disease is found in such distant sites as the lungs, central nervous system, surgical wounds and the kidney.

Endometriosis unquestionably affects millions of women (prevalence data would indicate about 5 million women in the USA alone) of reproductive age and, with the increasing use of hormone replacement therapy in the menopause, may continue to impact the lives of women following menopause—a time previously associated with spontaneous regression of clinical disease. The prevalence of the disease in women of reproductive age has been reported to range from 1% to 7% (Barbieri, 1990), while Moen (1987) and Moen & Muus (1991) have placed the prevalence at 1–18%. Much of this variability results from the fact that most series are based on observations of women undergoing surgery of many sorts with lack of baseline similarities between series. Other sources have placed the prevalence at between 1% and 18% when women are examined during laparoscopy (Moen, 1987; Moen & Muus, 1991). Other studies examining the prevalence in hospital records and other such data have placed the prevalence at between 1% and 15% (Cramer, 1987). Estimates of prevalence, as well as awareness of endometriosis, have risen in the last two decades, when laparoscopic diagnosis has made incidental recognition and confirmation of clinical suspicion of the disease easier and safer.

Endometriosis accounts for a significant proportion of infertility and pelvic and abdominal pain in young women. Recent focus on infertility and other women's health issues has led to an increase in the awareness of endometriosis as a significant clinical issue. With the appearance of support and educational groups concerned with the disease, there will continue to be an increase in reporting of this disease.

Clinical Manifestations

Endometriosis may be asymptomatic, but can also be the cause of serious clinical sequelae including dysmenorrhea and acute or chronic debilitating pain. The clinical symptoms characteristically occur on a monthly basis, typically tied to the menstrual cycle, and are probably induced by bleeding of the endometrial implants into non-uterine tissues.

Endometriosis may also present as asymptomatic infertility of both a mechanical and biochemical origin. Other common presentations include chronic fatigue, chronic pelvic pain, symptoms of ovarian mass and dyspareunia. Genito-urinary dysfunction and intrinsic and extrinsic bowel disease are among the rare and more serious complications of this disease.

On further examination, many patients with unexplained infertility will demonstrate underlying endometriosis (Surrey & Halme, 1989; Olive & Haney, 1986). Many studies have shown a correlation between the presence of endometriosis and infertility (Damewood, 1993). The cause of infertility is not always obvious, but both anatomical distortions due to ectopic endometrial tissue and local inflammatory factors interfering with normal ovarian and tubal function may be causative. Paradoxically, even the mild forms of endometriosis, often characterized by small peritoneal implants, have been associated with an increased incidence of infertility. Local secretion of inflammatory factors by these implants may provide a reason for infertility.

Endometriosis is one of the leading indications for surgery such as abdominal hysterectomy, bilateral oophorectomy and laparoscopy in young women worldwide. In addition, multiple surgical procedures are often conducted for pain and for therapy of adhesive disease in the pelvis leading to pain and infertility. Although controversial, endometriosis is considered by many to be an indication for assisted reproductive technology (ART) when it occurs in the presence of infertility refractory to other treatments.

Etiology

Considerable research effort is presently under way to understand the basic pathophysiology of endometriosis. Early theories attributed the presence of pelvic implants to retrograde menstruation (Sampson, 1927). However, studies have shown that while retrograde menstruation may be virtually universal, in only a small proportion (10–15% of women), implantation of these cells occurs in the pelvis, setting the stage for endometriosis to develop (Halme et al, 1984). This finding would suggest that factors other than retrograde menstruation must play a role in the evolution of this disease. The factors which lead to successful implantation and the development of the disease endometriosis have intrigued researchers. Recent data have implicated a number of factors necessary for successful implantation of endometrial tissue in a foreign environment, namely the peritoneal surface of the pelvic regions. Data suggest that large fragments of functional endometrium are necessary for successful implantation (Sillem et al, 1996) and that subsequent angiogenesis (Oosterlynck et al, 1993) is critical for growth of endometrial implants.

Other often quoted causes are genetic, autoimmune, congenital defects in the reproductive tract, and defective lymphatics. Recent studies are beginning to support evidence for the involvement of modulators of the immune system as playing a critical role in the establishment and growth of the ectopic endometrial tissue. Studies imply that endometriosis may in fact be a systemic disease (Dmowski, Braun & Gebel, 1991; Dmowski et al, 1995). Several studies have shown an abnormal humoral immune system in endometriosis, associated with alterations in the antibody mediated (Gleicher et al, 1987), with cell-mediated immunity also considered to play a role (Steele, Dmowski & Harmer, 1984; Dmowski, Steele & Baker, 1981; Oosterlynk et al, 1991). In fact, prednisolone appears to be helpful in increasing the fecundity of patients with endometriosis-induced infertility (Polak de Fried et al, 1993). Danazol, and not GnRH analogs, appears to affect the autoimmune system as one of its critical modes of action (El-Roeiy et al, 1988).

Therapeutic Approaches: Efficacy and Safety

Presently available therapies for endometriosis serve two purposes: to *alleviate* local and systemic symptoms and/or *treat* associated infertility. Current therapeutic regimens for endometriosis may be pharmacologic or surgical. Non-steroidal anti-inflammatory agents are used in cases of mild pain. More severe cases of pain, dysmenorrhea or dyspareunia are treated with pharmacologic suppression of the reproductive cycle, with GnRH analogs or by altering the steroidal milieu with steroid analogs such as danazol or progestogens. The latter agents will induce a menopausal state and result in complete suppression of the menstrual cycle. Surgical treatment with fulguration and destruction of the implants is usually performed during symptomatic phases of the disease or as part of the infertility work-up.

Danazol

Historically, danazol was the first product approved in the USA as an agent for specific treatment of endometriosis. Danazol is a synthetic steroid, an iso-oxazole derivative of ethisterone. The customary starting dose for moderate to severe disease is 800 mg given in two to four divided doses, although smaller doses as low as 200 mg/day are also given. Doses of 400–600 mg per day are common in Europe, where doses are titrated based on response and severity of disease.

Although the mechanism of action of danazol is not completely understood, it probably works by several modes of action. Danazol may induce anovulation and/or suppress gonadotropin release and thus ovarian steroidogenesis, but this effect may not be critical for its action, since studies have shown that serum levels of estradiol following treatment were not completely suppressed and furthermore this effect may be found at higher doses (Wood et al, 1975). Some studies have implied a direct mechanism of action on endometriotic tissue in addition to alteration of steroid metabolism and binding to steroid receptors. Furthermore, there is evidence that danazol, unlike other products, may in fact have an effect on the autoimmune disorder in endometriosis (El-Roeiy et al, 1988) and may be involved in inducing apoptosis of endometrial tissue.

When danazol is administered, circulating estrogens are modestly but uniformly decreased and there is a profound androgenic effect. This results in decreases in synthesis of liver-associated proteins such as SHBG and CBG. Androgen side effects such as acne, hirsutism, amenorrhea and voice change are common at clinically useful doses, and anabolic changes may include increased muscle mass and weight gain. Therapy may be chronic, but is usually limited to 6–9 months in duration. A vaginal ring containing danazol has been studied in Japan (Igarishi, 1990).

Gonadotropin-releasing Hormone Analogs

Several GnRH analogs are presently marketed for treatment of pain of endometriosis. Although these agents were frequently used off label in the late 1980s, the first product to be formally approved was intranasal nafarelin in 1989. The most common form of GnRH agonist currently used for treatment of endometriosis is depot leuprolide, an intramuscular form of the drug which is administered monthly. An implant containing gosarelin, another GnRH super-agonist, and an extended duration (3 months) depot leuprolide are also used for the disease (Crosignani et al, 1996). Additional agonists as well as generic equivalents are either in use or will soon be available in some markets.

Agonist analogs of GnRH work by overwhelming pituitary receptors for the native decapeptide. Endogenous, low concentration, pulsatile hormone production is replaced by constant high levels of drug. These levels are coupled with a longer lead to down-regulation of pituitary receptors and severe damping of FSH and LH production. Without pulsatile gonadotropin stimulation, ovarian estradiol production stops after the initial period of 'flare' (the first 1–2 weeks of treatment, which result in a stimulation of estradiol, eventually leading to suppression during treatment).

Three to six months of therapy are most commonly provided for infertility, but courses of nine months or longer are sometimes used for treatment of pelvic symptoms in the absence of a desire for pregnancy. Concomitant therapy with small doses of progestin, or progestin plus estrogen, are often used as 'add-back' therapies—replacing steroid synthesis lost following GnRH down-regulation.

Like danazol and oral contraceptives, GnRH agonists produce relief of pain and dysmenorrhea in 80–90% of cases of endometriosis, although therapy may decrease the number of visible implants. It has been well-documented that the number and size of implants does not directly correlate with severity of clinical symptoms. Studies have shown that secretory and glandular elements remain within the implants that have improved visually, regardless of treatment (Nisolle-Pochet et al, 1988). No clear-cut remission rates are available after the first course of treatment, although clinical studies have demonstrated that in some patients, remissions of clinical symptoms often last six months or longer after discontinuation of treatment. Pregnancy is also more likely to occur after a variety of medical or surgical treatments for endometriosis.

The development and testing of GnRH antagonists, a slightly different form of GnRH analog, also promises to provide us with new drugs to enhance the activity of administered gonadotropins. Like the agonists, antagonists are administered during long-term therapy for endometriosis, leiomyomata or ovulation induction for ART for the purpose of pituitary down-regulation. They have the advantage of not causing a 'flare' of gonadotropin activity, however, and are extremely potent. They may in time supplant GnRH agonists as our adjunctive therapies of choice for these disorders. Early generations of GnRH antagonists have been troubled by problems of stability and formulation and also potentially dangerous release of histamine. Newer forms of the neuropeptide promise improvements. Several GnRH antagonists are in late stage clinical trials for endometriosis, breast and prostate cancer therapy, and other indications in both the USA and Europe.

Gestrinone

Gestrinone, a steroid analog similar to danazol, is used in Europe and other countries outside Europe. A large multi-center comparative study conducted under the Gestrinone Italian Study Group compared the efficacy of six month treatment of gestrinone vs. leuprolide acetate and found a similar efficacy rate (Gestrinone Italian Study Group, 1996; Coutinho, 1982). Vaginal gestrinone has also been studied in endometriosis (Coutinho, 1988).

Progestins

Medically induced suppression of the reproductive axis can be accomplished by the use of continuous progestin, or continuous estrogen and progestin. Progestins may also directly inhibit growth of endometriotic tissue by stimulating terminal differentiation and eventually atrophy. Although not approved in the USA, many progestins otherwise used in HRT or contraception have been approved in Europe and other parts of the world specifically for endometriosis, often at high doses. The list is long, but medroxyprogesterone acetate, megestrol acetate and norethindrone acetate are among the most commonly used progestins. Progestin-alone therapy can be associated with menstrual abnormalities, including amenorrhea and significant breakthrough bleeding. Addition of estrogens can stabilize the endometrium, but can also theoretically impair progestin efficacy. Progestin-alone therapy for endometriosis has not achieved regulatory or clinical success in the USA. Continuous or cyclic combined oral contraceptive use remains one of the most popular forms of therapy for endometriosis.

Other Steroidal Agents

Tissue-selective progestins, or antiprogestins, are also being developed for endometriosis. Other tissue-selective progestins, such as mifepristone and Onapristone, are under investigation as anti-endometriosis agents (Van Look & von Hertzen, 1995; Kettel et al, 1996). The mechanism of antiprogestin action is currently unknown but could include the suppression of ovarian steroid synthesis, anti-estrogen-like activities in some reproductive cell targets, or the presence of a weak progestin agonist activity. Tissue-selective estrogens, anti-estrogens, may have potential utility (Kadaba & Simpson, 1990) although they have not been studied extensively in endometriosis therapy (Haber & Behelak, 1987). Raloxifene and other tissue-selective estrogens are presently being studied for this indication. Several types of inhibitors of steroid conversion (e.g. aromatase inhibitors) and non-steroidal estrogen receptor antagonists are also under development as agents for this disease. While they lack the profound side effects profiles of danazol, GnRH antagonists and high-dose progestins, concern about metabolic parameters and hepatic toxicity has clouded early trials with these agents.

Research on Etiology and Therapeutics

As described previously, current therapies for endometriosis do not address a specific underlying disease process. The cost of lost work, surgical interventions, and infertility therapies alone justify the exploration of long-term medical alternatives and attempts at identifying prevention and cure of underlying disease.

Previously, discussions of etiology focused on the possible retrograde flow of menstrual tissue via the fallopian tubes into the pelvic cavity and subsequent growth in patients with endometriosis. However, there is now growing evidence that, while retrograde menstruation may be more common than previously thought, only a small proportion of women succumb to the full-blown syndrome of pain, disseminated peritoneal disease, ovarian masses and intra-abdominal adhesions. Other factors must be critical to the receptivity and growth of ectopic endometrial tissue.

Recent investigations have demonstrated at least two important factors leading to the disease entity: the presence of a receptive environment in the pelvis which allows for growth of endometriotic tissue, and the intrinsic nature of the endo-metrium in women with the disease. Elevated levels of cytokines and other immune-related products are abundant around endometrial tissue and may be found in the peritoneal fluid of women with advanced disease. Other evidence points to altered immune system function, both locally and systemically, in endo-metriosis (Dmowski, 1991). This has been discussed at length in a previous section. In fact, addition of methylprednisolone has been shown to improve in vitro fertilization and implantation in women with endometriosis-induced infertility (Polak de Fried et al, 1993). The exact nature of the alterations are still not well known, but ongoing investigations are focused on identifying endometriosis-related antigens or antibodies for non-invasive diagnosis. Identification of endometriosis-specific antigens can also possibly lead to immune therapy and further our under-standing of this enigmatic disorder.

Cytokines found in high levels locally in endometrial tissue may contribute to the pain of endometriosis and may also contribute to the infertility (Braun et al, 1992). Therapies aimed at cytokine action or reduction of inflammatory processes that lead to adhesion formation are therefore being evaluated in pre-clinical models. Further investigation into these phenomena are needed.

Approach to Efficacy Studies

The two clinical endpoints which have been utilized in endometriosis studies are decrease in implant volume and relief of pain (dysmenorrhea, dyspareunia and/or chronic pelvic pain). Certainly relief of pain is an acceptable clinical end point, but the correlation between decrease in implants and a definitive clinical end point such as relief of pain or enhanced fertility has not been well established.

Because of the numbers of subjects needed to demonstrate efficacy, outcomes related to successful treatment of endometriosis-related infertility have not been well studied. It is not clear whether treatment with GnRH analogs or danazol improves long-term fertility rates. This crucial question needs to be addressed with further research.

Many studies have recently tried to combine several categories of drugs in order to overcome the severe side effects associated with the products. A popular type of administration has attempted to add steroids in low doses to women on GnRH analogs (Edmonds, 1996; Surrey, 1995). A small study evaluated the efficacy of adding tibolone (a novel steroid with estrogenic and progestogenic properties) to gosarelin and demonstrated relief of some of the menopausal symptoms and potential bone protection (Taskin et al, 1997). These regimens have met with some success and are now used extensively in Europe and the USA. In Europe, 25 mg estradiol patches are combined with medroxyprogesterone (5 mg). This regimen has resulted in decreased bone density without loss of efficacy, but long-term follow-up of the disease is still not known.

Although initial clinical efficacy end point studies were based on 6 months of treatment, recent data have shown that 3 months of treatment may be equivalent to the longer, 6 months' treatment (Hornstein et al, 1995). Re-treatment studies have been conducted, again for shorter time periods, such as 3 months (Hornstein et al, 1997).

UTERINE FIBROIDS (LEIOMYOMAS)

Prevalence and Epidemiology

Leiomyomas, benign tumors of the smooth muscle of the uterus, are common and can be present in up to 50% of women in some autopsy series. Prevalence rates increase with age, as do the size and number of these tumors: 10–20% in women aged 30, 40% in women aged 40 and up to 50% in women 50 years of age or more (Buttram & Reiter, 1981). They are thought to be more common amongst Afro-American women.

Clinical Manifestations

Uterine fibroids can occur in almost any part of the sub-serous, interstitial and sub-mucous parts of the myometrium. In addition, fibroids may be found in the cervix, the extra-uterine ligaments (broad and round) and, rarely, as multiple nodular neoplasms thoughout the peritoneal cavity (leiomyomatasis peritonei disseminata). Although the prevalence is quite high, in many women these tumors cause few or modest symptoms and the women are unaware of the presence of the leiomyomas. However, as women get older, these tumors tend to become symptomatic, and can often cause serious gynecological problems in women over the age of 30 (Cramer, 1992).

When fibroids become symptomatic, the clinical manifestation will often depend on the anatomical location of the fibroid. The following symptoms are among the more common:

- Excessive menstrual or intermenstrual bleeding.
- Moderate to severe menstrual pain.
- Infertility or recurrent pregnancy loss.
- Disturbances in urination or defecation.
- Pre-term labor or late pregnancy complications (dystocia, post-partum hemorrhage).
- Pelvic pain.
- Polycythemia.

Symptoms can vary from mild to severe and life-threatening. Clinically significant abnormal uterine bleeding, most often manifest as menorrhagia or as intermenstrual bleeding, can occur. Uterine enlargement can be asymptomatic, but often will cause significant pelvic pain and can lead to other problems such as ureter or bowel obstruction. Dependent on the location, uterine fibroids can be associated with infertility or repeated miscarriages.

Therapeutic Approaches: Efficacy and Safety

Surgical Treatment of Myomas

In spite of their common occurrence, therapeutic approaches to leiomyomas have not changed significantly over the last few decades and surgical correction remains the primary approach to treatment for clinically significant fibroids. Fibroids are the single most common diagnosis cited for hysterectomies, especially around the perimenopause when the bleeding episodes associated with the tumors can be especially troubling. In women still in their reproductive years, a more conservative approach to removing significant myomas but leaving the uterus as intact as possible (myomectomy) is an increasingly popular option.

Myomectomies are usually performed using traditional abdominal surgical approaches, but if myomas are small or singular, other techniques are being used increasingly to minimize surgical procedures. Laparoscopy has been used with mixed success on both clinical and aesthetic grounds. Hysteroscopy is used to remove those myomas found within the uterine cavity and can also be used effectively to treat infertility and bleeding due to space-occupying intra-uterine lesions. Other non-medical approaches used to treat myomas include electro-cautery or laser debulking, but these are utilized by few centers with limited success beyond more traditional therapies.

Non-surgical Treatment of Myomas

Like the treatment of endometriosis, most of the currently available therapies for myomas work by inducing a hypo-estrogenic state. No drugs are currently approved for the treatment of myomas in the USA, although some countries outside the USA have approved the use of GnRH agonists as short-term or pre-surgical therapy. Several studies have shown that the analogs decrease the size of myomas (Friedman et al, 1989, 1991; Adamson, 1992). This decrease in size is considered to be primarily related to the estrogenic suppressive properties of analogs (Friedman, 1990). There can be individual variation in response to fibroids and studies have demonstrated that within a month, the ability of analogs to decrease fibroid size can be determined (Friedman, 1992). Similar to studies on endometriosis patients treated with add-back therapy, such an approval has also been studied in patients with fibroids (Friedman, 1993).

The GnRH agonists are used primarily as a pre-operative adjunct to reduce the size of the tumors prior to surgical procedures, to decrease blood loss during surgery or to reduce serious bleeding manifestations. Use of such therapy has become increasingly widespread, although some controversy still exists as to its ultimate cost-effectiveness. Furthermore, studies have shown that there can be difficulty in removing enucleation of myomas surgically after analog treatment (Deligdisch, Hirschmann & Altchek, 1997). These drugs are not useful for long-term therapy since the tumors invariably grow back when the drug is discontinued.

Progestins and antiprogestins have also been utilized to control bleeding and decrease the size of the fibroids, but these approaches have had mixed success, as has the use of danazol. Trans-vaginal, trans-abdominal and endoscopic injection of myomas with a variety of agents, including chemotherapeutic agents, has not become a popular mode of therapy.

Approach to Efficacy Studies

An approach to efficacy studies must evaluate the important clinical manifestations of a disease. Two clinical end points which have been studied for myomas include decrease in menorrhagia and metrorrhagia and decrease in the anemias often associated with these bleeding disorders. Other than with submucous leiomyomas, which probably bleed because of their close proximity to the mucosa and vulnerability to changes during menstruation, the exact cause of increased bleeding with myomas is not completely understood. Increased uterine vascularity, often marked, is a hallmark of the uterus with large or multiple leiomyomata. Disruption of the normal contractility of the uterus and stretching of uterine blood vessels, leading to fragility, have been implicated. In addition, some myomas can bleed internally, resulting in tumor necrosis and ultimate fibrous tissue formation and calcification. These non-contractile tumors may also contribute to an abnormal anatomy. Whatever the reason, bleeding is a common manifestation of myomas and can be associated with significant morbidity, especially in perimenopausal women.

Many studies outlined above have clearly demonstrated that analogs decrease the size of fibroids. However, because the myomatous condition is a chronic condition in women, a short decrease in size of fibroids has not been previously deemed by the USA FDA to be an adequate clinical end point for approval of this class of drugs for this indication. For this reason, an indisputable clinical end point justifying the risk of treatment was needed.

Improvement in Anemia

One of the hard clinical end points considered acceptable for regulatory approval concerned the improvement of anemia associated with bleeding fibroids and, furthermore, the patients' ability to bank their own blood for surgery. Bleeding is a common manifestation of myomas, with both menorrhagia and/or menometror-rhagia, leading to symptomatic problems. Furthermore, bleeding can be significant enough to cause anemia (Christiansen, 1993). This makes surgery a difficult procedure, especially because it is precisely women with severe bleeding who may indeed require surgical correction for myomas.

Drugs effective in controlling the bleeding associated with the tumors add value to the treatment of myomas. GnRH analogs have been shown to be effective treatment, and in severely anemic women may improve hematocrit and make the women better surgical candidates. Clinical studies evaluating bleeding often use approaches similar to those taken with study of oral contraceptives, viz. daily diaries together with some measure of the amount of bleeding.

In order to evaluate the efficacy of analogs to decrease bleeding and anemia, comparative studies have been conducted with a positive control in women who were placed on iron alone. In one such controlled study (Benagiano et al, 1996), goserelin was found to have significant advantages when given with iron, compared to iron therapy given alone.

Decrease in Bleeding and Blood Loss During Surgery

Evaluation of decrease in bleeding during surgery is considerably more difficult because of the subjective nature of the study. In some studies, analogs have been shown to decrease bleeding during surgery (Stovall, 1993; Lumdsen et al, 1994; Miller & Frank, 1992). Evaluation of changes in total uterine volume and individual myoma size are important secondary end points in registration studies in Europe, although in the USA, the FDA has requested different clinical end points for approval.

Known Etiology and Research on Etiology and Therapeutics

Uterine fibroids, in large measure, arise from a monoclonal, smooth muscle cell line, almost always well differentiated and distinctly encapsulated. Even when these tumors grow to very large sizes, their growth pattern and mitotic characteristics maintain a benign status, implying a non-carcinogenic, non-mitotic factor resulting in their growth (Anderson & Barbieri, 1995). Hypotheses relating to the non-mitotic growth of leiomyomas revolve around both a retention of sensitivity to estrogen, or an abnormal responsiveness to estrogen-stimulated growth factors and/or disturbed auto-control of cellular growth and tissue architecture.

Leiomyoma cells have been shown to have a greater capacity to bind estrogen than normal myomas and, in addition, appear to have a greater binding capacity for estrogen throughout the menstrual cycle compared to normal tissue, especially in the follicular phase (Rein et al, 1990a). This continuous cyclic responsivity could account for continuous growth. Further evidence of estrogen responsiveness is demonstrated by the rapid shrinking of these tumors during GnRH therapy, when estrogen is completely suppressed, and their rapid re-growth on stopping this therapy. Furthermore, these tumors often shrink during the menopause. Progesterone receptors (both A and B) have also been demonstrated to be over-expressed in these tissues (Brandon, Bethers & Strawn, 1993).

Greater responsiveness to estrogen could result in local expression of higher levels of estrogen gene expression factors, such as growth factors, resulting in further growth of leiomyomas. Studies have shown that leiomyomatous tissue secretes more IGF-I and IGF-II than normal tissue in in vitro systems (Rein et al, 1990b). IGF-I receptors are also expressed in leiomyomas, implicating an autocrine effect and involvement in local responsiveness to growth factors. Other growth factors whose expression, responsiveness and receptors levels have been found in leiomyomatous tissues include epithelial growth factor (EGF; Yeh, Rein & Nowak, 1991) and parathyroid hormone-related peptide (PTH-RP; Weir et al, 1994). Their roles in leiomyoma growth are not as well established as IGF-I.

Interestingly, myomas can also be endocrine glands in their own right and have been known to secrete hormones such as erythropoietin, leading to polycythemia in rare cases. Recent studies have led to a growing understanding of the cellular and genetic mechanisms and the endocrinology of these tumors.

Although research into the factors controlling growth of fibroid tumors is continuing in some centers, no specific therapeutic approaches are clearly in sight and must await further understanding of the local and systemic factors contributing to their growth and to an understanding of the genetic basis of myomas, including identifying susceptible genes.

INFERTILITY

Prevalence and Epidemiology

Infertility is a major public health issue in developed nations and is compounded by voluntary delay in pregnancy and the high incidence of sexually transmitted diseases (STDs). When defined as the inability to conceive after 12 months of intercourse without contraception, approximately 2.4 million couples (about 10%) in the USA are considered infertile. The overall incidence of infertility has remained relatively unchanged over the last three decades. Other figures have quoted higher incidence rates: 15–20% of women or 6–8 million women (Medical and Healthcare Marketplace, 1993). About 35% of infertility has been attributed to the male, another 35% to the female and 30% to both.

Clinical Manifestations

Involuntary infertility is generally defined as greater than 18 months of attempts at pregnancy without success. This definition must be modified, however, to fit the social and medical situation of the couple. Older couples, for example, may be under significantly greater time pressure to conceive, and work-up for causes and treatment of infertility would typically be instituted earlier rather than later. Couples suspected or known to have specific problems should be evaluated before subjecting them to extended and fruitless attempts at conception.

General factors which impact the ability to conceive are age and frequency of sexual relations (Gast, 1994; Gindoff & Jewelewicz, 1986). The concept of half-time ($t^{1/2}$) for pregnancy is used to indicate the duration of time necessary for 50% of a given population of couples to conceive. An unselected population of couples who are 25 years of age will have a $t^{1/2}$ of 5.5 months to conception. For each additional 5 years of maternal age, the mean duration to pregnancy will approximately double. There is a smaller but nonetheless significant effect of advancing maternal age. Thus, the incidence of infertility increases with advancing age. About 1 in 7 couples are infertile in the 30–34 age range. That number will increase to 1 in 5 at age 35–39 and to over 1 in 4 beyond age 40.

Frequency of sexual relations likewise can have a profound effect on the conception process. Couples having sexual relations once weekly or less will have a much lower conception rate than those having relations twice weekly. Couples engaging in sexual intercourse 3–4 times weekly (or more) will maximize the rate at which pregnancies occur. It is one of many infertility-related myths that having sexual relations every other day during the expected week of ovulation will optimize the conception process. This is only true in cases where frequency of sexual relations is inadequate. It can lead to the potentially disastrous and dysfunctional sexual pattern of planning sex for the business-like purpose of conception, or the clustering of intercourse to the peri-ovulatory period, while ignoring it during the remainder of the month.

Even with a comprehensive and carefully performed infertility evaluation, 10% of infertile couples will have no apparent explanation for their inability to conceive. Similarly, at least 10–25% of couples with apparently satisfactory correction of detected infertility factors will not achieve pregnancy within 1 year of appropriate therapeutic intervention.

Infertility can be treated by either augmenting in vivo fertilization or by in vitro fertilization (IVF) or other assisted reproductive technologies (ARTs) with the underlying pathology dictating the appropriate action. The absence of anatomical defects allows for in vivo fertilization. Treatment of the underlying disease, such as anovulation or endometriosis, can often lead to pregnancy, but for a certain percentage of women, further procedures such as IVF would be needed. IVF remains the last resort for many couples who are unable to conceive using more conservative techniques, but the success rate in IVF specifically is not high per se; only 25–40% of women will become pregnant with each attempt. Furthermore, the actual 'take-home-baby-rate' is often only 10–20% under optimal conditions.

Known Etiology

Major causes of infertility are as follows:

- Cervical/immunologic factors.
- Ovulatory factors, such as:
    (a) Polycystic ovarian disease syndrome and other anovulatory disorders.
    (b) Prolactin-secreting tumors.
- Tubal damage due to STD, IUD, previous ectopic pregnancies, surgery.
- Endometriosis.

- Endometrial factors such as:
  - (a) Inadequate luteal phase.
  - (b) Endometrial synechiae or damage.
  - (c) Uterine leiomyomas.
- Male factor infertility.
- Unexplained infertility.

Cervical Factors

The cervix is one of the most complex and multifunctional organs in the human body. Mucus produced by the endocervical glands serves three major purposes: (a) filtering and acquisition of sperm from the seminal pool in the posterior vaginal fornix; (b) retention of sperm in the cervical crypts for their 'timed-release' into the reproductive tract throughout the peri-ovulatory period; and (c) a 'gatekeeper' function—excluding sperm and other non-functional vaginal detritus from the upper reproductive tract during those times of the cycle when it is unlikely or biologically unfavorable for pregnancy to occur. Cervical mucus production is under hormonal control and thus is coordinated with simultaneous events occurring in the endometrium, ovary and fallopian tubes. These events are carefully and deliberately interlocked to ensure that pregnancy is not a random event. Estrogen is the stimulus for the cervical glands to produce mucus. As ovulation nears and levels of estrogen increase rapidly, cervical mucus changes from a thick, scant, and hostile environment to sperm, to a thin, copious, acellular matrix that is a permissive milieu for sperm survival. Rapidly following ovulation, as progesterone production is rising, the cervical mucus returns to its thick, exclusionary state. If pregnancy occurs, the mucus will stay thick and remain as a bacteriostatic 'plug' in the cervix, eventually to be released at the onset of labor ('bloody show').

Failure of the cervix to respond to estrogen, drug therapies (such as clomiphene) or surgical damage to the cervix or its glands are examples of causes of cervical factor infertility.

Ovulatory Factors

Failure of ovulation and proper support of the endometrium and/or early pregnancy are the most common cause of female infertility. Fortuitously, ovulatory disruption is also one of the easiest causes to treat. Anovulation, inadequate luteal phase progesterone production, and possibly inadequate early pregnancy progesterone production are general categories of disorders that make up the broad class 'ovulatory failure'.

Polycystic ovarian syndrome (PCOS) and chronic anovulation are the most common forms of ovulatory failure. Elevation of serum androgens, gonadotropin imbalance (high levels of LH in the blood), and sonographic evidence of ovarian enlargement with multiple mid-size follicles are the most reliable diagnostic findings for PCOS. Chronic (idiopathic) anovulation is a diagnosis of exclusion.

Metabolic disorders can disrupt normal ovulation. Common metabolic defects leading to anovulation include thyroid dysfunction and hyperprolactinemia. Poorly controlled diabetes, collagen vascular and renal diseases can also cause ovulatory defects, but are usually clinically evident. Any severe debilitating systemic condition will disrupt normal ovulatory function. Metabolic dysfunction should be corrected with appropriate specific medications, e.g. bromocriptine, thyroid replacement, prior to the use of ovulation induction agents.

Luteal phase defect (LPD), a poorly understood phenomenon, may result in inadequately prepared endometrium for implantation. LPD is related to inadequate corpus luteum function after ovulation has occurred. LPD may be diagnosed by mid-luteal progesterone concentration (MLP), or endometrial biopsy (EB).

Tubal, Uterine and Peritoneal Factors

Disorders of reproductive tract anomalies of the female, either acquired or congenital, account for the failure of conception in about 1 in 7 infertile couples. Approximately 20% of all infertility problems are contributed to by a female pelvic factor.

Risk factors for pelvic problems include a history of prior abdominal or pelvic surgery, prior dilatation and curettage (D&C), prior pregnancy terminations, painful periods (dysmenorrhea) or painful intercourse (dyspareunia), prior IUD use, diethylstilbestrol exposure prior to birth, and history of prior pelvic infections or pelvic inflammatory disease. Patients with prior tubal pregnancies, a known history of endometriosis or certain gastro-intestinal problems are also at risk for pelvic problems. Problems involving the uterus that can lead to infertility as well as difficulties maintaining a pregnancy include congenital uterine anomalies, uterine fibroids and prior uterine surgery.

Male Factors in Infertility

Unlike the many treatments available for female-related infertility, management options for male factors is rudimentary at best. Male factor infertility includes sperm and seminal fluid factors. Sperm factors could be related to sperm count and/or sperm motility. Oligospermia (very low sperm count) and azospermia (absence of sperm) may be seen in the presence of congenital anomalies of the male reproductive tract, anatomic abnormalities (such as varicocele, vasectomy, or inadvertent interruption of the vas deferens during abdominal surgery), or can be found in the presence of metabolic defects and a variety of other causes. Other male factors which could lead to low sperm count and motility include certain drugs and chemical and heat exposure. The etiology of the majority of oligo-spermia and hypomotility in sub-fertile males remains obscure.

Seminal volumes can affect male infertility. Low seminal volume results in inadequate buffering capacity for sperm against the hostile low pH of the vaginal environment. Large seminal volumes lead to decreased sperm concentrations in the face of adequate numbers of total motile sperm per ejaculate.

Unexplained Infertility

Even with a comprehensive and carefully performed infertility evaluation, 10% of infertile couples have no apparent explanation for their inability to conceive. Similarly, at least 10–25% of couples with apparently satisfactory correction of detected infertility factors will not achieve pregnancy within 1 year of appropriate therapeutic intervention.

Therapeutic Approaches: Efficacy and Safety

Cervical Factors

If poor mucus persists throughout the peri-ovulatory period in at least two consecutive cycles, or if low sperm numbers or motility are observed during post-coital testing in the presence of adequate mucus and an adequate semen analysis, then intra-uterine insemination is the therapeutic modality of choice. Intra-uterine insemination has also been utilized as an empiric therapy in the presence of sperm antibodies in the male or female. Intra-uterine insemination or cervical capping may be of value in cases of male delivery disorders and, rarely, where loss of sperm motility is due to vaginal pH or other vaginal factors. Hormonal and other pharmacologic therapies (e.g. estrogen) have shown little or no additional thera-peutic benefit in controlled clinical trials of cervical factor infertility, but do produce higher pregnancy rates in cases of unexplained infertility.

Ovulatory Factors

The most common cause of female infertility is the failure to ovulate. Ovulation failure is also frequently seen in the general female population, where it is most appropriately managed with intermittent progestin interruption. The goal of the ovulation work-up is to carefully establish the diagnosis of anovulation, oligo-ovulation, or luteal phase defect. Metabolic causes, when present, must be identified and corrected. Finally, the physician should initiate an appropriate regimen of therapy to correct the problem.

Ovulation induction therapy should be reserved for situations in which the patient has an immediate desire for pregnancy. The medications available for ovulation induction fall into several categories. Clomiphene citrate (CC) and human menopausal gonadotropin (hMG) target the hypothalamic–pituitary–ovarian axis, creating controlled ovarian hyperstimulation. Dexamethasone, bromergocryptine and GnRH agonists are adjunctive agents utilized for a limited set of clinical conditions which perturb the normal female reproductive axis and ovary, respectively. Human chorionic gonadotropin (hCG) is an analog of luteinizing hormone (LH) which permits ovum release from mature follicles. Luteal phase progesterone supplementation is occasionally used in patients when therapy with the ovulation induction agents alone produces ovulation (as measured by ultrasound) but not adequate mid-luteal phase progesterone levels, or when treatment with clomiphene creates an 'out of phase' endometrium.

CC, given orally in doses of 50–200 mg/day for 5–7 days, and hMG are the cornerstones of such treatment. CC is a compound with both estrogenic and anti-estrogenic actions which belongs to the triphenylethylene class of non-steroid agents. The ultimate result of CC action is a temporary but marked increase in serum levels of FSH and LH. This hypergonadotropic milieu leads to increased follicular development by the ovary. The two most important side effects of CC therapy are ovarian hyperstimulation and multiple gestation. Both of these complications are far less frequent and far less severe than during therapy with menopausal gonadotropins. The incidence of ovarian hyperstimulation with CC is 5–10%. This hyperstimulation generally results from the failure of ovulation of individual ovarian follicles, producing predominantly cystic enlargement of the ovary. Multiple gestation also occurs in 4–8% of pregnancies conceived on CC. Multiple gestation following CC therapy almost always involves twin pregnancies. The incidence of triplets is no higher than in the general population and multiple births involving four or more babies are virtually unknown.

Other complications following CC therapy include hot flushes, vaginal dryness, deterioration of cervical mucus and development of luteal phase inadequacy. This latter complication may be treated with progesterone, but more commonly the patient is escalated to gonadotropin therapy. Retinal artery spasm is a serious and extremely rarely reported complication of therapy with this medication.

hMG, a defined mixture of LH and FSH derived from extraction of human menopausal urine, is the second-line therapy for induction of ovulation only in CC-resistant patients and is also used extensively in conjunction with assisted repro-ductive technologies and for treatment of unexplained infertility. Unlike CC, which requires an intact hypothalamic–pituitary–ovarian axis, hMG works directly on the ovary. The complications of hMG therapy are similar to those of CC. The incidence of ovarian hyperstimulation during hMG therapy is around 20%. About 10% of the hyperstimulation following hMG administration involves severe ovarian and systemic changes. Multiple gestation is also more frequent in patients undergoing hMG therapy. Up to 20% of pregnancies following hMG therapy are multiple gestations.

The half-life of the drug is relatively short and it is customarily delivered on a daily basis. Ovarian stimulation utilizing hMG is customarily initiated on the 2nd, 3rd or 4th day of the menstrual cycle. During an hMG cycle, appropriate monitoring, e.g. serum estradiol and ovarian ultrasound, is always indicated. These evaluations are generally performed at least every 2–3 days to monitor growth of the follicle. When the dominant follicles have reached 16–20 mm in size and estradiol is within the appropriate ovulatory range (500–1500 pg/ml), 10 000 units of hCG will be administered to permit the release of the ovum by mimicking the LH surge of the normal menstrual cycle. Recent approval of highly purified urinary follicle stimulating hormone (FSH) could result in replacement of hMG with FSH in many cases of ovulation induction and ART. Recombinant forms of LH and FSH and hCG are in late-phase trials worldwide.

Bromergocriptine is used in patients in whom hyperprolactinemia has been documented. Therapy with modest doses of bromocriptine (e.g. 2.5 mg orally, twice daily) will usually suffice to produce normoprolactinemia and the onset of normal ovulatory menstrual function generally follows normoprolactinemia by 4–8 weeks. In some women, normoprolactinemia alone will not produce ovulatory menses and adjunctive therapy with clomiphene (CC) should be initiated. Some authors advocate the empiric use of bromocriptine in normo-prolactinemic women who are not responding to standard CC therapy.

Hoffman & Lobo (1985) demonstrated that there is a group of women with hyperandrogenemia secondary to adrenal hyperfunction in whom CC alone does not produce effective ovulation. These women, who also have elevated levels of the weak adrenal androgen dehydroepiandrosterone sulfate (DHEA-S), respond well when small doses of corticosteroids, such as prednisone or dexamethasone, are administered primarily or in conjunction with CC.

In the last few years, GnRH agonists have become a popular adjunct to the use of hMG therapy. GnRH agonists for ovulation induction may be administered as a single daily 500–1000 μg subcutaneous injection (leuprolide) or as twice daily nasal sprays of 200 μg (nafarelin). In assisted reproductive technology (ART) patients there is a 10–20% incidence of premature LH surges and early luteinization of the developing follicles during hMG stimulation. GnRH agonist is often administered, beginning in the luteal phase of the cycle preceding hMG, to suppress endogenous gonadotropin secretion—thus preventing the premature ovulation event. Some ART programs use GnRH agonist as a 'flare' regimen. If used in the early follicular phase of the stimulation cycle, GnRH agonist has a stimulatory effect on gonadotropin secretion. This burst of LH and FSH provides for early stimulation of increased numbers of developing follicles which will subsequently be maintained by hMG.

Polycystic ovarian syndrome patients who are poorly responsive to hMG (e.g. excessive follicle formation, repeated hyperstimulation) may benefit from extended suppression of the hypothalamic–pituitary axis. Such suppression begins in the luteal phase of the preceding cycle and continues until after ovulation in the hMG treatment cycle. Once endogenous LH and FSH secretion is suppressed, hMG therapy may produce more normal ovarian responses.

Tubal/Endometrial/Peritoneal Factors

Treatment of tubal and peritoneal disease can be medical, surgical, or a combination of both. Certain pelvic abnormalities can be treated with medical therapy alone. A classic example of medical therapy of a pelvic factor is the treatment of certain (usually advanced) stages of endometriosis that may be treated by GnRH agonists, oral contraceptives, or androgens such as danazol—although in this group of women the abnormalities are more commonly treated surgically. The major drawback to medical therapy is the extended length of time (often 6–9 months) required for its completion.

Surgical therapy, including laparotomy, endoscopic laser vaporization, microsurgical tubal revision, and operative laparoscopy are used as primary therapy for pelvic adhesions and the more modest stages of endometriosis. Hysteroscopy and laparoscopy are the mainstays of infertility surgery and require considerable skill, since they are performed through a 'scope. Although endoscopic techniques have advanced dramatically over the past decade, at this time some surgical procedures are still best performed through a larger abdominal incision. Two excellent examples of this include reversal of a tubal ligation and cases of fibroid removal in which the fibroid involves a large portion of the uterine wall.

Combined medical and surgical therapy is becoming more popular for the management of potentially difficult surgical problems. GnRH agonist may be used as a pre- or post-operative tool in cases of severe (stage III or IV) endometriosis, and as a surgical adjunct prior to myomectomy.

Assisted Reproductive Technologies (ART)

The process of in vitro fertilization (IVF) was initially developed as a treatment for women with tubal infertility. Since the birth of Louise Brown in 1978, IVF has evolved to become a potential therapy for most infertility disorders. The development of techniques such as gamete intra-fallopian transfer (GIFT), zygote intra-fallopian transfer (ZIFT), and tubal embryo transfer (TET) have not only served to extend the usefulness of these assisted reproductive technologies (ART) to patients with at least one normal fallopian tube, but have also resulted in higher pregnancy rates in selected populations. The advent of micro-manipulation procedures, e.g. intra-cytoplasmic sperm injection (ICSI) has enabled us to treat severe male factor infertility that previously could only be treated by the use of donor sperm. The use of oocytes from appropriate donors has allowed us to effectively impregnate surgically castrate women, as well as patients near menopause or those with premature ovarian failure.

Male factor infertility. Male factor infertility is a relatively common problem and can be very difficult to treat, unlike the many options available for female infertility. The etiology of the majority of oligospermia and hypomotility in subfertile males remains obscure. Treatment of these conditions with medications, such as CC, hCG or testosterone, is generally unrewarding. Varicocele repair, as an effective technique for raising low sperm counts or increasing pregnancy rates, is controversial. The validity of intra-uterine insemination for the treatment of disorders of sperm count or motility is also unproved.

Medical therapy for the treatment of idiopathic male infertility has been uniformly disappointing. Anti-estrogens (CC, tamoxifen) are the most widely studied, and probably one of the most controversial treatments used (WHO, 1992; Abel et al, 1982; Sorbie & Perez-Marrero, 1984). While some studies have suggested an improvement in semen parameters following treatment with CC, no controlled study has shown an increase in pregnancy rates. hCG, hMG, or a combination of these agents have also been used to treat patients with male factor infertility. In a number of studies no consistent improvement in semen parameters or conception rates has been demonstrated with this therapy.

Artificial insemination using husband or partner's sperm (AIH) involves the delivery of sperm into the female reproductive tract by some means other than intercourse. These procedures require careful prediction of ovulation and insemination at the appropriate time in the cycle. Insemination can be accomplished using the partner's sperm or donor sperm by intra-uterine insemination (IUI; the injection of sperm directly into the uterine cavity), cervical cap insemination, or intra-cervical insemination.

Because semen contains a high concentration of prostaglandins, which could cause significant uterine cramping if injected into the uterus, semen must be washed prior to IUI. This method is designed to place motile sperm closer to the fallopian tube, where fertilization eventually occurs. Cervical cap insemination involves pouring the sperm and semen into a cap which is placed over the cervix much like a diaphragm, and allowed to stay in place for 4–6 hours before it is removed. This method allows motile sperm to swim up through the cervical canal and into the uterine cavity. Cap insemination is often used for donor insemination. Intra-cervical insemination involves the injection of semen into the cervical canal. The latter method tends to be less effective. Disorders of both high and low seminal volume are amenable to correction by artificial insemination. Because the highest concentrations of sperm are found in the first few drops of ejaculate, split collection of the semen from the 'high volume' male will yield a first fraction of high sperm concentration and low volume. This fraction may be used without 'washing' for cervical capping.

Assisted reproductive technologies (ART) have also been used to treat male infertility. In general, the rates of fertilization are lower in patients with severe sperm defects. However, once fertilization occurs, the pregnancy rates for male factor couples is roughly the same as that for couples with other diagnoses. Patients with male factor infertility should probably undergo a procedure in which fertilization can be documented, such as IVF, ZIFT or TET, as opposed to GIFT, in which fertilization cannot be confirmed unless pregnancy occurs. Micro-manipulation, used in conjunction with ART, can be a useful procedure in those patients with severe male factor infertility or in cases of unexplained fertilization failure or reduced rates of fertilization in IVF.

Another technique to produce pregnancy when the male is azoospermic, severely oligospermic, or carries an hereditary disease, is artificial insemination using donor sperm (therapeutic donor insemination, TDI). The decision to use donor sperm in place of husband or partner's sperm is often a difficult one and careful counseling should be part of the preparation for the procedure. Proper donor selection and very careful screening of semen samples for infectious diseases are critical.

Varicocele repair.   The incidence of a varicocele in healthy, fertile males is 10–15%. Recent studies suggest that varicoceles that can be felt on a physical examination probably do contribute to male infertility. Therefore, varicocele repair should be considered in a patient with a palpable varicocele *and* abnormal values from a semen analysis.

Unexplained infertility.   The first option offered to the couple who have been through the infertility work-up without identifying a cause for their inability to conceive, or who have corrected any abnormal findings for a period of at least 6 months, should be the discontinuation of the infertility work-up/therapy process. Long-term studies suggest that 50% of couples with unexplained infertility will conceive over a subsequent 5 year period in the absence of any therapeutic intervention. Combined with the active pursuit of adoption, this paints a happy picture for the couple with unexplained infertility who have been unsuccessful in their attempts at pregnancy and who have grown tired of the infertility process, or lack the financial ability to pursue the uncertain and often expensive options of empiric therapy.

Couples with unexplained infertility will sometimes benefit from the empiric use of superovulation and intra-uterine insemination (IUI). Therapy with menopausal gonadotropins and IUI will produce a 20% excess pregnancy rate in women undergoing stimulation for 3–6 cycles. As with all gonadotropin therapy, extensive monitoring of sonographic and hormonal parameters of the cycle is required.

Empiric use of ART for treatment of unexplained infertility has enjoyed tre-mendous popularity in the last decade. In vitro fertilization and embryo transfer (IVF-ET), GIFT and a wide variety of variations on the theme of ovum retrieval and anatomic replacement of gametes or embryos are an expensive—albeit effective—way to increase pregnancy rates in couples who have undergone the complete infertility work-up. Live birth rates of 15–25% per attempted ART cycle or 30–50% cumulatively (for couples who do three or more cycles) are common in good ART programs. Like empiric hormonal therapy, ART is an expensive undertaking, and currently is seldom covered under standard insurance plans.

Research on Etiology and Therapeutics

Many variables are encountered in IVF, including the number and maturity of oocytes, variability in incubation, underlying disorders, and post-implantation factors. In addition, with underlying disorders such as endometriosis or PCO, there are often local or hormonal factors which influence poor results. Age and sperm counts and quality also add their share of uncertainties.

Understanding local and systemic factors which influence oocyte development and implantation would greatly add to improvements in IVF rates. For instance, are local growth factors important in oocyte development, fertilization and growth of the embryo? How much progesterone is needed to support early pregnancy? What local endometrial factors influence successful implantation?

Approach to Efficacy Studies

Few drugs have sought indications for ART status alone, either in the USA or Europe. In general, pregnancy and delivery rates which are equivalent to or exceed those existing therapies are used as primary endpoints. Hormonal, sonographic and histologic end points can also be used as secondary indices of efficacy. Safety parameters for new agents for ART are, as always, carefully monitored. Reasonable numbers of pregnancies with a significant proportion of the offspring followed post partum to monitor for congenital anomalies or developmental difficulties are required.

Evaluation of ART outcomes is made more challenging because of the many etiologies of infertility leading to ART. Widely differing success rates at different ART centers, as well as those with different ART techniques (e.g. frozen embryo transfers, GIFT, ICSI) make use of control groups and appropriately powered statistical evaluation critical to decision making on ART agents.

HYPERANDROGENIC SYNDROMES AND POLYCYSTIC OVARIAN DISEASE

Prevalence and Clinical Manifestations

The vast majority of reproductive age women, about 85%, with hyperandrogenism/hirsutism will be found to have polycystic ovarian disease (PCO) or hyperthecosis (Maroulis, 1981; Hatch et al, 1981). PCO is a term used for a mixed bag of disorders, often manifested by chronic anovulatory states, hirsutism, insulin resistance, hyperandrogenism and obesity. These manifestations can be variable, with about 40–60% of patients demonstrating obesity, 50–90% of women with PCO can be oligomenorrheic and up to 55–75% can be infertile.

A common finding in patients with PCO is an elevated circulating serum concentration of LH, with low to normal FSH levels. PCO patients ovulate irregularly, resulting in the majority of women manifesting a chronic hyper-estrogenic state. The chronically elevated estradiol levels can result in endometrial hyperplasia syndromes, insulin resistance and infertility.

Although PCO accounts for a majority of complaints of hirsutism, excessive growth of 'sexual' hair in women is a common, though obviously non-fatal, problem. Hirsutism can also occur in the absence of hyperandrogenism. In these instances, a genetically predisposed sensitivity to normal circulating androgen levels probably accounts for the increase in hair growth or acne. Because hirsutism per se is considered to be primarily cosmetic, if this is the sole manifestation of PCO patients or in patients with idiopathic hirsutism, management and drug development for hirsutism, with rare exceptions such as patients with HAIR-AN (hirsutism–androgenism–insulin resistance–acanthosus nigricans) syndrome, has been a low priority in the past.

Acne is an inflammatory disease of the pilo-sebaceous duct and is characterized by the presence of inflamed lesions and blocked ducts, leading to infections and scarring. Acne is common in adolescence and usually resolves by the mid-20s. However, in adult states of hyperandrogenism, acne can appear de novo later in life. Chronic androgenic stimulation can result in hirsutism and acne, but almost never a virilized state in PCO syndrome. There is no direct correlation between circulating androgen levels and the degree of hirsutism, which may reflect differences in response by the primary androgen responsive end organ in women, namely the hair follicle (Lobo, Goebelsmann & Horton, 1983).

Although PCO tends to be the dominant cause of hyperandrogenism in young women, other causes of hyperandrogenism, such as androgen-secreting ovarian tumors or Cushing's syndrome, must be ruled out in women who complain of hirsutism or have other signs of androgen excess. Actual virilization, with clitoromegaly, temporal balding and other signs, signifies a serious underlying pathology and must be managed as such with proper diagnosis and treatment.

Known Etiology

The etiology of PCO is not known. The ovaries in this disorder are found to have multiple cysts, with hyperthecosis. The hyperthecosis results in hyperandrogenism. In addition to hyperandrogenism, abnormally high LH levels are found in PCO patients. The LH:FSH ratio is often in excess of 3:1. Anovulation leads to high unopposed estrogen levels, and unopposed estradiol (E2) levels are thought to act on the pituitary by increasing its sensitivity to luteinizing hormone-releasing hormone (LHRH) (Lobo et al, 1981) disrupting normal pulsatile LHRH release, and resulting in increased LH. In addition to its effect on LHRH neurons, estrogen, in the absence of progesterone, is also thought to alter dopaminergic and opiatergic influences on the hypothalamic LHRH centers (Quigley, Rakoff & Yen, 1989; Berga & Yen, 1989). Clomiphene, with its partial estrogen agonist activity, can induce a gonadotropin surge, with resultant ovulation in the PCO patient (Yen, Vela & Ryan, 1982) and progesterone administration can also reset an abnormal pulsatile center. FSH levels tend to be normal and this is believed to be due to the normal amounts of follicular inhibin found in PCO patients (Buckler et al, 1988).

PCO syndrome is characterized by a striking hyperinsulinemia which could partly contribute to the hyperandrogenism. Hyperinsulinemia and possible increases in IGF-I may also play a role in the increased pituitary sensitivity to LHRH (Adashi, Hsueh & Yen, 1981). Some studies have shown that reduction in insulin levels can decrease testosterone levels (Nestler et al, 1989). An increase in many androgenic hormones has been observed in PCO and the ovary is characterized by multiple cysts and thecal cell proliferation. Testosterone and its active metabolites and 17-keto steroids (DHEA, etc.) can all be elevated. Some of these androgens are converted peripherally to estradiol and estrone and contribute to the hyperestrogenic state. In addition, there could be an increase in circulating free estrogens, especially with decreases in SHBG found in a hyperandrogenic state (DeVane et al, 1975).

Therapeutic Approaches: Efficacy and Safety

Since the types of underlying disorders leading to hyperandrogenism can be quite diverse, and the etiology of PCO is not completely understood, therapeutic approaches in treating these disorders have focused on correcting symptoms. In general, the symptoms that are bothersome to patients are hirsutism/acne, amenorrhea or irregular bleeding, and infertility. General approaches to treatment of infertility are discussed above, but specific approaches to PCO patients are described in this section. Approaches to treating hirsutism/acne and irregular bleeding are described in this section. In addition, some of these women present with hyperprolactinemia and endometrial hyperplasia due to chronic unopposed estrogenization. The former can often be corrected with reduction in unopposed estrogenization by using oral contraceptives or by a short course in dopaminergic agonists such as bromocriptine. The latter is usually cleared by the administration of progestins to normalize and shed the endometrium, although persistent hyperplasia could be treated with more aggressive therapy. In addition, insulin resistance will correct with weight loss, treatment of hyperandrogenism or insulin therapy.

Infertility is a major concern of PCO patients. Because PCO patients in general are anovulatory, induction of ovulation is a necessary precursor to correction of infertility. CC can be helpful because it acts at the hypothalamus as a partial estrogen antagonist, re-establishing normal gonadotropin patterns and, in many patients, may initiate a normal cycle with ovulation. CC has been combined with dexamethasone (which induces suppression of adrenal androgens) for induction of ovulation in those subjects who have high adrenal androgen levels.

In those patients who fail with CC, a more traditional approach to assisted reproduction can result in a higher success rate. Pregnancy rates of 58–72% have been noted with the use of human menopausal gonadotropins (hMG) to induce ovum maturation (Tsapoulis, Zoulas & Comminos, 1978; Diamond & Wentz, 1979) and hCG to induce oocyte release. Use of FSH-rich or purified FSH preparations also contribute to successful pregnancy, since PCO patients have a low FSH:LH ratio. LHRH given in pulsatile fashion (Molloy, Hancock & Glass, 1985; Kelley & Jewelewicz, 1990), and LHRH analogs have also been used to promote ovulation in groups of PCO patients. The analogs can suppress endogenous cycles (Filicori et al, 1989). Following withdrawal of LHRH analogs, the patients have been shown to be either able to ovulate on their own or to be more responsive to CC.

Drug therapy for hirsutism has focused upon the use of oral contraceptives, the diuretic/anti-hypertensive spironolactone and, rarely, the corticosteroid preparations dexamethasone or prednisone. Anti-androgens have been studied for use in hirsutism. Spironolactone is an aldosterone antagonist with a structure similar to testosterone. It works through several mechanisms, including inhibiting endogenous androgen biosynthesis, binding to androgen receptors and acting as an anti-androgen. Used in proper doses, it is effective in up to 90% of subjects. Flutamide is a potent, non-steroidal anti-androgen without progestational activity. Several studies have shown that this agent may be helpful in treatment of hirsutism, in doses as low as 250 mg/day (Muderris et al, 1997; Cusan et al, 1994; Motta et al, 1991).

Cyproterone acetate (CPA), a progestogen with weak anti-androgen activity, acts as a competitive inhibitor of dihydrotestosterone, binding to its receptors, and reduces 5α-reductase activity in the skin. It also acts as an anti-gonadotropin and suppresses LH and subsequently ovarian androgen secretion. This product is approved in Europe, and is marketed alone, or in combination with ethinyl estradiol as an oral contraceptive, but is not available in this country. Studies attest to the efficacy of CPA-containing oral contraceptive with or without GnRH analogs, in treating androgenism associated with PCO (Acien et al, 1997). Finasteride, a potent 5α-reductase, has been studied for up to 1 year of treatment recently, noting significant reduction in hirsutism with no serious side effects (Moghetti et al, 1994; Castello et al, 1996; Wong et al, 1995; Ciotta et al, 1995). Ketoconazole has also been studied and found to be effective (Gokmen et al, 1996).

Another interesting concept in hirsutism unresponsive to standard therapies (Acien et al, 1997) is suppression of endogenous LH and FSH with a long-acting LHRH agonist, followed by replacement of estrogen and progestogen with the administration of oral contraceptives (Chang et al, 1983). This technique restores normal cycles while allowing regression of acne and excess hair growth.

Research on Etiology and Therapeutics

Current research efforts are limited by the low priority that the disorder has received from governmental agencies and lack of public awareness. Recent recognition of the multi-organ involvement of PCO has spurred an interest in evaluating the underlying disorder(s). Disorders of prolactin secretion and metabolism, the adrenal gland, the pancreas, insulin receptor structure and function, and other organ systems, including coagulation disorders and dyslipidemias, promise to expand our knowledge of the consequences of PCO. The possibility of an effective, non-intrusive form of therapy for dealing with this disease long-term (particularly if that therapy did not interfere with fertility) would be applicable to a large segment of the female population.

Recent studies have tried different therapeutic approaches. Since the hyperandrogenism may be related to higher levels of local 5α-reductase conversion of testosterone to dihydrotestosterone in androgen sensitive tissues, several investigators have studied the effect of finasteride, a 5α-reductase inhibitor, in hirsute women. In a placebo-controlled study, Ciotta et al (1995) gave 7.5 mg/day of oral finasteride for a period of 9 months to nine hirsute women. Compared to those given placebo, there was a significant decrease in hirsutism score in treated patients, with a marked decrease in serum dihydrotestosterone. Libido was not affected although some patients complained of headache and mild depression.

Ehrmann et al have attempted to treat the insulin resistance and hyperinsulinemia, which is a hallmark of this disease, with a new therapeutic agent, troglitazone, a novel insulin-sensitizing agent (Ehrmann et al, 1997). Troglitazone is a new agent that appears to improve insulin resistance and oral glucose tolerance found in Type II diabetics. In their study, Ehrmann et al found that they were able to achieve a marked attenuation of some of the insulin resistance in women with PCOS when treated for 12 weeks in this preliminary, uncontrolled study.

As mentioned in this section and the previous one, the therapeutic approaches under study treat the symptoms and signs of the disease. No specific therapeutic is under consideration for treating the underlying etiology, precisely because the underlying etiology is still not clearly understood at this time.

Approach to Efficacy Studies

This section will discuss primarily studies relating to hirsutism. No drugs are approved for hirsutism per se. All the drugs discussed above are approved for other indications and are often used for hirsutism.

No drugs are approved for the treatment of hirsutism or infertility exclusively applied to PCO syndromes. In general the drugs mentioned above have general indications regardless of underlying disorder. Since approaches to infertility studies have been reviewed earlier, and since no specific distinction has been made with regard to underlying disorders leading to infertility, these approaches will not be repeated again.

Systems describing normal and abnormal distribution of hair are often useful to distinguish mild vs. severe hyperandrogenism (Ferriman & Gallwey, 1961). Clinical studies on the efficacy of the drugs utilized in decreasing hair growth have primarily evaluated the growth velocity and thickness of terminal hair, the androgen-dependent type of hair. Measurement of both hair length and diameter, as well as photographs, have been used in evaluation.

DYSFUNCTIONAL UTERINE BLEEDING

Prevalence and Epidemiology

Bleeding during a normal menstrual cycle is universally accepted by women, but the occurrence of irregular menstrual bleeding is extremely troublesome for most women, even those with syndromes such as PCO who often experience irregular bleeding. Menorrhagia is a common and debilitating condition leading to consultation rates of 31 per 1000 women visits in one series (Morbidity statistics in general practice, 1981–82). This condition is most commonly found in women over the age of 35 and can be causal to close to a third of all hysterectomies performed in women of this age group.

Normal menstrual bleeding was defined in a population study by Hallberg et al (1966). Mean blood loss, given the difficulties of measuring blood loss accurately, was described as 35 ml for women between the ages of 15 and 50, with a coefficient of variation between individuals of 20–40%. Greater than 80 ml results in iron deficiency anemia in most women.

In healthy women with no underlying medical illnesses, non-menstrual bleeding could be described as abnormal uterine bleeding and when no obvious anatomical pathology can be noted, the term used is 'dysfunctional uterine bleeding' (DUB). DUB is necessarily a diagnosis of exclusion and is nearly always related to disruption of normal ovarian function; the uterine response to a lack of a normal cyclical secretion of hormones of a normally ovulating ovary. Since abnormal uterine bleeding due to anatomical reasons or disorders such as polyps or systemic pathologies is often treated surgically, this section will be devoted to the treatment modalities for DUB related to hormonal and non-anatomical disruptions of the normal menstrual cycle.

Known Etiology

Causes of abnormal uterine bleeding can be grouped into three main categories:

1. *Systemic illnesses*, e.g. coagulopathies, renal and hepatic diseases and many inflammatory conditions, can cause significant menorrhagia. The bleeding

often appears in context with other pathologies and can be a first presentation of the disease condition. Only a small proportion of menorrhagia is caused by systemic illnesses and if physician awareness of systemic causes for abnormal uterine bleeding is high, the diagnosis is not often difficult to make with the appropriate tests.

2. *Local anatomic pathology* should be thoroughly searched for, especially when the bleeding carries a menorrhagic pattern. Amongst the diseases that can cause abnormal uterine bleeding are myomata, often submucosal in location, adenomyosis, endometrial polyps, endometrial adenocarcinomas, IUDs and, rarely, myometrial hypertrophy or uterine vascular malformations (Frase, 1994). Although the treatment for some of these etiologies can be medical, often surgical interventions can be helpful.

3. *DUB*, a multi-source cause of abnormal bleeding, is a diagnosis of exclusion and thus, other causes should be searched for with appropriate endocrine testing. In DUB, bleeding can be excessive, prolonged or irregular. Any underlying etiology which disrupts the normal cyclical secretion of estrogen and progestin leading to normal endometrial shedding can result in DUB. Many diseases can cause such disruption; the major ones are as follows:

   • The most common cause of DUB is anovulatory bleeding, often due to polycystic ovarian disease, a hypothalamic cause of bleeding, described in detail in an earlier section of this chapter. Bleeding associated with PCO tends to be irregularly irregular and, while the underlying pathophysiology of PCO is not well understood, the final pathway of the bleeding is related to unopposed secretion of estrogen by the polycystic ovary. Anovulation results in failure of progesterone secretion. Under the constant influence of estrogen, the endometrium becomes fragile and hypertrophic, resulting in irregular shedding.

   • Dysfunctional uterine bleeding can result from other systemic causes of anovulation, such as the presence of a hyperprolactinemia, which can initially present with irregular bleeding or luteal phase defect.

   • Other unknown causes can be related to irregular endometrial shedding.

   • Excessive menstrual bleeding (menorrhagia) is often caused by fibroids.

   • Exogenous hormone therapies, such as oral contraceptives.

   • Endometriosis has been associated with a modestly increased incidence of abnormal vaginal bleeding.

Since DUB is primarily a sign of underlying disease, the treatment will necessarily depend on the underlying etiology.

Therapeutic Approaches: Efficacy and Safety

Primary approaches to therapy consist of proper diagnosis, including the evaluation for absence of non-systemic illnesses. A quick and easy to use diagnostic technique involves the administration of a progestin to make the diagnosis of absence or presence of endogenous estrogen. Following the administration of an appropriate progestin dose, a well-estrogenized endometrium will slough and the diagnosis is almost always anovulation and is usually secondary to PCO. If no withdrawal bleeding takes place, further tests are needed to define the absence of estrogen production. In the absence of a progestin withdrawal bleed, pregnancy should be always ruled out. Therapeutic approaches are related to the underlying etiology and the extent of bleeding.

Bleeding associated with ovulation, and amenable to non-surgical treatment, will usually be characterized by shortened or prolonged menstrual cycles. Polymenorrhea is either due to a shortened follicular phase or a shortened luteal phase, and is most often due to hypothalamic disruption of the normal menstrual cycle. When the follicular phase is very short, estrogen treatment can result in normalization of follicular phase and regularization of the cycle.

Shortened luteal phases are primarily due to an inadequate corpus luteum and respond to added progesterone during the luteal phase or (if pregnancy is desired) the use of CC in the first several days of the cycle. In both instances, oral contraceptives will provide a normalization of the cycle.

Bleeding due to submucosal fibroids represents an interesting challenge and its therapy is described in the section on clinical management of myomas. If withdrawal bleeding occurs with the use of progestins, as mentioned above, the cause of amenorrhea must be sought. Measurement of gonadotropins and ultrasound of the ovaries can assist in making the diagnosis of PCO.

The treatment of PCO will depend on understanding the underlying etiology, and in many instances the etiology is not completely understood. Oral contraceptives will regularize the cycle, as well as assist in removing other signs and symptoms of PCO, such as hyperandrogenism. OCs are obviously not appropriate therapy for women with PCO who are attempting to conceive. GnRH agonist has been studied and is indeed very effective in suppressing all menstrual bleeding, but can cause menopausal complaints and is not a long-term therapy (Thomas, Okuda & Thomas, 1991; Petruccol & Fraser, 1992).

In instances of pregnancy or pregnancy-related disorders, the intervention is usually surgical. Bleeding at ovulation may be self-limiting and not require any therapy. In addition, anatomical causes such as polyps may also require surgical treatment.

In clinical studies, other approaches have been tried to suppress menorrhagia. Bounduell, Walker & Calder (1991) compared danazol 200 mg/day to norethisterone. Danazol was more effective in suppressing bleeding.

DUB can also present either as an acute emergency with severe bleeding and/or with severe, chronic prolonged bleeding and anemia. The intent here is to attempt to stop the bleeding acutely to avoid any permanent surgical intervention. Progestins in high doses can be used when the bleeding is profuse and needs immediate medical attention. In this instance, progestogens such as NET can either be given intravenously in an acute situation or orally at about 5 mg every 6 hours for up to a month. If the bleeding is due to fibroids and cannot be controlled with progestogens, LHRH analogs, or with low-dose oral contraceptives, surgical treatment may be necessary. In cases which are refractory to all medical treatment, endometrial ablation can be considered, in which case, the use of LHRH agonists or danazol prior to endometrial ablation should be considered (Valle, 1993; Donnez et al, 1997).

Research on Etiology and Approach to Efficacy Studies

Causes of underlying conditions such as PCO are described elsewhere. This section will focus on research into the etiology of bleeding at the level of the endometrium. At the height of hormonal influence and just prior to shedding, the endometrium consists of three layers: the stratum basalis, the innermost layer, appears to be refractory to the action of progesterone and provides the rejuvenating source of endometrial glands throughout the menstrual cycle. This layer of endometrium appears to be sensitive to exposure to anti-progestins, e.g. RU-486. At menstruation, the two outermost layers are sloughed off: the stratum spongiosum containing tortuous secretory glands and few stromal cells and the outermost stratum compactum, which consists of hypertrophied, swollen, stromal cells.

Sloughing of the endometrium results from intense contractions of the spiral arterioles, leading to local ischemia and necrosis (Markee, 1940). Prostaglandins are believed to be involved in this vasospasm, in particular, prostaglandin F2α (Singh, Bacarini & Zuspan, 1975). Chamberlain et al (1991) studied two prostaglandin synthetase inhibitors, ethamsylate and mefenamic acid, in DUB and found that while both products worked better than other non-steroidal anti-inflammatory drugs (NSAIDs), mefenamic acid acted rapidly and reduced menstrual loss in the first month, but ethamsylate resulted in a better treatment for prolonged use.

Fibrinolytic activity has been noted to be increased in menstrual blood. For this reason, some investigators have given women tranexamic acid, an oral anti-fibrinolytic therapy, with success in reduction of menorrhagia (Gleeson et al, 1994).

Prostaglandins also appear to play an important role in endometrial hemostasis and dysmenorrhea. NSAIDs and anti-prostaglandin drugs have been used successfully in both reducing menstrual blood loss and decreasing molimenal pelvic cramping.

CONCLUSION

Although none of the diseases described above are life-threatening, as a group they nevertheless affect the quality of life for most afflicted women. Given the common prevalence of the many diseases described above, it is important that research continue on therapeutic modalities and on understanding pathophysiology. Continued research interest in this very diverse group of diseases needs to focus on understanding the etiology and genetics, and advancing the concept of therapeutics aimed at the disease, and not at suppressing or altering the endocrine system, as most present therapies do. In other words, present therapeutic approaches treat symptoms. In areas such as endometriosis, the recent advances in understanding basic pathophysiology may lead to diagnostic agents and therapies which are more focused. The commercial nature of assisted reproductive technologies promises to advance this treatment modality into continued research. Other common diseases such as polycystic ovarian disease and its attendant hirsutism could be helped with considerably more effort into research and therapeutics.

REFERENCES

Abel BJ, Carswell G, Elton R et al. Randomized trial of clomiphene citrate and vitamin C for male infertility. *Br J Urology* 1982; **54**: 78–4.

Acien P, Mauri M, Gutierrez M. Clinical and hormonal effects of the combination gonadotrophin-releasing hormone agonist plus oral contraceptive pills containing ethinyl-oestradiol (EE) and cyproterone acetate (CPA) versus the EE-CPA pill alone on polycystic ovarian disease-related hyperandrogenisms. *Human Reprod* 1997; **12**: 423–9.

Adamson GD. Treatment of uterine fibroids: current findings with gonadotropin-releasing hormone agonists. *Am J Obstet Gynecol* 1992; **166**: 746–51.

Adashi EY, Hsueh AJW, Yen SSC. Insulin enhancement of luteinizing hormone and follicle-stimulating hormone release by culture pituitary cells. *Endocrinology* 1981; **108**: 1141.

Anderson J, Barbieri RL. Abnormal gene expression in uterine leiomyomas. *J Soc Gynecol Invest* 1995; **2**: 663–72.

Barbieri RL. Etiology and epidemiology of endometriosis. *Am J Obstet Gynecol* 1990; **162**: 565.

Benagiano G, Kivinen ST, Fadini R et al. Zoladex (goserelin acetate) and the anemic patient: results of a multicenter fibroid study. *Fertil Steril* 1996; **66**: 223–9.

Berga SL, Yen SSC. Opiodergic regulation of LH pulsatility in women with polycystic ovary syndrome. *Clin Endoc* 1996; **30**: 177.

Bounduelle M, Walker JJ, Calder AA. A comparative study of danazol and norethisterone in dysfunctional uterine bleeding presenting as menorrhagia. *Postgrad Med J* 1991; **67**: 833–6.

Brandon DD, Bethers CL, Strawn ET. Progesterone receptor messenger ribonucleic acid and protein are over-expressed in human uterine leiomyomas. *Am J Obstet Gynecol* 1993; **169**: 78–85.

Braun DP, Gebel H, Muriana A et al. Differential endometrial cell (EC) proliferation in response to peripheral blood monocytes (PBM), peritoneal macrophages (PM) and macrophage-derived cytokines in patients with endometriosis (EN). Presented at the 48th Annual Meeting, The American Fertility Society, November, 1992, New Orleans, LA.

Buckler HM, McLachlan RI, MacLachlan VB et al. Serum inhibin levels in polycystic ovary syndrome: basal levels and responses to luteinizing hormone releasing hormone agonist and exogenous gonadotropin administration. *J Clin Endocrinol Metab* 1988; **66**: 798.

Buttram VC, Reiter RC. Uterine leiomyomatae: etiology, symptomatology, and management. *Fertil Steril* 1981; **36**: 433–45.

Castello R, Tosi F, Perrone F et al. Outcome of long-term treatment with the 5α-reductase inhibitor finasteride in idiopathic hirsutism: clinical and hormonal effects during a 1-year course of therapy and 1-year follow-up. *Fertil Steril* 1996; **66**: 734–40.

Chamberlain G, Freeman R, Price F et al. A comparative study of ethamsylate and mefenamic acid in dysfunctional uterine bleeding. *Br J Obstet Gynaecol* 1991; **98**: 707–11.

Chang RF, Laufer LR, Meldrum DR et al. Steroid secretion in polycystic ovarian disease after ovarian suppression by a long-acting gonadotropin releasing hormone agonist. *J Clin Endocrinol Metab* 1983; **56**: 897.

Christiansen JK. The facts about fibroids: presentation and latest management options. *Postgrad Med* 1993; **94**: 129–34.

Ciotta L, Cianci A, Calogero AE et al. Clinical and endocrine effects of finasteride, a 5α-reductase inhibitor in women with idiopathic hirsutism. *Fertil Steril* 1995; **64**: 299–306.

Coutinho EM. Treatment of endometriosis with Gestrinone (R-2323), a synthetic anti-estrogen, antiprogesterone. *Am J Obstet Gynecol* 1982; **144**: 895–8.

Coutinho EM, Azadian-Boulanger G. Treatment of endometriosis by vaginal administration of gestrinone. *Fertil Steril* 1988; **49**: 418–22.

Cramer DW. Epidemiology of endometriosis. In EA Wilson (ed.) *Endometriosis* 1987, pp 1–5; New York: Alan R. Liss.

Cramer DW. Epidemiology of myomas. *Semin Reprod Endocrinol* 1992; **10**: 3225–31.

Crosignani PG, de Cecco L, Gastaldi A et al. Leuprolide in a 3-monthly versus a monthly depot formulation for the treatment of symptomatic endometriosis: a pilot study. *Human Reprod* 1996; **11**: 2732–5.

Cusan L, Dupont A, Gomez J-L et al. Comparison of flutamide and spironolactone in the treatment of hirsutism: a randomized controlled trial. *Fertil Steril* 1994; **61**: 281–7.

Damewood MD. Endometriosis and infertility: physiological mechanisms and contemporary therapeutic considerations including GnRH agonists. *Semin Reprod Endocrin* 1993; **11**: 127.

Deligdisch L, Hirschmann S, Altchek A. Pathologic changes in gonadotropin-releasing hormone agonist analogue treated uterine leiomyomata. *Fertil Steril* 1997; **67**: 837–41.

DeVane GW, Cekala NM, Judd HL et al. Circulation of gonadotropins, estrogens, and androgens in polycystic ovary disease. *Am J Obstet Gynecol* 1975; **121**: 496.

Diamond MP, Wentz AC. Ovulation induction with human menopausal gonadotropins. *Obstet Gynecol* 1979; **135**: 122.

Dmowski WP, Braun D, Gebel H. The immune system in endometriosis. In: J Rock (ed.) *Modern Approaches to Endometriosis* 1991, p 97; New York: Kluwer.

Dmowski, WP, Rana N. Michalowska J et al. The effect of endometriosis, its stage and activity, and of autoantibodies on in vitro fertilization and embryo transfer success rates. *Fertil Steril* 1995; **63**: 555.

Donnez J, Vilos G, Gannon MJ et al. Goserelin acetate (Zoladex) plus endometrial ablation for dysfunctional uterine bleeding: a large randomized, double-blind study. *Fertil Steril* 1997; **68**: 29–36.

Edmonds DK. Add-back therapy in the treatment of endometriosis: the European experience. *Br J Obstet Gynaecol* 1996; **103** (suppl 14): 10–13.

Ehrmann DA, Schneider DJ, Sobel BE et al. Trogliatazone improves defects in insulin action, insulin secretion, ovarian steroidogenesis, and fibrinolysis in women with polycystic ovary syndrome. *J Clin Endocrinol Metab* 1997; **82**: 2108–16.

El-Roeiy A, Dmowski WP, Gleicher N et al. Danazol, but not gonadotropin releasing hormone agonist suppresses autoantibodies in endometriosis. *Fertil Steril* 1988; **50**: 864.

Ferriman D, Gallwey JD. Clinical assessment of body hair growth in women. *J Clin Endocrinol Metab* 1961; **21**: 1440–47.

Filicori M, Flamigni C, Campaniello E et al. The abnormal response of polycystic ovarian disease patients to exogenous pulsatile gonadotropin releasing hormone: characterization and management. *J Clin Endocrinol Metab* 1989; **69**: 825.

Frase IS. Menorrhagia—a pragmatic approach to the understanding of causes and the need for investigations. *Br J Obstet Gynaecol* 1994; **101**: 3–7.

Friedman AJ, Harrison-Atlas D, Barbieri RL et al. A randomized, placebo-controlled double-blind study evaluating the efficacy of leuprolide acetate depot in the treatment of uterine leiomyomata. *Fertil Steril* 1989; **51**: 251–6.

Friedman AJ, Lobel SM, Rein MS, Barbieri RL. Efficacy and safety considerations in women with uterine leiomyomas treated with gonadotropin-releasing hormone agonists: the estrogen threshold hypotheses. *Am J Obstet Gynecol* 1990; **163**: 1113–19.

Friedman AJ, Daly M, Juneau-Norcross M, Rein MS. Preduction of uterine volume reduction in women with myomas treated with gonadotropin-releasing hormone agonist. *Fertil Steril* 1992; **58**: 43–5.

Gast, MJ. Evaluation of the infertile couple. In AJ Jacobs, MJ Gast (eds) *Practical Gynecology* 1994, p 239; Norwalk, CT: Appleton and Lange.

Gestrinone Italian Study Group. Gestrinone versus a gonadotropin-releasing hormone agonist for the treatment of pelvic pain associated with endometriosis: a multicenter, randomized, double-blind study. *Fertil Steril* 1996; **66**: 911–19.

Gindoff PR, Jewelewicz R. Reproductive potential in the older woman. *Fert Steril* 1986; **46**: 989.

Gleeson JC, Buggy F, Sheppard BL, Bonnar J. The effect of tranexamic acid on measured menstrual loss and endometrial fibrinolytic enzymes in dysfunctional uterine bleeding. *Acta Obstet Gynecol Scand* 1994; **73**: 274–7.

Gleicher N, El-Roeiy A, Confino E, Friberg J. Abnormal autoantibodies in endometriosis: is endometriosis an autoimmune disease? *Obstet Gynecol* 1987; **70**: 115.

Gokmen O, Senoz S, Gulekli B, Isik AZ. Comparison of four different treatment regimes in hirsutism related to polycystic ovary syndrome. *Gynecol Endocrinol* 1996; **10**: 249–55.

Haber GM, Behelak, YF. Preliminary report on the use of tamoxifen in the treatment of osteoporosis. *Am J Obstet Gynecol* 1987; **156**: 582–6.

Hallberg L, Hoegdahl AM, Nilsson L, Rybo G. Menstrual blood loss: a population study. *Acta Obstet Gynecol Scand* 1966; **43**: 352.

Halme J, Hammond MG, Hulka JF et al. Retrograde menstruation in healthy women and in patients with endometriosis. *Am J Obstet Gynecol* 1984; **148**: 85.

Hatch R, Rosenfeld RL, Kim MH, Tredway D. Hirsutism: implications, etiology and management. *Am J Obstet Gynecol* 1981; **140**: 815.

Hoffman D, Lobo RA. Serum dehydroepiandrosterone sulfate and the use of clomiphene citrate in anovulatory women. *Fertil Steril* 1985; **43**: 196–9.

Hornstein MD, Yuzpe AA, Burry KA et al. Prospective randomized double blind trial of 3 versus 6 months of nafarelin therapy for endometriosis associated with pelvic pain. *Fertil Steril* 1995; **63**: 955–62.

Hornstein MD, Yuzpe AA, Burry KA et al. Retreatment with nafarelin for recurrent endometriosis symptoms: efficacy, safety, and bone mineral density. *Fertil Steril* 1997; **67**: 1013–18.

Igarishi M. A new therapy for pelvic endometriosis and uterine adenomyosis: local effect of vaginal and intra-uterine danazol application. *Asia-Oceania J Obstet Gynecol* 1990; **16**(1): 1–12.

Kadaba R, Simpson CW. Disparate effects of tamoxifen in rats with experimentally induced endometriosis. *Endocrinology* 1990; **126**: 3263–7.

Kelly AC, Jewelewicz R. Alternate regimens for ovulation induction in polycystic ovarian disease. *Fertil Steril* 1990; **54**: 195.

Kettel LM, Murphy AA, Morales AJ. Treatment of endometriosis with the antiprogesterone mifepristone (RU486). *Fertil Steril* 1996; **65**(1): 23–8.

Lobo RA, Granger L, Goebelsmann U, Mishell DR Jr. Elevations in unbound serum estradiol as a possible mechanism of inappropriate gonadotropin secretion in women with PCO. *J Clin Endocrinol Metab* 1981; **52**: 156.

Lobo RA, Goebelsmann U, Horton R. Evidence for the importance of peripheral tissue events in the development of hirsutism in polycystic ovary syndrome. *J Clin Endocrinol Metab* 1983; **57**: 393.

Lumsden MA, West CP, Thomas E et al. Treatment with the gonadotropin releasing hormone-agonist gosarelin before hysterectomy for uterine fibroids. *Br J Obstet Gynaecol* 1994; **101**: 438–42.

Markee JE. Menstruation in intraocular endometrial implants in the Rhesus monkey. *Contrib Embryol* 1940; **28**: 219.

Maroulis GB. Evaluation of hirsutism and hyperandrogenemia. *Fertil Steril* 1981; 273–305.

Miller RM, Frank RA. Zoladex (goserelin) in the treatment of benign gynecological disorders: an overview of safety and efficacy. *Br J Obstet Gynaecol* 1992; **99**: 37–41.

Moen, MH. Endometriosis in women at interval sterilization. *Acta Obstet Gynecol Scand* 1987; **66**: 451–4.

Moen MH, Muus KM. Endometriosis in pregnant and non-pregnant women at tubal sterilization. *Human Reprod* 1991; **6**: 697–702.

Moghetti P, Castello R, Magnani CM et al. Clinical and hormonal effects of the 5α-reductase inhibitor finasteride in idiopathic hirsutism. *J Clin Endocrinol Metab* 19981; **79**: 1115–21.

Molloy BG, Hancock KW, Glass MR. Ovulation induction in clomiphene-nonresponsive patients: the place of pulsatile gonadotropin releasing hormone in clinical practice. *Fertil Steril* 1985; **43**: 26.

Morbidity Statistics in general practice, 1981–1982 (Introduction to a symposium). *Br J Obstet Gynaecol* 1994; **101**: 1–2.

Motta T, Maggi G, Perra M et al. Flutamide in the treatment of hirsutism. *Int J Gynecol Obstet* 1991; **36**: 155–7.

Muderris II, Bayram F, Sahim Y et al. The efficacy of 250 mg/day flutamide in the treatment of patients with hirsutism. *Fertil Steril* 1996; **66**: 220–22.

Nestler JE, Barlascini CO, Matt DW et al. Suppression of serum insulin by diazoxide reduces serum testosterone levels in obese women with polycystic ovary syndrome. *J Clin Endocrinol Metab* 1989; **68**: 1027.

Nisolle-Pochet N et al. Histologic study of ovarian endometriosis after hormonal therapy. *Fertil Steril* 1988; **49**: 423–6.

Olive DL, Haney AF. Endometriosis-associated infertility: a critical review of therapeutic approaches. *Obstet Gynecol Surv* 1986; **41**: 538–55.

Oosterlynck DJ, Cornille FJ, Waer M et al. Women with endometriosis show a defect in natural killer activity resulting in a decreased cytotoxicity to autologous endometrium. *Fertil Steril* 1991; **56**: 45.

Oosterlynck DJ, Meuleman C, Sobis H et al. Angiogenic activity of peritoneal fluid from women with endometriosis. *Fertil Steril* 1993; **59**: 778–82.

Quigley ME, Rakoff JS, Yen SSC. Increased luteinizing hormone sensitivity to dopamine inhibition in polycystic ovary syndrome. *J Clin Endocrinol Metab* 1989; **52**: 231.

Petruccol OM, Fraser IS. The potential for the use of GnRH agonists for treatment of dysfunctional uterine bleeding. *Br J Obstet Gynaecol* 1992; **99**: 34–6.

Polak de Fried E, Blanco L, Lancuba S, Asch RH. Improvement of clinical pregnancy rate and implantation rate of in vitro fertilization–embryo-transfer patients by using methylprednisolone. *Human Reprod* 1993; **8**: 393.

Rein MS, Friedman AJ, Stuart JM, MacLaughlin DT. Fibroid and myometrial steroid receptors in women treated with gonadotropin-releasing hormone agonist leuprolide acetate. *Fertil Steril* 1990a; **53**: 1018–23.

Rein MS, Friedman AJ, Pandian MR, Heffner LJ. The secretion of insulin-like growth factors I and II by explant cultures of fibroids and myometrium from women treated with a gonadotropin-releasing hormone agonist. *Obstet Gynecol* 1990b; **76**: 388–94.

Sampson JA. Peritoneal endometriosis due to menstrual dissemination of endometrial tissue into the peritoneal cavity. *Am J Obstet Gynecol* 1927; **14**: 422–69.

Sillem M, Hahn U, Coddington CC III et al. Ectopic growth of endometrium depends on its structural integrity and proteolytic activity in the cynomolgus monkey (*Macaca fascicularis*) model of endometriosis. *Fertil Steril* 1996; **66**: 268–73.

Singh EJ, Bacarini IM, Zuspan FP. Levels of prostaglandin F2 alpha and E2 in human endometrium during the menstrual cycle. *Am J Obstet Gynecol* 1975; **121**: 1003.

Sorbie PJ, Perez-Marrero R. The use of clomiphene citrate in male infertility. *J Urol* 1984; **131**: 425–9.

Steele RW, Dmowski WP, Harmer DJ. Immunological aspects of human endometrosis. *Am J Reprod Immunol* 1984; **6**: 33.

Stovall TG. Gonadotropin-releasing hormone agonists: utilization before hysterectomy. *Clin Obstet Gynecol* 1993; **36**: 642–9.

Surrey ES, Halme J. Endometriosis as a cause of infertility. *Obstet Gynecol Clin North Am* 1989; **16**: 79.

Surrey ES. Steroidal and nonsteroidal 'add-back' therapy: extending safety and efficacy of gonadotropin-releasing hormone agonists in the gynecologic patient. *Fertil Steril* 1995; **64**: 673.

Taskin O, Yalcinoglu AI, Kucuk S et al. Effectiveness of tibolone on hypoestrogenic symptoms induced by gosarelin treatment in patients with endometriosis. *Fertil Steril* 1997; **67**: 40–45.

Thomas EJ, Okuda KJ, Thomas NM. The combination of depot gonadotropin releasing hormone agonist and cyclical hormone replacement therapy for dysfunctional uterine bleeding. *Br J Obstet Gynaecol* 1991; **98**: 1155–9.

Tsapoulis AD, Zoulas PA, Comminos AC. Observations on 320 infertile patients treated with human gonadotropin. *Fertil Steril* 1978; **29**: 492.

Valle RF. Endometrial ablation for dysfunctional uterine bleeding: role of GNRH agonists. *Int J Gynecol Obstet* 1993; **41**: 3–15.

Van Look PF, von Hertzen H. Clinical uses of antiprogestogens. *Human Reproduct Update* 1995; **1**: 19–34.

WHO (World Health Organization). A double-blind trial of clomiphene citrate for the treatment of idiopathic male infertility. *Int J Androl* 1992; **15**: 299–307.

Weir EC, Goad DI, Daifotis AG et al. Related over-expression of the parathyroid hormone related peptide gene in human leiomyomas. *Clin Endocrin Metab* 1994; **78**: 784–9.

Wong IL, Morris RS, Chang L. A prospective randomized trial comparing finasteride to spironolactone in the treatment of hirsute women. *J Clin Endocrinol Metab* 1995; **80**: 233–8.

Wood GP, Wu CH, Flickinger GL, Mikhail G. Hormonal changes associated with danazol therapy. *Obstet Gynecol* 1975; **45**: 302.

Yeh J, Rein M, Nowak R. Presence of messenger ribonucleic acid for epidermal growth factor (EGF) and EGF receptor demonstrable in monolayer cell cultures of myometria and leiomyomata. *Fertil Steril* 1991; **56**: 997–1000.

Yen SSC, Vela CP, Ryan KJ. Effect of clomiphene citrate in polycystic ovary syndrome: Relationship between serum gonadotropin and corpus luteum function. *J Clin Endocrinol Metab* 1982; **54**: 490.

9

Pre-term Labor and Birth

Phillip N. Rauk

University of Pittsburgh and Magee Women's Research Institute, Pittsburgh, PA, USA

Delivery before 37 weeks of pregnancy occurs in 10% of all pregnancies and accounts for as much as 80% of all neonatal morbidity and mortality. The pre-term birth rate is affected by age, ethnic background and socioeconomic status. The rate of pre-term birth among African-Americans is 18.7% compared with 8.7% in Whites (National Center for Health Statistics, 1991). Low socioeconomic status and poor education level carry a relative risk of pre-term birth of 1.2–1.5. Maternal nutritional status, pre-pregnancy weight, and weight gain during pregnancy also influence pre-term birth rates. The immediate causes of pre-term birth, however, include idiopathic factors, pre-term rupture of membranes, infection, multiple gestation, utero-placental ischemia, maternal disease and hemorrhage.

Despite improved tocolytic therapy and increased pregnancy surveillance, efforts to reduce the pre-term birth rate in the last 20 years have largely been unsuccessful. Neonatal mortality has dropped over the last 20 years secondary to improved care of the neonate. Survival from respiratory distress syndrome has increased markedly with the use of antenatal steroid therapy and neonatal surfactant administration. Large randomized, placebo-controlled trials of tocolytics demonstrate only a 48 h delay in delivery. The use of tocolytics for prolonging delivery to permit the administration of antenatal steroids and for transportation of the patient to a level III neonatal center is therefore justified and greatly increases neonatal survival. Tocolytics by necessity are used for the treatment of pre-term labor when it occurs, not as a prophylaxis against pre-term birth. No study has demonstrated a benefit from prophylactic use of oral tocolytic agents. Tocolytics are perhaps indicated in only 30% of cases of pre-term labor (for idiopathic causes and multiple gestation). Therefore, an expectation that tocolytics will reduce the pre-term birth rate is not supported by current research. This chapter will discuss mechanisms of uterine contractility and causes of pre-term labor amenable to tocolytic therapy. Drugs in current use and those in development are compared with respect to efficacy, side effects and administration. Basic research is discussed which could lead to new drug development over the next 20 years.

Drug Development for Women. Edited by V.V. Ragavan. © 1998 John Wiley & Sons Ltd.

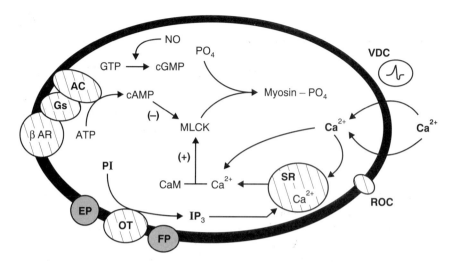

FIGURE 9.1 Mechanisms of myometrial contractility. βAR, β-adrenergic receptor; AC, adenylate cyclase; OT, oxytocin receptor; EP, PGE receptor; FP, $PGF_{2\alpha}$ receptor; SR, sarcoplasmic reticulum; ROC, receptor-operated calcium channel; VDC, voltage-dependent calcium channel; NO, nitric oxide; PI, phosphotidylinositol; IP_3, inositol triphosphate; CaM, calmodulin; MLCK, myosin light chain kinase; GS, GTP-binding protein-s. Adapted from Daftary, Rauk & Caritis (1992), by permission of Wiley-Liss

MECHANISM OF UTERINE CONTRACTILITY

Most tocolytics (magnesium sulfate, β-adrenergic agonists, calcium channel blockers) were developed to inhibit the contractile function of myometrial cells. Uterine contractility is controlled by both free intracellular calcium concentration as well as the phosphorylation of the contractile protein, myosin. Figure 9.1 shows the cellular pathways controlling myometrial cell contractility. In resting myometrium, free intracellular calcium is maintained at a very low concentration by two mechanisms: a membrane cyclic adenosine monophosphate (cAMP)-dependent calcium-magnesium ATPase, which transports calcium out of the cell, and a cAMP-dependent calcium ATPase, which sequesters calcium in the sarcoplasmic reticulum. A voltage-dependent calcium channel allows calcium to enter the cell following depolarization. Intracellular calcium stores in sarcoplasmic reticulum are released by increased intracellular inositol triphosphate. The oxytocin receptor, PGE_2 receptor (EP3) and $PGF_{2\alpha}$ receptor (FP) activate phospholipase C, resulting in hydrolysis of membrane-bound phosphotidyl inositol to inositol triphosphate and diacylglycerol (Ku et al, 1995; Asboth et al, 1996). Diacylglycerol activates protein kinase C as well as cellular lipases, resulting in the release of arachidonic acid from membrane phospholipids. Arachidonic acid is the precursor for prostaglandin synthesis.

Contractions in the myometrium result from the binding of the two contractile proteins, myosin (thick filaments) and actin (thin filaments). Increased free intracellular calcium binds to the regulatory protein, calmodulin. This calcium–calmodulin complex activates myosin light chain kinase (MLCK). The myosin protein is phosphorylated by MLCK and binds to actin, resulting in contractions. The binding of actin to myosin is broken by the dephosphorylation of myosin by its own ATPase activity.

Intracellular concentrations of cyclic adenosine monophosphate (cAMP) control contraction activity. cAMP is produced by the enzyme adenylate cyclase and degraded by the enzyme phophodiesterase. Adenylate cyclase activity is increased by the β-adrenergic receptor (BAR). Binding of agonist to BAR results in increased cAMP through G-protein-mediated activation of adenylate cyclase. cAMP inhibits contractions through phosphorylation and inactivation of MLCK and through a decrease in intracellular free calcium. The β-adrenergic receptor agonists, terbutaline and ritodrine, inhibit contractions by this mechanism.

MECHANISMS OF PRE-TERM BIRTH

Many maternal and fetal factors play a role in pre-term birth. The actual sequence of events leading to term birth in humans remains unknown. Several pathways leading to both pre-term and term birth have been extensively studied, including the role of oxytocin, prostaglandins and infection. Currently, some tocolytics have been chosen as an approach to blocking these pathways and they are therefore discussed in this chapter. Other mechanisms of pre-term birth, including the role of stress and fetal endocrine signaling, are not discussed.

Oxytocin

Oxytocin clearly plays a role in the maintenance, if not initiation, of both term and pre-term labor. There is little evidence to suggest that serum oxytocin concentrations increase prior to the onset of labor in humans; however, oxytocin may be produced locally in decidua (Leake et al, 1981; Thornton, Davison & Baylis, 1992). Oxytocin mRNA is increased five-fold in decidua coincident with the labor (Chibbar, Miller & Mitchell, 1993). Fuchs et al (1991), using a more sensitive assay of oxytocin, did demonstrate higher pulsatile concentrations of oxytocin in women in spontaneous labor vs. no labor.

Increasing sensitivity to oxytocin occurs at term largely as a result of increased receptors. Uterine oxytocin receptors increase in sheep, rat, rabbit and human pregnancy immediately prior to the onset of labor (Ikeda, Shibata & Yamamoto, 1987; Alexandrova & Soloff, 1980; Fuchs et al, 1984). This increased uterine sensitivity to oxytocin is also observed in patients who deliver pre-term. In a retrospective analysis of oxytocin challenge tests among complicated pre-term pregnancies, uterine sensitivity to oxytocin increases prior to the onset of pre-term labor and delivery (Takahashi et al, 1980). These authors suggest accelerated sensitivity to oxytocin as a mechanism of pre-term labor in these patients. Bossmar et al (1994), in a similar group of pre-term patients, demonstrated an increase in oxytocin receptors in patients delivering pre-term. This rise was the same as that observed in patients in term labor and correlated well with the sensitivity of isolated uterine strips to oxytocin contraction in vitro.

Oxytocin most likely has a dual role in the initiation of labor both through direct action on myometrium and through the synthesis of decidual prostaglandins. Decidual prostaglandins not only increase myometrial sensitivity to oxytocin but stimulate uterine contractions. Oxytocin receptors are present on cultured amnion, chorion and decidua (Soloff & Hiuko, 1993; Fuchs, Husslein & Fuchs, 1981; Benedetto et al, 1990). These receptors have the same affinity for oxytocin as myometrial receptors. The concentrations of receptors are highest in pre-term labor and in early labor. Oxytocin stimulation of receptors in amnion and decidua leads to PGE_2 and $PGF_{2\alpha}$ release, respectively (Soloff & Hinko, 1993; Wilson, Liggins & Whittaker, 1988; Fuchs, Husslein & Fuchs, 1981).

Prostaglandins

Prostaglandins are believed to contribute to the initiation of both pre-term and term labor. Prostaglandins are produced in the amnion, chorion, decidua and myometrium. The amnion produces PGE_2, while chorion and decidua produce both PGE_2 and $PGF_{2\alpha}$. Myometrium produces PGE_2, $PGF_{2\alpha}$ and prostacyclin. During labor, both term and pre-term, amniotic fluid concentrations of all prostaglandins increase (Casey & MacDonald, 1988). The decidua appears to play a major role in uterine prostaglandin production. In the setting of pre-term labor with infection, decidual prostaglandin production increases through the induction of prostaglandin H-synthase (PGHS-2). The signal which initiates increased decidual prostaglandin production at term is unknown.

Infection

Intra-amniotic infection and chorio-amnionitis account for as much as 20% of all cases of pre-term labor (Romero et al, 1989c). A report of 11 studies looking at amniocentesis in the setting of pre-term labor identified positive cultures in 16.1% (range 0–48%) (Romero & Mazor, 1988). In fact, in those cases where labor was refractory to tocolysis, as many as 65% of amniotic fluid cultures were positive. The pathophysiology of infection-mediated pre-term labor has been extensively studied. Intra-amniotic infection is associated with the production of inflammatory cytokines by decidua, chorion and amnion. These cytokines, specifically interleukin-1 (IL-1), tumor necrosis factor alpha (TNFα), and interleukin-6 (IL-6), are found in high concentrations in amniotic fluid in the setting of intra-amniotic infection and pre-term labor (Romero et al, 1989a, c, 1990; Hillier et al, 1993). An increase in amniotic cytokines and PGE_2 is strongly associated with positive amniotic culture and also with pre-term delivery within 7 days of amniocentesis. Lack of detection of IL-1 is associated with a delay in delivery for greater than 7 days (Hillier et al, 1993).

Several in vitro studies have shown that decidual tissue produces IL-1, $TNF\alpha$ and IL-6 in response to bacteria and lipopolysaccharide (Romero et al, 1989b, 1990; Casey et al, 1989). These cytokines are believed to initiate labor via the local production of uterotonic prostaglandins, PGE_2 and $PGF_{2\alpha}$ (Mitchell, Trautman & Dudley, 1993; Bry & Hallman, 1992; Lundin-Schiller & Mitchell, 1990; Molnar, Romero & Hertelendy, 1993). This increase in prostaglandin production is secondary to induction of the inducible form of PGHS-2 (Slater et al, 1995; Hirst et al, 1995; Gibb & Sun, 1996). The above studies clearly establish a direct link between intra-amniotic infection, cytokine production, prostaglandin production and pre-term labor. Although the combined effect of many cytokines is involved in the sequence of events leading to pre-term labor with intra-amniotic infection, the data from animal studies suggest that IL-1 alone is able to induce pre-term delivery.

TOCOLYTIC AGENTS CURRENTLY IN USE

Tocolytics have been developed either to decrease uterine contractions by blocking the contractile mechanism (β-adrenergic agonists, magnesium sulfate, calcium channel blockers) or interfering with the production or action of known contractile agonists (prostaglandin synthase inhibitors) and oxytocin receptor antagonists. Generally, tocolytic efficacy is balanced by undesirable maternal and fetal side effects. These side effects may be reduced by altered dosing and administration but currently limit the effectiveness of all tocolytic agents.

β-Adrenergic Agonists

Currently, the β_2-receptor agonist, ritodrine, is the only FDA-approved drug for the treatment of pre-term contractions. The β_2-agonists also include the drugs salbutamol, terbutaline and hexoprenaline. Two types of β-receptors are present in human tissues. The β_1-receptors predominate in the heart, intestine and adipose tissues, while β_2-receptors predominate in the myometrium, vascular smooth muscle, pancreas and bronchioles. It is the β_2 action of ritodrine which accounts for the uterine relaxant, metabolic and blood pressure-lowering properties of the drug. Ritodrine is not a pure β_2-agonist. The β_1 action accounts for the tachycardia and increased stroke volume associated with ritodrine administration. On binding ritodrine, the cell surface β_2-receptor binds the GTP binding protein G_s. The G_s protein activates the membrane-bound enzyme adenylate cyclase, resulting in increased intracellular cAMP. cAMP inhibits the action of myosin light chain kinase, thus preventing the phosphorylation of myosin and the myosin–actin interaction which results in uterine smooth muscle contractions. The concentration of free intracellular calcium is also lowered through calcium sequestration in sarcoplasmic reticulum. Although the β_2 are potent inhibitors of smooth muscle contraction, continued use results in tachyphylaxis to the drug through both desensitization and down-regulation. Desensitization is acute and occurs through receptor phosphorylation by protein kinase A and results in uncoupling of the receptor from the enzyme adenylate cyclase. This process is rapidly reversible with removal of the agonist (Hausdorff, Caron & Lefkowitz, 1990). After more prolonged exposure to agonist the receptor becomes phosphorylated by β-adrenergic receptor kinase and ultimately is sequestered and removed from the cell surface. Both processes result in decreased effectiveness in the agonist to block uterine contractions. Changes in dosing and administration of these agents may delay tachyphylaxis and improve efficacy.

Clinical Efficacy

Few studies have proven β-agonist to be effective in reducing neonatal mortality and morbidity. Perhaps the largest trial to date on tocolytic efficacy was conducted by the Canadian Preterm Labor Investigators' Group (1992). This study was a randomized prospective placebo-controlled trial of ritodrine for the treatment of pre-term labor in 708 women at 20–35 weeks' gestation. The primary outcome to be tested was perinatal mortality. The study did not demonstrate any benefit of ritodrine compared with placebo in perinatal mortality, pre-term birth, low birth weight or neonatal morbidity. The study did, however, demonstrate a significant delay in delivery at both 24 and 48 hours. Based on this data, ritodrine is effective at delaying delivery for a time sufficient to administer steroid therapy for lung maturation. The meta-analysis of randomized placebo-controlled trials of King et al (1988) reached the same conclusion as the Canadian Trial.

Adverse Side Effects

Adverse maternal side effects limit the use of ritodrine and are responsible for the discontinuation of β-agonist therapy in 14% of subjects in the Canadian Trial. The majority of side effects result from the unwanted β_1 action of the drug. Palpitations (53.4%), chest pain (7.7%), cardiac arrhythmias (2%) and dyspnea (15.1) limit the use of ritodrine in a large number of patients. Secondary to the metabolic action of this drug, both hypokalemia (39.2%) and hyperglycemia (30.1%) are common but rarely necessitate potassium replacement or insulin infusion. Nausea, vomiting, tremor and headache are also common. All these side effects are dose-dependent and occur at the highest infusion rates of the drug. All are rapidly reversible with discontinuation of the infusion. Perhaps the two most significant side affects attributed to ritodrine are suspected myocardial ischemia and pulmonary edema.

Benedetti (1983) reported EKG changes (S-T segment depression, T-wave flattening, and prolonged Q-T interval) consistent with myocardial ischemia in some patients. No associated changes in cardiac enzymes have been found in these patients (Hendricks, Keroes & Katz, 1986). Pulmonary edema has been reported in as high as 5% of patients but occurred in only 0.3% of patients in the Canadian Trial. Fetal side effects of ritodrine are uncommon. A single retrospective evaluation of intraventricular hemorrhage in neonates exposed to β-agonist found an increased incidence with an odds ratio of 2.47 (Groome et al, 1992). The Canadian Trial, however, demonstrated no difference in neonatal intraventricular hemorrhage, respiratory distress syndrome, hypoglycemia, hypotension or seizures.

Although ritodrine is the primary parenteral β-agonist used for tocolysis, terbutaline remains the principal oral agent for maintenance therapy. Dosing is empirical at 5 mg every 4–6 hours. There is limited information on the efficacy of prolonged therapy for prevention of recurrent pre-term labor. Similarly, maintenance therapy with subcutaneous terbutaline therapy by pump has been studied in patients who do not respond to conventional therapy (Lam et al, 1988). Moise et al (1992) demonstrated limited success with this therapy in 13 women. Pulsatile administration of terbutaline by pump may prevent tachyphylaxis but has not been of proven benefit in preventing pre-term birth.

Pharmacology, Dosing and Administration

There is considerable variation in plasma concentrations of ritodrine among pregnant women. Based on available pharmacokinetic data and information of tachyphylaxis, Caritis et al (1990) have proposed a protocol for administration different from the manufacturer's recommendation. The infusion starts at a dose of 50 μg/min and increases 50 μg/min every 20 min until tocolysis is achieved or side effects result. The infusion is then lowered by 50 μg/min every 30 min to the lowest dose which results in continued tocolysis. With this regimen a lower dose of drug is infused, resulting in fewer side effects and equal efficacy. Caritis, Chiao & Kridgen (1991) have also recommended intermittent pulsatile infusion of ritodrine to reduce the incidence of tachyphylaxis to the drug.

Ongoing Clinical Research

Aside from novel strategies for administering β-agonist, such as pulsatile therapy, to both reduce side effects and limit tachyphylaxis, new drug development has focused on more β_2-specific agents. Hexoprenaline was first introduced as a tocolytic in 1976 (Lipshitz, Ballie & Davey, 1976). Hexoprenaline raises the pulse rate to a lesser degree than other β-agonists and is as effective in reducing contractions (Lipshitz & Lipshitz, 1984). Hankins & Hauth (1985), in a study of the cardiovascular effects of several β-agonists in dogs, concluded that hexoprenaline had the least heart rate and arrhythmogenic affect, while terbutaline administration had the most profound increase in heart rate and arrhythmias. Despite these improvements in safety profile, hexoprenaline has not been approved for use as a tocolytic agent in the USA.

Magnesium Sulfate

Magnesium sulfate is the primary drug used for tocolysis in the USA today. This choice has largely been made based on safety issues rather than efficacy data. The mechanism by which magnesium sulfate inhibits uterine contractions has not been well studied. Magnesium sulfate has been shown to decrease intracellular calcium in bronchial smooth muscle via a block in voltage-dependent calcium channels (Kumasaka et al, 1996). Magnesium sulfate also inhibits oxytocin-induced Ca^{2+} influx into myometrial cells (Mizuki et al, 1993). The effect of magnesium on sarcoplasmic reticulum calcium stores is unknown.

Clinical Efficacy

The use of magnesium sulfate for tocolysis was first reported by Steer & Petrie (1977); however, conclusions on the efficacy of magnesium sulfate based on this study cannot be made secondary to small sample size and inadequate definition of pre-term labor. Only two studies have been performed comparing magnesium sulfate with placebo. Cotton et al (1984) compared magnesium sulfate with terbutaline and placebo in 54 patients and showed no difference in efficacy at 48 h. In a similar study by Cox, Sherman & Leveno (1990), 156 patients were randomized to magnesium sulfate vs. placebo. No difference was seen between magnesium sulfate and placebo in delay of delivery, birth weight or neonatal morbidity and mortality. Both studies have been criticized for the use of inadequate doses of magnesium sulfate. Three studies have compared magnesium sulfate with β-agonist and found no difference in prolongation of pregnancy (Beall et al, 1985; Hollander, Nagey & Pupkin, 1987; Wilkins et al, 1988). Although oral magnesium sulfate has been studied as a tocolytic, no study to date has enrolled sufficient patients to adequately compare oral therapy with placebo or terbutaline.

Adverse Side Effects

Common side effects reported among women receiving magnesium sulfate at therapeutic doses (plasma concentrations of 5.5–7.5 mg/dl) include flushing, hypotension, headache, nausea, emesis, blurred vision, palpitations, lethargy and dry mouth (Elliott, 1985). Toxicity is related to serum magnesium concentration. At 8–12 mg/dl deep tendon reflexes become lost. At 12–15 mg/dl respiratory depression occurs and at 30 mg/dl cardiac arrest occurs. Pulmonary edema has been reported in less than 2% of patients. Fetal side effects of magnesium sulfate are minimal. Fetal serum magnesium concentrations are comparable to maternal concentrations at 3 h of infusion (Hallak et al, 1993). High neonatal serum concentrations may cause transient hypoventilation and hypotonia but are often limited and resolve within 24–48 h. Long-term (greater than 6 weeks) intravenous magnesium sulfate therapy has been associated with abnormal neonatal bone mineralization which resolves by 2 months of life (Santi, Henry & Douglas, 1994).

Pharmacology, Dosing and Administration

Magnesium sulfate is administered as an intravenous infusion for the treatment of pre-term labor. Following a bolus infusion of 6 g, maintenance infusions are adjusted from 2 g/h to as high as 5 g/h to achieve cessation of contractions. Magnesium sulfate clearance is solely by renal excretion and therefore plasma concentrations are altered by impaired renal function. Toxicity can be followed either clinically or by measuring serum magnesium concentrations. At plasma concentrations of less than 7 g/dl, tocolysis is usually achieved and side effects are minimal.

Indomethacin

Indomethacin belongs to a family of non-steroidal anti-inflammatory drugs (NSAIDs) whose mechanism of action is the inhibition of the enzyme prostaglandin H-synthase (PGHS). PGHS converts arachidonic acid released from cell membrane phospholipids to the prostaglandin intermediate, prostaglandin endoperoxide (PGG_2). PGG_2 is further converted to the thromboxanes, prostacycline, and the uterotonic prostaglandins, PGE_2 and $PGF_{2\alpha}$. PGHS exists in two isoforms, the constitutively expressed form, PGHS-1 and the inducible form, PGHS-2. PGHS-2 is induced in tissues following exposure to bacteria as well as inflammatory cytokines, specifically IL-1. Uterine tissues express both forms of PGHS; however, the relative contribution each makes to prostaglandin production by both decidua and myometrium changes in both pre-term and term labor. Several studies demonstrate no change in the abundance of the PGHS-1 isoform during labor and a dramatic increase in the inducible form of PGHS-2 (Hirst et al, 1995; Slater et al, 1995; Gibb & Sun, 1996). These studies suggest that with the onset of labor prostaglandins are produced predominately by the action of PGHS-2 by both fetal membranes and myometrium. Indomethacin is an inhibitor of both PGHS-1 and PGHS-2 but its action on PGHS-1 is 10–100 times greater than PGHS-2. Indomethacin therefore blocks labor through the slowly reversible inhibition of both isoforms of PGHS in uterine tissues.

Clinical Efficacy

Two randomized placebo-controlled trials have compared the efficacy of indomethacin compared with placebo. In the first trial, Zuckerman et al randomized 36 patients in pre-term labor between 25 and 35 weeks gestation to either indomethacin at 100 mg/day or placebo (Zuckerman et al, 1984). Indomethacin was more effective in delaying delivery by at least 7 days compared with placebo, 85% undelivered with indomethacin vs. 17% with placebo. Similarly, Niebyl et al (1980) enrolled 32 patients in pre-term labor in a placebo-controlled trial of indomethacin. The outcome to be tested was failure of tocolysis. Twenty percent of the indomethacin-treated patients failed, compared with 66% of placebo-treated controls.

Adverse Side Effects

Severe fetal side effects currently limit the use of indomethacin as a tocolytic agent. Fetal side effects limiting the use of indomethacin are principally ductal constriction and oligohydramnios. Neonatal side effects include an increased incidence of necrotizing enterocolitis and intraventricular hemorrhage. The most comprehensive evaluation of ductal constriction was performed by Moise et al (1988). Of 13 fetuses studied between 26 and 31 weeks' gestation, ductal constriction was detected in 50% by fetal echocardiography. The constriction in all cases was reversed by 24 h following discontinuation of the drug. Three fetuses, however, had persistent tricuspid regurgitation for up to 40 h after discontinuation. This regurgitation is secondary to either elevated right ventricular pressures or tricuspid valve papillary muscle dysfunction. Ductal constriction also appears to be a gestational age-dependent effect. Tulzer et al (1992) reported the incidence of ductal constriction as 61% between 31 and 34 weeks, 43% at 27–30 weeks, and 0% at less than 27 weeks, the overall rate being 38%.

NSAIDs all have an adverse effect of renal function. In adults, indomethacin decreased creatinine clearance by 13% and renal blood flow by 23% (Bergamo et al, 1989). Prostaglandins are also known to inhibit the central release of antidiuretic hormone (ADH) and antagonize the action of ADH at the renal tubules. Both of these effects may explain the occurrence of oligohydramnios with indomethacin administration. Fetal urine output decreases after indomethacin administration. Kirshon et al (1988), using ultrasound to measure fetal bladder volume and bladder emptying, estimated fetal urine output. Fetal urine output decreased from 12 ml/min to 2 ml/min by 5–12 h of indomethacin therapy and returned to baseline at 24 h after therapy. A decrease in neonatal creatinine clearance has also been observed in infants exposed to antenatal indomethacin within 48 h of delivery (Heijden et al, 1988). Wurtzel (1990) reported oligohydramnios in 30% of fetuses exposed to average daily dose of indomethacin of 117 mg/day. Oligohydramnios is reversible on discontinuation of the drug.

Recently two retrospective studies of indomethacin exposure antenatally have demonstrated an increase in neonatal necrotizing enterocolitis (NEC). Confirmed cases of NEC occurred in 19% of infants exposed to indomethacin compared with 2% in gestation-age-matched controls (Norton et al, 1993). Major et al (1994) reported an incidence of NEC of 20% compared with 9% in infants exposed to indomethacin antenatally within 24 h of delivery. The increased incidence of NEC is also associated with duration of therapy. Necrotizing enterocolitis occurred in 26.4% of infants exposed to indomethacin for greater than 48 h compared with 4.1% after less than 48 h of exposure. The mechanism of increased NEC is unknown but is most likely secondary to decreased mesenteric blood flow, a block in autoregulation of oxygen consumption by the bowel, and temporary ischemia (Norton et al, 1993). Infants exposed to indomethacin also have an increased incidence of grades II–IV intracranial hemorrhage, 28% in the indomethacin-treated group vs. 9% in controls (Norton et al, 1993). This is secondary to an increase in grade II hemorrhage of 21% vs. 6% in the indomethacin and control groups, respectively.

Pharmacology, Dosing and Administration

Indomethacin is available as both 25 mg and 50 mg tablets and rectal supposi-tories. Peak drug concentrations from both oral and rectal administration occur in 30–120 min (Hellenberg, 1981). The inhibition of prostaglandin production, as measured by platelet thromboxane concentrations, reaches a peak after only 5 min and persists up to 24 h after a single oral dose of indomethacin (Cagossi et al, 1992). Fetal indomethacin concentrations parallel those of the mother and are independent of gestational age (Moise et al, 1990). The plasma half-life in the newborn is 11–20 h compared with 12 h in the non-pregnant adult and accounts for the prolonged period of side effects observed in neonates recently exposed to indomethacin in utero (Evans et al, 1979).

The observed fetal and neonatal adverse outcomes are associated with duration of indomethacin exposure as well as dose and gestational age at exposure. For this reason, indomethacin is currently recommended for only 48 h of therapy and at a gestation age of less than 34 weeks. Discontinuation of therapy is recommended once delivery is anticipated, as neonatal adverse effects are associated with recent exposure. Observed ductal constriction and oligohydramnios rarely occur during the first 48 h of therapy and are reversible within 24 h of discontinuation of the drug. Limiting the dose of indomethacin to 25 mg every 6 h exposes the fetus and neonate to less drug and may result in fewer serious side effects.

Ongoing Clinical Research

With the discovery of two isoforms of PGHS, new drug development has focused on specific inhibition of PGHS-2. Clinical conditions in women which require the uses of current PGHS inhibitors such as aspirin, ketoprofen, ibuprofen and indomethacin, include arthritis, menorrhagia and dysmenorrhea. The inhibition of PGHS-2 accounts for the desired anti-inflammatory and analgesic properties of these drugs. The inhibition of PGHS-1 by these drugs accounts for the unwanted side effects, including gastric and renal damage (Mitchell et al, 1994). It is likely that the undesired fetal and neonatal side effects of indomethacin are directly the result of PGHS-1 inhibition in the fetal ductus arteriosus, kidney and intestinal and brain arterioles. The efficacy of indomethacin as a tocolytic is most likely secondary to the inhibition of PGHS-2 in the fetal membranes and myometrium.

Selective inhibitors of PGHS-2 are currently being tested in animals and in Phase I trials in humans for the treatment of arthritis. NS-398 has been shown to inhibit PGHS-2 selectively and have equal anti-inflammatory and analgesic effects as indomethacin with no effect on PGHS-1 inhibition (Futaki et al, 1994). NS-398 also inhibits both PGE_2 and $PGF_{2\alpha}$ production by the guinea pig uterus and endometrium during the estrous cycle when PGHS-2 is maximally expressed (Naderali & Poyser, 1996). Prostacyclin, which relaxes human uterine muscle production, is not inhibited. Should the selective PGHS-2 agents be safe in humans, they may prove to be effective new tocolytic agents with less adverse fetal and neonatal side effects.

Nifedipine

Nifedipine belongs to a class of drugs known as calcium channel blockers. These agents block the voltage-dependent calcium channels in smooth and cardiac muscle. Both nifedipine and nicardipine block uterine contractions by reducing intracellular calcium concentrations.

Clinical Efficacy

Information on the efficacy of nifedipine is limited as no randomized placebo-controlled trials have been conducted. Several randomized comparative trials with ritodrine and magnesium sulfate have been conducted. Ferguson et al (1990) compared nifedipine with ritodrine in 66 women in pre-term labor. Delivery was delayed for 48 h in 85% and for 7 days in 70% nifedipine compared with the delay with ritodrine in 72% for 48 h and 63% for 7 days. Glock & Morales (1993) compared ritodrine with magnesium sulfate in 80 women in pre-term labor. Both agents delayed delivery beyond 48 h by 92%. Oral terbutaline and nifedipine were also compared for maintenance therapy. Nifedipine was equally as effective as terbutaline in preventing recurrence, 26% vs. 24%, and in delaying delivery beyond 34 weeks in 62% and 68%, respectively.

Adverse Side Effects

The side effects of nifedipine are primarily on the maternal cardiovascular system. A decrease in mean systolic blood pressure of 8.6% and diastolic blood pressure of 15.7% without a significant change in heart rate occurs in pregnant women receiving a single 10 mg dose of nifedipine (Thaler et al, 1991). Ferguson et al (1989a) also reported a drop in blood pressure of less than 10%. The reduction in blood pressure is secondary to arteriolar vascular relaxation. Reflex increase in heart rate secondary to catecholamine release may occur following significant hypotension. The fetal effects of nifedipine are unknown. A single study in sheep demonstrated a 15% reduction in fetal arterial oxygen in conjunction with maternal hypotension after maternal nifedipine administration (Harake et al, 1989). Two studies in humans using fetal umbilical and maternal uterine arterial Doppler measurements failed to demonstrate a reduction in uteroplacental or fetal umbilical blood flow (Mari et al, 1989; Thaler et al, 1991).

Pharmacology, Dosing and Administration

Nifedipine is available in 10 and 20 mg tablets and capsules. Rapid absorption occurs with peak drug levels within 30 min of administration. The drug is more rapidly cleared by pregnant women compared with males (McAllister, 1986; Ferguson et al, 1989b). Based on this data, as well as the cardiovascular effects of the drug, current dosing is between 10 and 20 mg initially followed by 10–20 mg every 4–6 h for maintenance therapy. Given the limited data on fetal effects of nifedipine its use for tocolysis has been confined to patients who fail either magnesium sulfate or ritodrine therapy.

ADJUNCTIVE ANTIBIOTICS

As occult infection accounts for as much as 20% of pre-term labor with intact membranes, several studies have recommended the use of antibiotics in conjunction with tocolytic agents. Nine placebo-controlled prospective studies have evaluated antibiotics for the treatment of pre-term labor with intact membranes (McGregor et al, 1986; McGregor, French & Seo, 1991; Winkler et al, 1988; Morales et al, 1988; Newton et al, 1989, 1991; Norman et al, 1994; Romero et al, 1993; Gordon et al, 1995). Various antibiotics have been used including erythromycin, ampicillin, unasyn, clindamycin, metronidazole and cefizoxime. Only one study has shown a decrease in pre-term birth rate (Morales et al, 1988). The largest trial enrolled 277 women randomized between ampicillin/amoxicillin or erythromycin (Romero et al, 1993). Positive amniotic fluid cultures were found in 5.9% of the participants. The study was prematurely stopped secondary to a lower than expected rate of pre-term birth in the placebo group. The study failed to show a prolongation in pregnancy or reduction in pre-term birth rate. No study to date has demonstrated a decrease in neonatal morbidity or mortality with adjunctive antibiotics in pre-term labor with intact membranes.

Oxytocin Receptor Antagonist

Oxytocin receptor antagonists have been considered for tocolysis for the last 30 years. Only recently has large-scale production of selective oxytocin receptor antagonist been achieved. Based on the information provided earlier in this chapter supporting oxytocin receptor involvement in pre-term labor, these agents are potentially ideal tocolytics and likely to be available for clinical use within 5 years. Oxytocin receptor antagonists offer a distinct advantage over the previously described tocolytics. As only fetal membranes, uterine myometrium, kidney and breast tissue contain significant oxytocin receptors, oxytocin receptor antagonists are highly selective for uterine tissues with limited anticipated adverse side effects. Oxytocin receptor antagonists act to bind the oxytocin receptor without generating the intracellular signaling leading to contractions. The action of locally produced oxytocin on fetal membrane prostaglandin production and myometrial contractions is thereby blocked. Atosiban, the most extensively studied antagonist, is a pure reversible competitive inhibitor of the oxytocin receptor. Binding of atosiban to the receptor does not result in receptor down-regulation as occurs with oxytocin itself (Phaneuf et al, 1994). This is advantageous as discontinuation of tocolysis may be necessary for maternal and/or fetal indications. Oxytocin may be used immediately for both labor induction and prevention of post-partum hemorrhage.

Clinical Efficacy

Oxytocin receptor antagonists were first studied clinically in 1984 (Akerlund et al, 1987). In 13 women in pre-term labor between 27 and 35 weeks' gestation intravenous infusion of the oxytocin receptor analog resulted in complete cessation of contractions. Goodwin et al (1994) enrolled 120 women in pre-term labor between 20 and 36 weeks in a randomized, placebo-controlled trial of intravenous atosiban for 2 h. Atosiban resulted in a mean percentage decrease in contraction frequency of 55.3% compared with 26.7% in control subjects. The first open-labeled trial of atosiban in pre-term labor demonstrated a cessation of uterine contractions in 62.3% of patients. Atosiban has been compared with placebo in two trials. Atosiban resulted in a significant delay of delivery at 24 (OR = 1.93) and 48 (OR = 1.62) h and 7 (OR = 1.70) days compared with placebo (Sibai et al, 1997). The study, however, did not demonstrate a delay in median time to delivery. Atosiban use subcutaneously following successful intravenous therapy is significantly better than placebo at reducing the time to recurrent labor (Sanchez-Ramos et al, 1997). This effect was most pronounced at less than 28 weeks' gestation.

Adverse Side Effects

Oxytocin receptor antagonists have few side effects given the limited tissue distribution of the oxytocin receptor. Among the 62 patients enrolled in the initial study of atosiban, no adverse side effects were reported (Goodwin et al, 1996). In the two placebo-controlled trials of atosiban, the incidence of side effects including headache, nausea, vomiting, dizziness, constipation and back pain were comparable to placebo controls. Only injection site irritation was higher among atosiban-treated patients. No cardiovascular alterations are reported with atosiban. Placental passage of atosiban is 12% and has no effect on fetal acid/base status (Valenzuela et al, 1995).

Pharmacology, Dosing and Administration

Dosing of atosiban was determined in a dose ranging study comparing five treatments (Goodwin et al, 1996). The recommended dose is a 6.75 mg bolus followed by 300 μg/min for 3 h and 100 μg/min for 18 h. This was the minimal effective dose resulting in rapid cessation of contractions and continued maintenance inhibition of contractions for 24 h.

FUTURE DRUG DEVELOPMENT

Nitric Oxide Analogs

Recently research in animals and humans has proposed nitric oxide (NO) as an endogenous uterine relaxant. Nitric oxide is produced in myometrial cells by the action of nitric oxide synthase. The action of NO results in increased cyclic GMP in myometrial cells which results in uterine relaxation (Buhimschi et al, 1995). Nitric oxide activity and NO production has been shown to decrease at term in some studies (Natuzzi et al, 1993; Sladek et al, 1993; Yallampalli, Garfield & Byam-Smith, 1993). The use of NO donors for uterine relaxation in humans is scarce. A single study of inhaled amyl nitrite blocked oxytocin-mediated but not spontaneous contractions in women in labor at term (Kumar, Zourlas & Barnes, 1965). Amyl nitrate and intravenous nitrogylcerine relaxes the uterus post partum (Hendricks et al, 1992; Altabef, Spencer & Zuberg, 1992; DeSimone, Norris & Leighton, 1990). Only one placebo-controlled trial of nitroglycerin has been conducted (Lees et al, 1994). As nitric oxide donors may have profound blood pressure-lowering effects, these agents may produce cardiovascular side effects, limiting their use as tocolytics. Further work confirming the efficacy of nitric oxide donors in blocking pre-term uterine contractions is needed before such agents are used as tocolytics.

Cytokine Antagonists

As previously discussed, infection accounts for 20% of all pre-term labor. Decidual cytokine release, specifically IL-1 and IL-6, and increased decidual prostaglandin production result in pre-term contractions. The extent to which infection may stimulate labor is modulated by the decidual production of anti-inflammatory cytokines, specifically IL-1 receptor antagonist (IL-1ra) and transforming growth factor β (TGFβ). The IL-1ra is a naturally occurring cytokine which binds the IL-1 receptor and antagonizes the action of IL-1 both in vivo and in vitro. IL-1ra prevents shock and death in rabbits due to lipopolysaccharide and bacteria (Ohlsson et al, 1990; Wakabayashi, 1991). IL-1ra at 100-fold greater concentration than IL-1 is also produced in humans following endotoxin injection (Granowitz et al, 1991). Endogenous IL-1ra production prevents death and shock secondary to infection. IL-1ra therapy may be a useful clinical adjunct to antibiotics for the treatment of infection in humans. IL-1ra appears to play a similar role in infection-mediated pre-term labor. Amniotic fluid contains higher levels of IL-1ra than any other fluid in the body (Romero et al, 1994). The levels increased throughout gestation and in pre-term labor associated with infection but not in term labor associated with infection. Several studies show that IL-1ra is produced by decidua, chorion and amnion with and without stimulation by IL-1, TNFα and LPS (Fidel et al, 1994a). In mice the induction of pre-term birth with IL-1 is completely blocked by co-administration of 100-fold excess IL-1ra (Romero & Tartakovsky, 1992b). In the rhesus monkey model of infection-induced pre-term labor, concentrations of both IL-1 and IL-1ra increases in amniotic fluid (Witkin et al, 1994). Early in infection, IL-1ra blocks the action of IL-1 and animals do not labor. With worsening infection IL-1 production exceeds IL-1ra production, resulting in increased contractions and subsequent pre-term delivery. IL-1ra most likely blocks infection through the down-regulation of PGHS-2 and decidual prostaglandin production (Bry, Lappalainen & Hallman, 1993; Porreca et al, 1996). These data suggest that treatment of pre-term labor in the setting of early infection may be successful using antibiotics in combination with IL-1ra. Whether sufficient IL-1ra can be delivered to the uterus by system administration is not known. Clinical trials in humans are needed to demonstrate the safety of IL-1ra administration before trials in pregnancy can be initiated.

REFERENCES

Akerlund M, Stromberg P, Hauksson A et al. Inhibition of uterine contractions of premature labor with an oxytocin analogue. Results from a pilot study. *Br J Obstet Gynaecol* 1987; **94**: 1040–44.

Alexandrova M, Soloff MS. Oxytocin receptors and parturition. I. Control of oxytocin receptor concentration in the rat myometrium at term. *Endocrinology* 1980; **106**: 730–35.

Altabef KM, Spencer JT, Zinberg S. Intravenous nitrogylcerin for uterine relaxation of an inverted uterus. *Am J Obstet Gynecol* 1992; **166**: 1237–8.

Asboth G, Phaneuf S, Europe-Finner GN et al. Prostaglandin E_2 activates phospholipase C and elevates intracellular calcium in cultured myometrial cells: involvement of EP1 and EP3 receptor subtypes. *Endocrinology* 1996; **137**: 2572–9.

Beall M, Edgar B, Paul R et al. A comparison of ritodrine, terbutaline and magnesium sulfate for the suppression of preterm labor. *Am J Obstet Gynecol* 1985; **153**: 854–9.

Benedetti T. Maternal complications of parenteral beta sympathomimetic therapy for preterm labor. *Am J Obstet Gynecol* 1983; **145**: 1.

Benedetto MT, De Cicco F, Rossiello F et al. Oxytocin receptor in human fetal membranes at term and during labor. *J Steroid Biochem* 1990; **35**: 205–8.

Bergamo RR, Cominelli F, Kopple JD, Zipser RD. Comparative acute effects of aspirin, diflunisal, ibuprofen and indomethacin on renal function in healthy man. *Am J Nephrol* 1989; **9**: 460–63.

Bossmar T, Akerlund M, Fantoni G et al. Receptors for and myometrial response to oxytocin and vasopressin in preterm and term human pregnancy: effects of the oxytocin antagonist atosiban. *Am J Obstet Gynecol* 1994; **171**: 1634–42.

Bry K, Hallman M. Transforming growth factor-β opposes the stimulatory effects of interleukin-1 and tumor necrosis factor on amnion cell prostaglandin E_2 production: implication for preterm labor. *Am J Obstet Gynecol* 1992; **167**: 222–6.

Bry K, Lappalainen U, Hallman M. Interleukin-1 binding and prostaglandin E_2 synthesis by amnion cells in culture: regulation by tumor necrosis factor-α, transforming growth factor-β, and interleukin-1 receptor antagonist. *Biochim Biophs Acta* 1993; **1181**: 31–6.

Buhimschi I, Yallampalli C, Dong YL, Garfield RE. Involvement of a nitric oxide–cyclic guanosine monophosphate pathway in control of human uterine contractility during pregnancy. *Am J Obstet Gynecol* 1995; **172**: 1577–84.

Cagossi M, Salgarello M, Patrignani P, Salgarello G. Effects of various prostaglandin synthesis inhibitors on the tone of the lower esophageal sphincter in man. *Eur J Pharmacol* 1992; **43**: 303–5.

Canadian Preterm Labor Investigators' Group. Treatment of preterm labor with beta-adrenergic agonist ritodrine. *N Engl J Med* 1992; **327**: 308–12.

Caritis SN, Chiao JP, Kridgen P. Comparison of pulsatile and continuous ritodrine administration: effects on uterine contractility and β-adrenergic receptor cascade. *Am J Obstet Gynecol* 1991; **164**: 1005–12.

Caritis SN, Venkataraman R, Darby MJ et al. Pharmacokinetics of ritodrine administered intravenously: recommendations for changes in current regimen. *Am J Obstet Gynecol* 1990; **162**: 429–37.

Casey ML, Cox SM, Beutler B et al. Cachectin/tumor necrosis factor-α formation in human decidua: potential role of cytokines in infection-induced preterm labor. *J Clin Invest* 1989; **83**: 430–36.

Casey ML, MacDonald PC. Biomolecular processes in the initiation of parturition: decidual activation. *Clin Obstet Gynecol* 1988; **31**: 533–52.

Chibbar R, Miller FD, Mitchell BF. Synthesis of oxytocin in amnion, chorion, and decidua may influence the timing of human parturition. *J Clin Invest* 1993; **91**: 185–92.

Cotton D, Strasser H, Hill L et al. Comparison of magnesium sulfate, terbutaline, and placebo for the inhibition of preterm labor. *J Repro Med* 1984; **29**: 92–7.

Cox S, Sherman L, Leveno K. Randomized investigation of magnesium sulfate for prevention of preterm birth. *Am J Obstet Gynecol* 1990; **163**: 767–72.

Daftary AR, Rauk PN, Caritis SN. A pharmacokinetic approach to preterm labor inhibition. *J Matern Fetal Med* 1992; **1**: 104–16.

DeSimone CA, Norris MC, Leighton BL. Intravenous nitroglycerin aids manual extraction of a retained placenta. *Anesthesiology* 1990; **73**: 787.

Elliott JP. Magnesium sulfate as a tocolytic agent. *Contemp Obstet Gynecol* 1985; **June**: 49–61.

Evans MA, Bhat R, Vidyasager D et al. Gestational age and indomethacin elimination in the neonate. *Clin Pharmacol Ther* 1979; **26**: 746–51.

Ferguson J, Dyson D, Holbrook R et al. Cardiovascular and metabolic effects associated with nifedipine and ritodrine tocolysis. *Am J Obstet Gynecol* 1989a; **161**: 788.

Ferguson J, Schultz T, Pershe R et al. Nifedipine pharmacokinetics during preterm labor tocolysis. *Am J Obstet Gynecol* 1989b; **160**: 1485–90.

Ferguson J, Dyson D, Schultz T, Stevenson D. A comparison of nifedipine and ritodrine for the treatment of preterm labor. *Am J Obstet Gynecol* 1990; **163**: 150.

Fidel PL, Romero R, Ramirez M et al. Interleukin-1 receptor antagonist (IL-1ra) production by human amnion, chorion, and decidua. *Am J Reprod Immunol* 1994a; **32**: 1–7.

Fuchs A-R, Husslein P, Fuchs F. Oxytocin and the initiation of human parturition. II. Stimulation of prostaglandin production in human decidua by oxytocin. *Am J Obstet Gynecol* 1981; **141**: 694–7.

Fuchs A-R, Fuchs F, Husslein F, Soloff MS. Oxytocin receptors in the human uterus during pregnancy and parturition. *Am J Obstet Gynecol* 1984; **150**: 734–41.

Fuchs A-R, Romero R, Keefe D et al. Oxytocin secretion and human parturition: pulse frequency and duration increase during spontaneous labor in women. *Am J Obstet Gynecol* 1991; **165**: 1515–23.

Futaki N, Takahashi S, Yokoyama M et al. NS-398, a new anti-inflammatory agent, selectively inhibits prostaglandin G/H sythase/cyclooxygenase (COX-2) activity in vitro. *Prostaglandins* 1994; **47**: 55–9.

Gibb W, Sun M. Localization of prostaglandin H synthase type 2 and mRNA in term human fetal membranes and decidua. *J Endocrinol* 1996; **150**: 497–503.

Glock JL, Morales WJ. Efficacy and safety of nifedipine versus magnesium sulfate in the management of preterm labor: a randomized study. *Am J Obstet Gynecol* 1993; **169**: 960–64.

Goodwin TM, Paul R, Sliver H et al. The effect of the oxytocin antagonist atosiban on preterm uterine activity in the human. *Am J Obstet Gynecol* 1994; **170**: 474–8.

Goodwin TM, Valenzuela GJ, Silver H et al. Dose ranging study of the oxytocin receptor antagonist in the treatment of preterm labor. *Obstet Gynecol* 1996; **88**: 331–6.

Gordon M, Samuels P, Johnson F et al. A randomized, prospective study of adjunctive ceftizoxime in preterm labor. *Am J Obstet Gynecol* 1995; **172**: 1546–52.

Granowitz EV, Santosi AA, Poutsiaka DD et al. Production of interleukin-1-receptor antagonist during experimental endotoxaemia. *Lancet* 1991; **338**: 1423–4.

Groome LJ, Goldenberg RL, Cliver SP et al. Neonatal periventricular–intraventricular hemorrhage after maternal beta-sympathomimetic tocolysis. *Am J Obstet Gynecol* 1992; **167**: 873–9.

Hallak M, Berry SM, Madincea F et al. Fetal serum and amniotic fluid magnesium concentrations with maternal treatment. *Obstet Gynecol* 1993; **81**: 185–8.

Hankins G, Hauth JC. A comparison of the relative toxicities of β-sympathomimetic tocolytic agents. *Amer J Perinatol* 1985; **2**: 338–46.

Harake B, Gilbert RD, Ashwal S, Power GG. Nifedipine: effects on fetal and maternal hemodynamics in pregnant sheep. *Am J Obstet Gynecol* 1989; **157**: 1003–8.

Hausdorff WP, Caron MG, Lefkowitz RJ. Turning off the signal: desensitization of β-adrenergic receptor function. *FASEB J* 1990; **4**: 2881–9.

Heijden AJ, Provoost AP, Nauta J et al. Renal function impairment in preterm neonates related to intrauterine indomethacin exposure. *Pediatr Res* 1988; **24**: 644–8.

Hellenberg L. Clinical pharmacokinetics of indomethacin. *Clin Pharmacokinet* 1981; **6**: 245–58.

Hendricks S, Keroes J, Katz M. Electrocardiographic changes associated with ritodrine-induced maternal tachycardia and hypokalemia. *Am J Obstet Gynecol* 1986; **154**: 921.

Hendricks SK, Ross B, Colvard MA et al. Amyl nitrite: use as a smooth muscle relaxant in difficult preterm cesarean section. *Am J Perinatol* 1992; **9**: 289–92.

Hillier SL, Witkin SS, Krohn MA et al. The relationship of amniotic fluid cytokines and preterm delivery, amniotic fluid infection, histologic chorioamnionitis, and chorioamnion infection. *Obstet Gynecol* 1993; **81**: 941–8.

Hirst JJ, Teixeira FJ, Zaker T, Olson DM. Prostaglandin endoperoxide-H synthase-1 and -2 messenger ribonucleic acid levels in human amnion with spontaneous labor onset. *J Clin Endocrinol Metab* 1995; **80**: 517–23.

Hollander D, Nagey D, Pupkin M. Magnesium sulfate and ritodrine hydrochloride: a randomized comparison. *Am J Obstet Gynecol* 1987; **156**: 631–7.

Ikeda M, Shibata Y, Yamamoto T. Rapid formation of myometrial gap junctions during parturition in the unilaterally implanted rat uterus. *Cell Tissue Res* 1987; **248**: 297.

King J, Grant A, Keirse M, Chalmers I. Beta-mimetics in preterm labor: an overview of the randomized clinical trials. *Br J Obstet Gynaecol* 1988; **95**: 211–22.

Kirshon B, Moise KJ, Wasserstrum N et al. Influence of short-term indomethacin therapy on fetal urine output. *Obstet Gynecol* 1988; **72**: 51–3.

Ku CY, Qian A, Wen Y et al. Oxytocin stimulates myometrial guanosine triphosphatase and phospholipase-C activities via coupling to $G_{\alpha-q/11}$. *Endocrinology* 1995; **136**: 1509–15.

Kumar D, Zourlas PA, Barnes AC. In vivo effect of amyl nitrite on human pregnant uterine contractility. *Am J Obstet Gynecol* 1965; **91**: 1066–8.

Kumasaka D, Lindeman KS, Clancy J et al. $MgSO_4$ relaxes porcine airway muscle by reducing Ca^{2+} entry. *Am J Physiol* 1996; **270**: L469–74.

Lam F, Gill P, Smith M et al. Use of the subcutaneous terbutaline pump for long-term tocolysis. *Obstet Gynecol* 1988; **72**: 810–13.

Leake RD, Weitzman RE, Glatz TH, Fisher DA. Plasma oxytocin concentrations in men, nonpregnant women, and pregnant women before and during spontaneous labor. *J Clin Endocrinol Metab* 1981; **53**: 730–33.

Lees C, Campbell S, Jauniaux E et al. Arrest of preterm labour and prolongation of gestation with glyceryl trinitrate, a nitric oxide donor. *Lancet* 1994; **343**: 1325–6.

Lipshitz J, Ballie P, Davey DA. A comparison of the uterine beta-2-adrenoreceptor selectivity of fenoterol, hexoprenaline, ritodrine and salbutamol. *S Afr Med J* 1976; **50**: 1969–72.

Lipshitz J, Lipshitz EM. Uterine and cardiovascular effects of fenoterol and hexoprenaline in prostaglandin $F_{2\alpha}$-induced labor in humans. *Obstet Gynecol* 1984; **63**: 396–400.

Lundin-Schiller S, Mitchell MD. Prostaglandin production by human chorion laeve cells in response to inflammatory mediators. *Placenta* 1991; **12**: 353–63.

Major CA, Lewis DF, Harding JA et al. Tocolysis with indomethacin increases the incidence of necrotizing enterocolitis in the low-birth-weight neonate. *Am J Obstet Gynecol* 1994; **170**: 102–6.

Mari G, Kirshon B, Moise KJ et al. Doppler assessment of the fetal and uteroplacental circulation during nifedipine therapy for preterm labor. *Am J Obstet Gynecol* 1989; **161**: 1514–18.

McAllister RG. Kinetics and dynamics of nifedipine after oral and sublingual doses. *Am J Med* 1986; **81**: 2–5.

McGregor JA, French JI, Reller LB et al. Adjunctive erythromycin treatment for idiopathic preterm labor: results of a randomized double-blind, placebo-controlled trial. *Am J Obstet Gynecol* 1986; **154**: 98–103.

McGregor JA, French JJ, Seo K. Adjunctive clindamycin therapy for preterm labour: results of a double-blind placebo controlled trial. *Am J Obstet Gynecol* 1991; **165**: 867–75.

Mitchell JA, Akarasereenont P, Thiemermann C et al. Selectivity of nonsteroidal anti-inflammatory drugs as inhibitors of constitutive and inducible cyclo-oxygenase. *Proc Natl Acad Sci USA* 1994; **90**; 11693–7.

Mitchell MD, Trautman MS, Dudley DJ. Cytokine networking in the placenta. *Placenta* 1993; **14**: 249–75.

Mizuki J, Tasaka K, Masumato N et al. Magnesium sulfate inhibits oxytocin-induced calcium mobilization in human puerperal myometrial cells: possible involvement of intracellular free magnesium concentration. *Am J Obstet Gynecol* 1993; **169**: 134–9.

Moise K, Ou C, Kirshon B et al. Placental transfer of indomethacin in human pregnancy. *Am J Obstet Gynecol* 1990; **162**: 549–54.

Moise KJ, Huhta JC, Sharif DS et al. Indomethacin in the treatment of premature labor: effects on the fetal ductus arteriosus. *N Engl J Med* 1988; **318**: 327–31.

Moise KJ, Sala DJ, Zurawin RK et al. Continuous subcutaneous terbutaline pump therapy for premature labor: safety and efficacy. *Southern Med J* 1992; **85**: 255–60.

Molnar M, Romero R, Hertelendy F. Interleukin-1 and tumor necrosis factor stimulate arachidonic acid release and phospholipid metabolism in human myometrial cells. *Am J Obstet Gynecol* 1993; **169**: 825–9.

Morales WJ, Angel JL, O'Brian WF et al. A randomized study of antibiotic therapy in idiopathic preterm labor. *Obstet Gynecol* 1988; **72**: 829–33.

Naderali EK, Poyser NL. Effect of a selective prostaglandin H synthase-2 inhibitor (NS-398) on prostaglandin production by guinea-pig uterus. *J Reprod Fertil* 1996; **108**: 75–80.

National Center for Health Statistics. *Advance Report on Final Natality Statistics, 1989. Monthly Statistics Report* 1991, vol. 40; Hyattsville, MD: US Public Health Service.

Natuzzi ES, Ursell PC, Harrison M et al. Nitric oxide synthase activity in the pregnant uterus decreases at parturition. *Biochem Biophys Res Comm* 1993; **194**: 1–8.

Newton ER, Dinsmoor MJ, Gibbs RS. A randomized blinded placebo controlled trial of antibiotics in idiopathic preterm labor. *Obstet Gynecol* 1989; **74**: 562–6.

Newton ER, Shields L, Ridgeway LE III et al. Combination antibiotics and indomethacin in idiopathic preterm labor: a randomized double-blind clinical trial. *Am J Obstet Gynecol* 1991; **165**: 1753–9.

Niebyl JR, Blake DA, White RD et al. The inhibition of premature labor with indomethacin. *Am J Obstet Gynecol* 1980; **136**: 1014–19.

Norman K, Pattinson RC, de Souza J et al. Ampicillin and metronidazole treatment in preterm labor: a multicenter randomised controlled trial. *Br J Obstet Gynaecol* 1994; **101**: 404–8.

Norton ME, Merrill J, Cooper BAB et al. Neonatal complications after the administration of indomethacin for preterm labor. *N Engl J Med* 1993; **329**: 1602–7.

Ohlsson K, Bjork P, Bergenfeldt M et al. Interleukin-1 receptor antagonist reduces mortality from endotoxin shock. *Nature* 1990; **348**: 550–52.

Phaneuf S, Asboth G, MacKenzie IZ et al. Effect of oxytocin antagonists on the activation of human myometrium in vitro: atosiban prevents oxytocin-induced desensitization. *Am J Obstet Gynecol* 1994; **171**: 627–34.

Porreca E, Reale M, Di Febbo C et al. Down-regulation of cyclooxygenase-2 (COX-2) by interleukin-1 receptor antagonist in human monocytes. *Immunology* 1996; **89**: 424–9.

Romero R, Avila C, Santhanam U, Sehgal PB. Amniotic fluid interleukin 6 in preterm labor. *J Clin Invest* 1990; **85**: 1392–1400.

Romero R, Brody DT, Oyarzun E et al. Infection and labor. III. Interleukin-1: a signal for the onset of parturition. *Am J Obstet Gynecol* 1989a; **160**: 1117–23.

Romero R, Gomez R, Galasso M et al. The natural interleukin-1 receptor antagonist in the fetal, maternal, and amniotic fluid compartments: the effect of gestational age, fetal gender, and intrauterine infection. *Am J Obstet Gynecol* 1994; **171**: 912–21.

Romero R, King Y, Brody DT et al. Human decidua: a source of interleukin-1. *Obstet Gynecol* 1989b; **73**: 31–4.

Romero R, Manogue KR, Mitchell MD et al. Infection and labor. IV. Cachectin-tumor necrosis factor in the amniotic fluid of women with intra-amniotic infection and preterm labor. *Am J Obstet Gynecol* 1989c; **161**: 336–41.

Romero R, Mazor M. Infection and preterm labor. *Clin Obstet Gynecol* 1988; **31**(3): 553–61.

Romero R, Sibai B, Caritis S et al. Antibiotic treatment of preterm labor with intact membranes: a multicenter randomized double-blinded placebo-controlled trial. *Am J Obstet Gynecol* 1993; **169**: 764–74.

Romero R, Tartakovsky B. The natural interleukin-1 receptor antagonist prevents interleukin-1 induced preterm delivery in mice. *Am J Obstet Gynecol* 1992b; **167**: 1041–5.

Sanchez-Ramos L, Valenzuela G, Romero R et al. A double-blind placebo-controlled trial of the oxytocin recepter antagonist atosiban (Antocin™) in maintenance therapy in patients with preterm labor. Abstract 69, Society of Perinatal Obstetricians; *Am J Obstet Gynecol* 1997; **176**(1, part 2): S30.

Santi MD, Henry GW, Douglas GL. Magnesium sulfate treatment of preterm labor as a cause of abnormal neonatal bone mineralization. *J Pediatr Ortho* 1994; **14**: 249–53.

Sibai BM, Romero R, Sanchez-Ramos L et al. A double-blind placebo-controlled trial of an oxytocin receptor antagonist atosiban (Antocin™) in the treatment of preterm labor. Abstract 2, Society of Perinatal Obstetricians; *Am J Obstet Gynecol* 1997; **176**(1, part 2): S2.

Sladek SM, Regenstein AC, Lykins D, Roberts JM. Nitric oxide synthase activity in pregnant rabbit uterus decreases on the last day of pregnancy. *Am J Obstet Gynecol* 1993; **169**: 1285–91.

Slater DM, Berger LC, Newton R et al. Expression of cyclo-oxygenase types 1 and 2 in human fetal membranes at term. *Am J Obstet Gynecol* 1995; **172**: 77–82.

Soloff MS, Hinko A. Oxytocin receptors and prostaglandin release in rabbit amnion. *Ann NY Acad Sci* 1993; **689**: 207–18.

Steer C, Petrie R. A comparison of magnesium sulfate and alcohol for the prevention of premature labor. *Am J Obstet Gynecol* 1977; **129**: 1–4.

Takahashi D, Diamond F, Bieniarz J et al. Uterine contractility and oxytocin sensitivity in preterm, term, and post-term pregnancy. *Am J Obstet Gynecol* 1980; **136**: 774–9.

Thaler I, Weiner Z, Manor D, Itskovitz J. Effect of calcium channel blocker nifedipine on uterine artery flow velocity waveforms. *J Ultrasound Med* 1991; **10**: 301–4.

Thornton S, Davison JM, Baylis PH. Plasma oxytocin during the first and second stages of spontaneous human labour. *Acta Endocrinol* 1992; **126**: 425–9.

Tulzer G, Gudmundsson S, Tews G et al. Incidence of indomethacin-induced human fetal ductus arteriosus constriction. *J Matern Fetal Invest* 1992; **1**: 267.

Valenzuela GJ, Craig J, Bernhardt MD, Holland ML. Placental passage of the oxytocin receptor antagonist atosiban. *Am J Obstet Gynecol* 1995; **172**: 1304–6.

Wilkins I, Lynch L, Mehalek K et al. Efficacy and side effects of magnesium sulfate and ritodrine as tocolytic agents. *Am J Obstet Gynecol* 1988; **159**: 685–9.

Wilson T, Liggins GC, Whittaker DJ. Oxytocin stimulates the release of arachidonic acid and prostaglandin $F_{2\alpha}$ from human decidual cells. *Prostaglandins* 1988; **35**(5): 771–80.

Winkler M, Baumann L, Ruchhaberle KE, Schiller EM. Erythromycin therapy for subclinical intrauterine infections in threatened preterm delivery—a preliminary report. *J Perinatal Med* 1988; **16**: 253–6.

Witkin SS, Gravett MG, Haluska GJ, Novy MJ. Induction of interleukin-1 receptor antagonist in rhesus monkeys after intraamniotic infection with group B streptococci interleukin-1 infusion. *Am J Obstet Gynecol* 1994; **171**: 1668–72.

Wurtzel D. Prenatal administration of indomethacin as a tocolytic agent: effect on neonatal renal function. *Obstet Gynecol* 1990; **76**: 689–92.

Yallampalli C, Garfield RE, Byam-Smith M. Nitric oxide inhibits uterine contractility during pregnancy but not during delivery. *Endocrinology* 1993; **133**: 1899–902.

Zuckerman H, Shalev E, Gilad G, Katzuni E. Futhur study of the inhibition of premature labor by indomethacin: Part II. Double-blind study. *J Perinatol* 1984; **12**: 25–9.

10

Drug Development for Pregnancy

Gautum Chaudhuri[1], George P. Giacoia[2] and Sumner Y. Yaffe[2]

[1]*UCLA School of Medicine, Los Angeles, CA, and* [2]*National Institutes of Health, Bethesda, MD, USA*

One of the most neglected areas in clinical pharmacology and pharmaceutical research involves the study of therapeutic drug use in pregnancy. As a consequence, only a handful of drugs have been approved by the FDA for use during pregnancy. Nonetheless, drug prescribing during pregnancy occurs at a great frequency for the management of maternal disease. The complexities of drug use in pregnancy revolve around the distinctly different metabolic and physiologic attributes of the mother and the fetus which occur during pregnancy. There is a specific set of alterations that occur in the pregnant state, both in the mother and in the fetus, and these vary according to the stage of gestation. For the mother, these involve progressive changes in the intravascular volume and body water, renal blood flow and changes in hepatic enzymes, which in turn will modulate the effects of drugs during pregnancy. Many drugs will cross the placental barrier in significant amounts and will be available for action on and distribution within the fetus. The placenta is a metabolically active organ that can participate in the biotransformation of xenobiotics. The distribution and handling of drugs by the fetus depends on the stage of fetal maturation and these variables may play a role in fetal response to the drug.

To understand how the disposition and effects of drugs are altered during pregnancy, knowledge of their pharmacokinetics and pharmacodynamics is necessary (Krauer, Krauer & Hytten, 1984). *Pharmacokinetics* involves the complex interaction of absorption, distribution, binding or localization in tissues, transformation and elimination of a drug. These factors determine the drug concentration at receptor sites. *Pharmacodynamics* is concerned with the mechanism(s) and final outcome of the biochemical and physiological effects of drugs. Pharmacodynamics therefore determines the clinical effects and the therapeutic outcome. Quantitation of clinical effects is usually more complicated than quantitation of plasma drug concentrations, but for many drugs there is considerable clinical and pharmacological evidence of a close relation between the concentration of a drug in body fluids and its effects.

Drug Development for Women. Edited by V.V. Ragavan. © 1998 John Wiley & Sons Ltd.

Physiological functions which determine the disposition of drugs may show large individual differences due to numerous factors, including genetics, sex, age, body weight, diet, intake of other drugs and smoking and may also be modified in many ways by disease. Pregnancy, in particular, is characterized by progressive and widespread morphological and physiological changes of such a degree as to mimic pathological states; similar parameters which would be considered to be within normal limits in non-pregnant women may reflect pathological conditions in pregnancy. The complexities of drug disposition in the pregnant woman occur not only because the organism which is to be treated has become a highly intricate unit consisting of the mother and the product of conception, but also because this integrated system undergoes continuous specific changes as pregnancy advances, which may significantly alter the absorption and disposition of drugs and thereby influence their pharmacological effects. It is sometimes erroneously assumed that, for therapeutic purposes, a pregnant woman is no more than a non-pregnant woman with a passive fetus attached. In fact, every component of pharmacokinetics may be progressively modified by morphological and physiological changes which characterize pregnancy. It is also important to realize that the placenta is not a barrier to the transfer of drugs from the mother to her fetus and that the placenta has its own specific functional characteristics of drug disposition particularly related to drug metabolism. The major reason for drug therapy in pregnancy is based on maternal rather than on embryonic or fetal requirements and the fetus is in most cases an unintentional and possibly non-benefiting recipient. The susceptibility to a drug may be entirely different in the mother and fetus and hence there is the possibility that a drug may prove devastating for the embryo or the fetus but harmless or favorable for the mother. Therefore, the possible effects elicited by drugs in the developing organism and the potential risks to the offspring (the fetus, the newborn, or even after some latency the child or the adult), have to be considered.

The decision of whether a drug should be used during pregnancy should depend on the probability of an eventual beneficial effect for the mother and/or for the conceptus; a lack of benefit or, worse, the likelihood of adverse drug effect should dissuade one from using the drug. Unfortunately, while these principles may appear very simple, in practice there are enormous difficulties. Information on drug disposition and pharmacokinetics in human pregnancy is fragmentary and insight into pharmacodynamics virtually incomplete. The reason for this lack of information is that, ethically, drugs can only be given for a clinical need, so that standardized experimental conditions are difficult to achieve. Equally, access to the human fetal–placental unit is restricted for technical, ethical and legal reasons, and samples of body fluids from the product of conception can usually be taken only at delivery. Animal experiments are only of limited value since human reproductive physiology, particularly placental function, differs in so many respects from that of other species that the relevance of animal data is always in doubt.

REASON FOR THE NEED FOR DRUG THERAPY IN PREGNANCY

The great majority of pregnancies are normal and therefore, ideally, pregnant women should usually be prescribed only a small number of drugs for specific medical indications. In reality, a large number of drugs are taken by pregnant women, prescribed for the treatment of the many symptoms that are characteristic of the normal pregnancy. Maternal disease may endanger the developing conceptus and the identification of high-risk mother and fetus is important, since adequate management, including the use of drugs, can significantly improve the obstetric outcome. Theoretically, the fetus may thereby become exposed to a double risk, that from the maternal disease and that from the drugs used to treat it. It is impossible to guarantee absolute safety from drug exposure, but it would mean denying treatment and benefits of treatment to the pregnant woman.

INFLUENCE OF PHYSIOLOGICAL CHANGES IN PREGNANCY ON DRUG HANDLING

Every component of pharmacokinetics is modified, and progressively so, by the continuous morphological and physiological changes associated with pregnancy (Krauer, Krauer & Hytten, 1980).

Ingestion

Pregnancy has considerable influence on compliance, where women sometimes refuse to take any drugs during pregnancy on the grounds that the fetus might be harmed. Other reasons for not being compliant are because the common symptoms of nausea and heartburn and vomiting may reject any drug that is taken.

Absorption

Gastric Function

The stomach empties more slowly and gut motility is retarded, so that gastrointestinal transit is prolonged by 30–50% (Davison, Davison & Hay, 1970; Parry, Shields & Turnbull, 1970). This could reduce the rate and completeness of drug absorption. This theory may not be completely borne out in practice and may therefore be less important from a drug development point of view. With the possible exception of digoxin (Luxford & Kellaway, 1983), drug absorption does not appear to be appreciably changed until the very end of pregnancy when, largely because of opiate administration, sluggish gastric emptying postpones drug responses and a parenteral route of administration is preferred (Nimmo, Wilson & Prescott, 1975). Gastric emptying appears to be delayed in pregnancy particularly if a high-osmolality liquid meal is taken (Lind & Hytten, 1969) and conspicuously delayed in labor, particularly in association with narcotic analgesics (Nimmo, Wilson & Prescott, 1975) and possibly also with antacids, so that drugs may be erratically absorbed and may, with repeated doses, accumulate in the stomach and possibly result in toxic doses when the stomach empties.

Function of the Small Intestine

The small intestine shares the general sluggishness of the gut in pregnancy, so that transit time is prolonged, and in some cases this is considerable (Parry, Shields & Turnbull, 1970). There is no evidence that this has any influence on drug absorption but, in theory, slower mixing and slower passage of intestinal contents could lead to more prolonged contact with the absorbing surface and thus to more complete absorption. For drugs whose elimination is saturable (concentration-dependent), delayed absorption will tend to minimize the saturation phenomena. On the other hand, for drugs which are metabolized in the gut wall, such as chlorpromazine (Dahl & Strandjord, 1977), less of the parent drug will reach the systemic circulation and bioavailability will be reduced. During drug development, it is therefore important to know whether a given drug is metabolized in the gut wall.

In conditions where transit time is artificially shortened, as, for example, after surgical removal of a large amount of small intestine (Montgomery & Pincus, 1955), or following jejunal ileostomy for the treatment of obesity (Olon et al, 1976), pregnancy may exert a beneficial effect in reducing motility and affording more time for absorption. Many pregnant women take regular supplements of iron salts and there may be a high iron concentration in the gut contents. Salts of aluminum, magnesium and calcium are also commonly taken. It is therefore important to realize that these could chelate and interfere with absorption of drugs such as tetracycline (Neuvonen, 1976).

Epidural Space

Demerol placed in the epidural space is much more rapidly absorbed in pregnancy than in the non-pregnant woman and its concentration in blood differs little from a direct intravenous injection (Husemeyer et al, 1981). The difference between the pregnant and non-pregnant state in this context is presumably due to greatly increased vascularity in the epidural space during pregnancy, and any of the drugs instilled there would be liable to rapid absorption also. The dosage of drugs administered by this route therefore needs to be adjusted during pregnancy.

DISTRIBUTION OF DRUGS DURING PREGNANCY

Drug distribution is related to body composition and in pregnancy the absorbed drug is diluted in a greatly increased but highly variable distribution volume. Moreover, the distribution of drug molecules throughout the body depends on their lipid solubility (which determines transfer across lipid membranes and uptake by adipose tissue), and their inclination to bind to proteins in either plasma or extravascular tissue. Once equilibrium distribution has occurred, the apparent volume in which the drug is distributed is the proportionality constant relating the amount of drug in the body compared with the drug concentration measured in the plasma: it has no reality in terms of organ or body fluid compartments. Drugs with small apparent volumes of distribution are those with low lipid solubility and those which bind heavily to plasma proteins, while those with large volumes of distribution are highly lipid-soluble and are often heavily bound to tissue protein (Mucklow, 1986).

In pregnancy, total body water increases by up to 8 liters (Hytten & Leitch, 1971) and plasma volume by 50% (Piraui, Campbell & MacGillivray, 1973). The concentration of plasma albumin (to which most acidic drugs, such as phenytoin, are bound) falls by 5–10 g/l (Rebond et al, 1963) and endogenous ligands such as free fatty acids compete with drugs for binding sites on both albumin and α_1-acid glycoprotein (to which basic drugs, such as propranolol, bind). The average pregnant woman eating normally stores between 3 and 4 kg of body fat, largely in subcutaneous depots (Hytten & Leitch, 1971). Such a store is associated with an average weight increase of about 12 kg for the whole pregnancy and it is likely that weight gains substantially more or less than the average 12 kg will have a disproportionate effect on body fat storage. Thus, a woman who in an otherwise normal pregnancy gains only 8 kg of body weight may store little or no fat; one who gains 20 kg may well have accumulated 10 kg of fat. Fat is gained in the first two trimesters of pregnancy with little further increase in late pregnancy. There is a tendency for fat to be mobilized in the last trimester of pregnancy, with an increase in the plasma of free fatty acids and glycerol (McDonald-Gibson, Young & Hytten, 1975). The large accumulation of fat by many pregnant women will provide a greatly increased storage area for fat-soluble substances and has been used to explain, for example, the more pronounced postanesthetic somnolence after thiopentone due to slow release from this reservoir.

The implications of these changes in body composition, all of which will influence the apparent volume of distribution and, hence, plasma drug concentration, are likely to be greatest for drugs of relatively low lipid solubility that are highly bound to plasma protein (e.g. anticonvulsants, benzodiazepines). An increased distribution volume will reduce peak plasma drug concentration after a dose and will retard drug elimination (i.e. half-life will be longer) unless there is a simultaneous increase in clearance by metabolism or excretion. The mathematical relationship between these parameters is given by the following equation:

$$\text{half-life} = \frac{\text{volume of distribution}}{\text{clearance}} \times \log c^2$$

The consequences of a reduction in plasma protein binding per se are, at first sight, surprising. Less binding, for whatever reason, results in a larger fraction of unbound drug: these molecules are free to escape from the circulation to be distributed more widely to exert pharmacological effects, and to be eliminated by metabolism or excretion. Greater elimination prevents an increase in tissue concentration. In pregnancy, the net result of the gradual increase in unbound fraction, together with remodulation, results in a lower total drug concentration in plasma (Mucklow, 1986). The therapeutic range of concentration for drugs whose use is monitored by measurements of total plasma concentration must be adjusted downwards if their binding changes during pregnancy; phenytoin is the classical example (Perucca & Crema, 1982).

Maternal cardiac output increases about 30–50% during pregnancy (Katz, Karliner & Renik, 1978), with the mean increase being about 33% from a non-pregnant level of 4.5 l/min to a pregnancy maximum of approximately 6 l/min (Hytten & Lind, 1973); according to these authors, cardiac output is maximal by 10 weeks' gestation. Other investigators (Elkayam & Gleicher, 1982) state that the rising cardiac output is most rapid during the first trimester but that smaller increments continue to a peak at about 20–24 weeks. There is almost universal agreement now that cardiac output remains maximal until delivery. The increase in cardiac output in pregnancy is distributed to the various circulatory beds. The uterine circulation shows a steady increase throughout pregnancy to reach a maximum at term of about 500 ml/min (de Swiet, 1980). The renal plasma flow increases markedly and quite early in pregnancy. The effective renal plasma flow (ERPF) is increased 75% over non-pregnant levels to a mean value of 840 ml/min by 16 weeks' gestation (Dunlop, 1981). This increase is maintained until the late third trimester, when a small but significant decline in ERPF occurs. The late pregnancy fall in ERPF has been well demonstrated in subjects studied serially in both sitting and left lateral recumbent positions. Like ERPF, glomerular filtration rate (GFR) measured by insulin clearance increases early in pregnancy with increases demonstrated by 5–7 weeks; by the end of the first trimester, GFR is 50% higher than in the non-pregnant state (Dunlop, 1981). This increase is maintained until the end of pregnancy; there is no late pregnancy fall in GFR as occurs with ERPF. The endogenous creatinine clearance is greatly increased in pregnancy and values of 150–200 ml/min are normal. As with GFR, the increase in creatinine clearance begins by 5–7 weeks' gestation, is maximal by the end of the first trimester, and is maintained at maximum levels until after delivery (Dunlop, 1981). Thus, the clearance of drugs which are excreted unchanged (such as gentamicin and digoxin) is directly proportional to the clearance of creatinine. During pregnancy, higher doses of the drug and/or more frequent administration of the drug may therefore be necessary if the drug is cleared by the kidney.

DRUG METABOLISM

Water-soluble drugs escape reabsorption from the renal tubule after glomerular filtration and are eliminated in an unchanged form. Lipid-soluble drugs have to be rendered more polar by metabolism prior to excretion in bile or urine. This is achieved most commonly by oxidation (e.g. hydroxylation, demethylation) or by conjugation (e.g. with glucuronide, or sulfate). The overall activity of drug-metabolizing enzyme systems is reflected by the urinary excretion of endogenous waste products, such as 6-β-hydrocortisol and D-glucaric acid, which are useful indirect indices. In pregnancy, increased excretion of these products (Frantz, Katz & Jailer, 1960; Davis et al, 1973) and histological evidence of hyperplasia of the endoplasmic reticulum in liver cells imply that drug metabolism is induced and progesterone is held responsible in large part (Mucklow, 1986). Indeed, the increase in the two isoforms of flavin-containing monoxygenase isoforms during mid- and late human gestation appears to be regulated by progesterone (Lee et al, 1995). Earlier animal studies had shown a pregnancy-induced depression in hepatic microsomal enzyme activity (Dean & Stock, 1975).

New knowledge on the metabolism of drugs given during pregnancy suggests that pregnancy may be associated with more complex alterations in drug metabolizing enzymes than had been previously thought. The metabolism of carbamazepine and phenytoin provides an interesting example of this complexity. Both carbamazepine and phenytoin are biotransformed following similar pathways. They are first oxidized to form phenolic compounds and arene oxides (epoxides) in different proportions; the former predominates with phenytoin and the latter with carbamazepine. The epoxides are subsequently hydrolized to phenolic derivatives that are conjugated mostly with glucuronic acid. During pregnancy the microsomal oxidation of carbamazepine to its 10, 11 epoxide more than doubles, but subsequent biotransformation increases only by 25%. Consequently, the epoxide derivative accumulates. It is important to note that carbamazepine epoxide retains the pharmacologic activity of the parent compounds. In contrast, although the initial metabolism of phenytoin is also increased and intermediary metabolites accumulate, they are devoid of pharmacologic effect (Bernus, Hooper & Eadie, 1997).

Although metabolism of drugs also occurs in both the placenta and the fetal liver, the relative contribution made by these organs to the clearance of drugs from the maternal body is thought to be small. However, it would be important during drug development to assess the metabolism of drugs by the placenta and if possible to assess the amount of active drug that passes to the fetus. It will also be important to assess whether the fetus has the capability to dispose of the active drug in order to prevent adverse effects of the drug or its metabolite on the fetus.

Receptor Sensitivity

There are very few studies that have assessed whether the sensitivity of maternal receptor tissue to drugs is altered in pregnancy. The magnitude of drug response is wholly dependent upon the number of drug molecules reaching the target tissue, and any differences which may be apparent between the pregnant and the non-pregnant woman may result from changes in drug handling.

USE OF SPECIFIC DRUGS DURING PREGNANCY

Antibiotics

Ampicillin

Ampicillin is one of the most widely used and studied drugs with respect to its pharmacokinetics in pregnancy. Philipson (1979) measured the volume of distribution and half-life for intravenous ampicillin in women requiring treatment during pregnancy. These women were subsequently re-evaluated for these pharmacokinetic indices following the completion of pregnancy, allowing each woman to serve as her own control. The use of these parameters suggests that by term the initial concentration of ampicillin is almost half the initial concentration in the non-pregnant state following an intravenous bolus of 500 mg. The plasma concentration of ampicillin decreases more rapidly during pregnancy because the rate of elimination of the drug is increased. If therapeutic responses to ampicillin requires that the area under the curve (AUC) in pregnant patients should be the same as that in non-pregnant patients following ampicillin administration, the dose will have to be increased. The doses of ampicillin at 10, 20, 30 and 40 weeks of gestation that will produce the same AUC as in the non-pregnant state given 500 mg of ampicillin are 770, 823, 892 and 953 mg (Philipson, 1977, 1978). If treatment is by intermittent bolus dosing of 500 mg every 8 h, the effect of pregnancy on increased rate of elimination and increased volume of distribution are quite apparent. By 10 weeks of gestation, the maximum and minimum ampicillin plasma concentrations are less than two-thirds the concentration in the non-pregnant state. By term, the maximum and minimum ampicillin plasma concentrations are approximately half the concentrations obtained in non-pregnant women. Therefore, one has to double the dose of ampicillin in pregnant women at term so that the plasma levels of ampicillin are equal to that of 'normal non-pregnant women' (Philipson, 1977, 1978).

Cephalosporins

Unlike that seen with ampicillin, administration of cephaloridine at different doses to both pregnant and non-pregnant women did not produce any difference in the serum levels (Barr & Graham, 1967). On the other hand, cephazolin given at a particular dose to pregnant women produced lower serum concentrations than that observed in non-pregnant adults following a similar dose (Bernard et al, 1977). The rate of elimination of ceftriazone from the fetal compartment is close to that of maternal serum but, in contrast to other beta-lactam antibiotics, the drug does not accumulate in the amniotic fluid (Kafetzis et al, 1983).

In one study, 1 g of ceftriaxone was given intravenously during Cesarean section. Adequate blood levels were found in the mother but the fetal blood levels were low (Lang, Shalit & Segal, 1993). Cefoperazone is of interest because, in contrast to other cephalosporins, the drug is eliminated primarily by the biliary tree. In one report the administration of cefoperazone to term pregnant women at the time of Cesarean section resulted in larger V_d values and lower C_{max} concentration than have been found in non-pregnant subjects (Gonik, Feldman & Pickering, 1986).

Clindamycin

The data are very variable according to the different studies that have been undertaken. It is likely that serum levels of clindamycin in pregnant women are similar to those which have been reported in a non-pregnant population using the same dosage regimen (Weinstein, Gibbs & Gallagher, 1976).

Aminoglycosides

When similar doses of gentamicin were administered to both pregnant and non-pregnant women, the serum levels in pregnant women were consistently lower than those observed in non-pregnant individuals (Daubenfeld, Madde & Hirsch, 1974).

Penicillin V (Phenoxymethylpenicillin)

Penicillin V has been studied during pregnancy and altered pharmacokinetics has been found when compared to non-pregnant women. Elimination rates from plasma are faster and C_{max} and AUC are lower in pregnant women compared to non-pregnant women (Heikkila & Erkkola, 1993).

Anticonvulsants

Steady state plasma concentration of phenytoin and carbamazepine falls after the first trimester and rises again in the post-partum period. The oral bioavailability of these drugs is not reduced during pregnancy (Lander et al, 1984). There is a doubling of the clearance of phenytoin by metabolism, with a fall in unbound (as well as total) phenytoin concentration (Lander et al, 1977). The unbound concentration, or alternatively the salivary concentration, of phenytoin should be measured every few weeks so that the need for an increase in the daily dosage can be assessed (Mucklow, 1986). The plasma concentrations of valproic acid fall considerably during the third trimester because of an increase in both the metabolic clearance and the distribution volume (Nau et al, 1982), but the clinical relevance is difficult to ascertain as no definitive correlation between plasma concentration and the effect has been shown for this drug. There is a dearth of information on the pharmacokinetics and safety during pregnancy of the new antiepileptic drugs, vigabatrin, lamotrigine and gabapentin.

A number of reports in the literature relate the use for anticonvulsant drugs during pregnancy to hemorrhage in the newborn, presumably because of vitamin K deficiency. The mechanism by which certain anticonvulsants (phenytoin, phenobarbital and carbamazepine) adversely affect vitamin K metabolism has not been fully unraveled. It has been postulated that these drugs induce an increase in oxidative enzymes and thereby increase the degradation of vitamin K1. Maternal vitamin K1 concentration has been low in women on anticonvulsant therapy (Cornelisson et al, 1993). The prenatal administration of vitamin K to prevent deficiency remains controversial (Anai et al, 1993). Nevertheless, it should be routinely administered to the newborn before hospital discharge.

Meperidine

The pharmacokinetics of meperidine are entirely opposite to that of ampicillin with the rate of elimination significantly decreased rather than increased in pregnancy (Krauer & Krauer, 1977; Nation, 1980). The volume of distribution for meperidine also decreases during gestation. It is therefore important to remember that, at all stages of pregnancy, the plasma concentration curves following a single bolus dose are above the non-pregnant curve. As meperidine clearance is lower in pregnancy, the effect of multiple doses will also be more pronounced. It is therefore necessary to decrease the dose required for therapeutic effect. This is especially relevant as meperidine crosses the placenta and produces a dose-dependent neonatal depression.

Antihypertensives

Chronic hypertension, gestational hypertension and pre-eclampsia are the most common medical disorders of pregnancy (Sibai, 1996). Distinction between these disorders is important, since pre-eclampsia generally does not respond well to conventional antihypertensive medications. The use of antihypertensives in women with gestational hypertension remains controversial, especially since the outcome of these patients is relatively good without treatment. Methyldopa is the most common drug used to treat chronic hypertension during pregnancy. There is no consensus for the treatment of severe hypertension in pre-eclampsia. Hydralazine is considered by many the drug of choice. Concern about fetal distress associated with its use prompted investigators to use alternative medications, including labetolol, nifedipine and pindolol. Several randomized trials comparing hydralazine with other drugs failed to demonstrate the purported increase of fetal side effects with hydralazine (Sibai, 1996; Fenakel et al, 1991).

The pharmacokinetics of antihypertensive drugs can be affected in pregnancy in various ways. These could be due to factors modifying absorption, volume of distribution, protein binding, as well as elimination. The absorption of methyldopa was reduced by 73% when it was administered with ferrous sulfate and by 61% when given in combination with ferrous glucuronide (Campbell, Paddock & Sundaram, 1988). As iron supplements are very widely used during pregnancy, this should be kept in mind. In the third trimester of pregnancy, there is an increase in the non-esterified free fatty acids and this may displace drugs from their albumin binding sites (Notarianni, 1990). As plasma protein concentration is already reduced during pregnancy, this will tend to further raise the unbound fraction of the drug. Most antihypertensives, however, are weak bases and are therefore principally bound with high affinity and low capacity to α_1-acid glycoprotein, the level of which does not consistently change during pregnancy (Krauer, Dayer & Anner, 1984). Excretion of drugs can also be affected during pregnancy. The renal plasma flow almost doubles in early pregnancy and glomerular filtration rate is also significantly increased. Therefore, in mild to moderate hypertension without associated renal lesions, renal blood flow may be similar to that seen in normotensive pregnancies or raised even further. However, pre-eclampsia is associated with edema and renal blood flow is about 20% below normal pregnancy levels. This could lead to a reduction in drug clearance. Also, in pre-eclampsia there is marked retention of water leading to edema and this increases the potential volume of distribution.

Antirheumatic Drug Treatment

Knowledge of the risks to the fetus of antirheumatic drugs during pregnancy is quite limited and reports are highly variable. The effect of non-steroidal anti-inflammatory drugs (NSAIDs) in the treatment of active rheumatic disease have been clearly shown for acetylsalicylic acid and indomethacin. Data on the fetal effects of diclofenac, sulindac and ibuprofen is sparse and inconclusive (Ostesen, 1994). No information on the effects of newer compounds, such as fenemates and oxicans, is currently available.

The inhibition of prostaglandin synthesis common to many of the NSAIDs is responsible for the occasional adverse effects seen. The latter has been implicated as a cause for intestinal perforation (Giacoia, Azubuike & Taylor, 1993).

For pregnant patients requiring steroids, both prednisone and prednisolone are recommended. The reason for this preference is that the placenta metabolizes prednisolone to an inactive metabolite and the fetal liver has a limited capacity to convert prednisone to its active metabolite. These mechanisms serve to protect the fetus.

Slow-acting antirheumatic drugs for the treatment of rheumatoid arthritis are rarely, if ever, indicated during pregnancy.

Hydroxychloroquine is occasionally used for the treatment of pregnant patients with active systemic lupus erythematosus (SLE). The placental transfer of hydroxychloroquine, however, has not been adequately studied.

Antiviral Drugs

As HIV infections become more prevalent in women, the use of antiretroviral drugs during pregnancy assumes greater importance. Unfortunately there is a paucity of information concerning the use of these drugs in pregnant women. There are currently eight FDA approved drugs for the treatment of HIV infections: five nucleoside analogs and three protease inhibitors.

Zidovudine (ZDV) is the drug most studied. Both animal and in vitro perfused human placenta studies have shown that ZDV readily crosses the placenta barrier (Lopez-Anaya et al, 1991; Lieber et al, 1990). Zidovudine pharmacokinetics have been evaluated in a limited number of pregnant women with AIDS. No significant differences were found in total body clearance and half-life between pregnant and non-pregnant adults (O'Sullivan et al, 1993). In contrast, the results of a recent study in pregnant baboons and the analysis of the sparse paired data available in humans revealed a significant increase in ZDV clearance during pregnancy (Garland et al, 1996). So far, no accumulation of ZDV in fetal tissues have been found. The ZDV half-life in the newborn was found to be significantly prolonged when compared with the mother. This finding most likely reflects the decreased rate of glucuronidation in the fetus and newborn.

A randomized, double-blind controlled clinical trial to evaluate the safety and efficacy of ZDV given to pregnant women has been conducted by the AIDS Clinical Trial Group (Connor et al, 1994). The estimation of viral transmission rate was found to be 27.7% in the placebo group and 7.9% in the ZDV group (Connor & Mofenson, 1995). The only toxicity observed in the offspring was a transient anemia. Because women enrolled in this trial had a relatively mild disease, another trial is under way in pregnant women with compromised immunologic status. Because of the striking decrease in viral transmission, ZDV is now recommended for use in pregnant women with AIDS. Limited information is available regarding the use of other antiretroviral drugs in pregnancy. Preclinical studies of didanosine (ddI) in the macaque has shown that the drug undergoes significant placental metabolism (Pereira et al, 1995); consequently, only about 50% of the drug was transported to the fetal circulation. The protease inhibitor, saquinavar, has been shown to be non-toxic in animal studies but has limited placental transmission. Nevirapine, a drug with rapid antiviral effect and wide tissue distribution, is being evaluated in a phase I pharmacokinetics study during labor and in the newborn. It is hoped that its use may prevent HIV perinatal transmission during or close to delivery.

The use of acyclovir to treat life-threatening maternal infections associated with herpes simplex or varicella zoster remains problematic. Definite data about safety and efficacy is lacking, although the literature cites several instances of its successful use (Smego & Asperilla, 1991; Lotsham, Keegan & Gordon, 1991). Limited specific pharmacokinetics of acyclovir in pregnant patients have been reported (Frenkel et al, 1991). In comparison to healthy non-pregnant patients receiving acyclovir, mean plasma concentrations are lower. Amniotic fluid levels two to eight times higher than those in maternal plasma have been reported (Frenkel et al, 1991). Because of the limited number of patients with life-threatening herpes or varicella infections and the difficulty in performing appropriate antiviral studies during gestation, no definitive recommendations for the use of acyclovir in pregnancy can be made.

Psychotropic Drugs

It has been estimated that 35% of pregnant women receive psychotropic drugs (Goldberg & Nissim, 1994). As with other drugs used during pregnancy, there is a lack of controlled studies and solid data. The physiologic changes that occur during pregnancy influence the disposition of psychotropic drugs. Protein binding of tricyclic antidepressants, benzodiazepines and neuroleptics is decreased, with a consequent increase in the free fraction of the drugs. At standard doses the blood levels of domipramine and imipramine decrease during pregnancy (Wisner, Perel & Wheeler, 1993). This decrease toward the end of pregnancy may result from the expansion of the plasma volume by the third trimester or an increased activity of some liver microsomal enzymes and renal clearance rates. The necessary dose may have to be increased significantly.

There are currently no data concerning the effects of pregnancy on the plasma concentration of selective re-uptake inhibitors, bupropion, trazodone, sertraline or other antidepressants.

Diazepam is almost entirely oxidized (demethylated) and its major metabolite, nordiazepam, does not exhibit any change in hepatic clearance. The serum concentrations achieved following administration of this drug to pregnant women are lower compared with non-pregnant women and this is because of an increase in the volume of distribution. Oxazepam is eliminated largely by conjugation with glucuronic acid and clearance increases sufficiently to reduce half-life. However, there is no evidence to justify any consistent alteration in the doses of these benzodiazepines used during pregnancy.

During pregnancy there is a fall in the plasma lithium concentration compared with the non-pregnant state (Schou, Amdisen & Sheenstrap, 1973). This is because the renal clearances of lithium and of creatinine are increased to a similar extent during pregnancy. It is therefore important to monitor the serum concentration of lithium and, if necessary, to increase the daily dosage. One should decrease the lithium dosage immediately following delivery, as the renal clearance reverts rapidly to a non-pregnant value and maternal lithium concentration may rise to toxic levels unless the dose is reduced at the onset of labor. Few long-term follow-up data are available on children exposed to psychotropic drugs during pregnancy. A major caveat of these studies has been the lack of a comparison group. Recently, however, a study compared a group of children exposed to antidepressant drugs during pregnancy with a control group of children with no history of antenatal exposure to drugs (Nulman et al, 1997). The study group had been exposed to fluoxetine or tricyclic antidepressants. Exposure to either one of these drugs did not affect the IQ, or language and behavioral development measured during preschool years. This subject requires greater study before definitive conclusions can be drawn on the safety of these drugs for use during pregnancy.

Pulmonary Pharmacology

The absorption of drugs administered by inhalation may be influenced by the physiologic changes that occur during pregnancy. The increased pulmonary blood flow, coupled with hyperventilation and increased tidal volume, may increase the absorption of inhalants (Montella, 1992). This possibility has not been documented by systematic studies. The short-term inhalation of a maximum dose of albuterol did not affect fetal heart rate or aortic velocities in the fetus (Rayburn et al, 1994).

The chronotropic response to adrenergic agonists may be affected by complications of pregnancy. Indeed, a study found a greater chronotropic response to an intravenous bolus of isoproterenol in pre-eclamptic women (Leighton, Norris & De Simone, 1990). This different response may be due to differences in the number and function of adrenergic receptors. Recent evidence suggests that the decreased vascular responsiveness that occurs in pregnancy may be due to a physiologic decrease in the number or function of adrenergic receptors (Smiley & Finister, 1996).

Bronchial asthma occurs in 4–8% of pregnancies. It is known that acute asthma during pregnancy is potentially dangerous to the fetus and that patients with inadequate inhaled anti-inflammatory treatment are more prone to develop acute asthma. Adequate clinical management of asthma during pregnancy is of high priority. A large randomized controlled trial is currently in progress at the National Institutes of Health.

Corticosteroids facilitate the effect of β-agonists on cAMP production and decrease the activity of inflammatory cells. Beclamethasone has been considered the inhalational steroid of choice for the treatment of asthma in pregnancy (Barron & Left, 1993) and to prevent exacerbations (Wendel et al, 1996). The safety of inhaled corticosteroids in pregnancy remains to be determined. The direct administration of β-adrenoreceptor agonists and corticosteroids results in low systemic blood levels and thus reduces fetal xenobiotic exposure.

Among the decongestants, pseudoephedrine should be preferred because, in contrast to other α-adrenergic compounds, it does not affect maternal blood pressure or fetal blood flow velocities (Smith et al, 1990) and has a high therapeutic index.

Theophylline protein binding is lower in the third trimester of pregnancy compared to non-pregnant women. The plasma clearance and volume of distribution for theophylline are reduced in pregnancy and plasma half-lives are generally increased. This would require more frequent monitoring of drug levels during pregnancy (Connelly et al, 1990).

PLACENTAL DRUG TRANSFER

Most of the studies on drug transport across the placenta are based on animal models. Unfortunately, extrapolation of these data to humans is limited by the variety of species used and differences in placental morphology and function. Drug transfer across the human placenta has been studied by in vivo techniques, mostly on pregnancies that were terminated after a drug was given, or by in vitro techniques. A number of mechanisms of placental transfer have been described: diffusion, active or facilitated transport, phagocytosis, membrane discontinuity and electrochemical gradient. Diffusion transport is the most important mechanism. The placental transfer of specific drugs has been extensively reviewed (Pacifi & Nottoli, 1995) and it will not be detailed here.

Because the placenta is a metabolically active organ, concern has been expressed regarding its role in the biotransformation of drugs. It is believed, however, that except for steroids, the placenta is not an important organ for inactivation of drugs before they reach the fetal circulation (Pacifi & Nottoli, 1995).

Pharmacological Treatment of the Fetus—Pharmacological Considerations

The pharmacokinetic parameters that govern the disposition of drugs in the fetus are complicated by the changing physiologic characteristics of the fetus and mother and placenta throughout gestation.

Drugs reach the fetus primarily across the placenta. Other avenues of fetal drug absorption may occur across the fetal skin and by fetal swallowing. The excretion of drugs by the fetal kidneys into the amniotic fluid may permit fetal accumulation for those compounds that are readily absorbed by the fetal gastro-intestinal tract.

The distribution of drugs in the fetal compartment is influenced by the changes in body composition that occur during gestation and the binding characteristics of circulating blood proteins. Body water decreases throughout gestation, while fat deposition increases during the last trimester of pregnancy. These marked changes in body composition may alter the distribution of drugs regardless of their fat partition coefficients. The lower concentration of fetal blood proteins and their decreased binding affinities for drugs may influence drug effects by the relative increase in the concentration of unbound drug. The activities of drug-metabolizing enzymes varies according to the stage of fetal development and the specific metabolic pathway.

Fetal Therapy

Despite the complexities of the maternal–placental–fetal unit, the fetus has been the recipient of drug therapy. In most instances drugs have been delivered by the maternal circulation, although direct administration (intravenous by cordocentesis, intraperitoneal or intramuscular) have also been used.

Drug treatment for fetal arrhythmias is increasingly used, especially for tachyarrhythmias. Digoxin has been the drug most commonly used for atrial flutter (AF) and supraventricular tachycardia (SVT). The increased digoxin maternal clearance requires high doses to achieve fetal therapeutic effect (Azancot-Benistry et al, 1992). The two-fold increase in digoxin clearance cannot be explained by the increase in glomerular filtration that occurs in pregnancy. Recently, a multidrug resistant protein has been implicated as a mediator for digoxin secretion by the renal tubular cells (Ito et al, 1993). This P-glycoprotein appears to be induced during pregnancy (Arceci et al, 1988). Interpretation of the data on placental transfer of digoxin is complicated by cross-reactivity of endogenous digoxin-like substance (EDLS) in digoxin immunoassays. About half the reported cases with fetal AF or SVT respond to digoxin monotherapy. The failure rate is higher in the hydropic fetus. Recently combined maternal and fetal intramuscular digoxin therapy has been shown to improve control of SVT in hydropic fetuses (Parilla, Straburger & Socol, 1996). Limited success has been reported by the direct fetal injection of anti-arrhythmic drugs by other routes: intravenous, intraperitoneal or intra-amniotic (Gembrach, Hansman & Bald, 1988). The high rate of treatment failures with digoxin monotherapy has prompted the use of other anti-arrhythmic drugs, either alone or in combination with digoxin. Verapamil and propranolol have been used for this purpose, although propranolol appears to be ineffective. Quinidine and procainamide have also been used in a few cases, with limited success. Recent reports on the use of flecainide in fetal arrhythmias are encouraging (Perry, Ayres & Carpenter, 1991; Allan et al, 1991). The negative inotropic effects of the drug, however, may limit its use. Likewise, although amiodarone seems effective in cases of recalcitrant tachycardia, concern about fetal thyroid dysfunction (Azancot-Benistry et al, 1992) precludes its routine use.

The term 'congenital adrenal hyperplasia' denotes a group of enzyme defects of adrenal steroidogenesis with autosomal recessive inheritance. In more than 90% of cases it is caused by 21-hydroxylase deficiency. The therapeutic approach is the suppression of fetal androgen production by maternal glucocorticoid therapy, to prevent fetal virilization and androgen-related behavioral changes in the offspring.

Worldwide, more than 300 pregnancies have been treated (Speiser & New, 1994). Dexamethasone is considered the drug of choice. Therapy is started when pregnancy is diagnosed and continues until term in affected pregnancies. Treatment failures have been ascribed to non-compliance, incomplete treatment or inadequate dosage (Forest, David & Morel, 1993). Maternal drug intolerance is related to the duration of therapy. A higher incidence of drug intolerance has been reported in women treated until term than in those receiving a short course of therapy (Forest & Door, 1993).

Fetal thyrotoxicosis is another condition amenable to transplacental pharmacologic therapy. The diagnosis is usually based on fetal tachycardia with fetal growth retardation or a history of a previously affected infant. Because the clinical signs may be unreliable, confirmation by testing fetal thyroid function is necessary (Wallace, Couch & Ginsberg, 1995). The treatment of fetal thyrotoxicosis is based on the ability of thionamide to cross the placenta and inhibit fetal thyroid hormone synthesis. Both propylthiouracil (PTU) and methimazole cross the placenta and inhibit fetal thyroid function, but no correlation exists between daily maternal dosages of either drug and fetal effect (Momotani et al, 1986).

There are differences in the maternal–fetal pharmacokinetics of methimazole and PTU. Methimazole, being a more polar compound than PTU, crosses the placenta more readily. Conversely, PTU has a slow fetal clearance rate and a prolonged fetal effect (Gardner et al, 1986).

Another role of fetal therapy has been in the treatment of intra-uterine infections: antibacterial, viral (see above) and parasitic. For certain infections (HIV and *Streptococcus* Group B) both the mother and infant are the pharmacologic targets; in others (e.g. toxoplasmosis) the fetus is primarily the intended recipient. Knowledge of the fetal pharmacokinetics and tissue distribution is important. For example, fetal brain damage is the most feared complication of congenital toxoplasmosis. Spiramycin has been used to prevent fetal infection in affected pregnant women. Unfortunately, although it is frequently stated that penetration of spiramycin into the cerebrospinal fluid is poor, the available evidence is inadequate (Shoondermark-Van de Ven, 1994).

In summary, empiric findings still prevail in the area of fetal pharmacology. The heterogeneity of the conditions, lack of pharmacologic studies and difficulty in monitoring fetal drug concentrations complicate the assessment of the efficacy and safety of the different modes of fetal therapy.

CONCLUSIONS

Physicians who treat pregnant women frequently prescribe medications that have never been approved by the FDA for obstetric patients. Furthermore, most studies dealing with the pharmacokinetics of drugs have used male subjects. The lack of obstetric labeling is the direct result of lack of research and clinical trials of drugs involving pregnant subjects. This situation mirrors a similar problem in the pediatric age group. In obstetric patients the problem is compounded by concerns regarding the effects of drugs on fetal organogenesis. Pharmaceutical companies are reluctant to perform the studies required for labeling for legal and economic reasons. The lack of knowledge concerning pharmacokinetics and pharmacodynamics in pregnancy is even more serious in abnormal pregnancies.

The recent regulatory changes promulgated by the FDA for pediatric patients should be extended to the obstetric population. Clinical trials should include non-pregnant subjects in parallel designs to ascertain the gender differences in the pharmacokinetics of drugs and the effects of physiologic adaptations that occur during pregnancy. Pregnant patients should also be restudied after parturition. While the pharmacokinetics of drugs in the mother can be easily performed, studies of drug disposition in the human fetus are more problematic because of the difficulty of monitoring fetal blood levels. As with pediatric patients, population pharmacokinetics may provide useful information. The use of a physiologically-based pharmacokinetics model deserves further study (Lueke, Wosilat & Pearce, 1994).

Current efforts to include more women in clinical research studies may lead to the recognition that obstetric studies need to be included at all levels of drug development.

REFERENCES

Allan LD, Chita SK, Sharland GK et al. Flecainide in the treatment of fetal tachycardia. *Br Heart J* 1991; **65**: 468.

Anai TY, Hirota J, Yoshimatsu J et al. Can prenatal vitamin K1 (phylloquinone) supplementation replace prophylaxis at birth? *Obstet Gynecol* 1993; **81**: 251–4.

Arceci RJ, Croop JM, Horwitz SB et al. The gene encoding multidrug resistance is induced and expressed at high level during pregnancy in the secretory epithelium of the uterus. *Proc Natl Acad Sci USA* 1988; **85**: 4350.

Azancot-Benistry A, Jacqz-Aigrain E, Guirguis NM et al. Clinical and pharmacologic study of fetal supraventricular tachyarrhythmias. *J Pediat* 1992; **121**: 608.

Barr W, Graham R. Placental transmission of cephaloridine. *Postgrad Med J* 1967 (suppl): 101–4.

Barron WM, Left AR. Asthma in pregnancy. *Am Rev Respir Dis* 1993; **147**: 510–11.

Bernard B, Thielen P, Garcia-Cazares SJ et al. Maternal–fetal pharmacology of cephatrizine in the first 20 weeks of pregnancy. *Antimicrob Agents Chemother* 1977; **12**: 231–6.

Bernus I, Hooper RG, Eadie MJ. Effects of pregnancy on various pathways of human antiepileptic drug metabolism. *Clin Neuropharmacol* 1997; **20**: 13–21.

Campbell N, Paddock V, Sundaram R. Alteration of methyldopa absorption, metabolism and blood pressure control caused by ferrous sulphate and ferrous glucuronate. *Clin Pharmacol Therap* 1988; **43**: 381–6.

Connelly JJ, Ruo TI, Frederiksen MC et al. Characterization of theophylline binding to serum proteins in pregnant and non-pregnant women. *Clin Pharmacol Therap* 1990; **47**: 68–72.

Connor EM, Mofenson LM. Zidovudine for the reduction of perinatal human immunodeficiency virus transmission: pediatrics AIDS Clinical Trials Group Protocol 076. *Pediatr Infect Dis J* 1995; **14**: 536–41.

Connor EM, Sperling RS, Gelber R et al. Reduction of maternal infant transmission of human immunodeficiency virus type I with zidovudine. *N Engl J Med* 1994; **331**: 1173–80.

Cornelissen MR, Steegers-Theunissen A, Kolle L et al. Increased incidence of neonatal vitamin K deficiency resulting from maternal anticonvulsive therapy. *Am Obstet Gynecol* 1993; **168**: 923–7.

Dahl SG, Strandjord RE. Pharmacokinetics of chlorpromazine after single and chronic dosage. *Clinical Pharm Therap* 1977; **21**: 437–48.

Daubenfeld O, Madde H, Hirsch HA. Transfer of gentamicin to the foetus and the amniotic fluid during a steady state in the mother. *Archiv Gynecol* 1974; **217**: 233–40.

Davis M, Simmons CJ, Dordoni B et al. Induction of hepatic enzymes during normal pregnancy. *J Obstet Gynecol Br Commonw* 1973; **80**: 690–94.

Davison JS, Davison MC, Hay DM. Gastric emptying time in late pregnancy and labour. *J Obstet Gynecol Br Commonw* 1970; **77**: 37–41.

Dean ME, Stock BH. Hepatic microsomal of drugs during pregnancy in the rat. *Drug Metab Dispos* 1975; **3**: 325–31.

Dunlop W. Serial changes in renal haemodynamics during normal human pregnancy. *Br J Obstet Gynaecol* 1981; **88**: 1.

Elkayam U, Gleicher N. Cardiovascular physiology of pregnancy. In Elkayam U, Gleicher N (eds) *Cardiac Problems in Pregnancy. Diagnosis and Management of Maternal and Fetal Disease* 1982, p 5; New York: Alan R. Liss.

Fenakel K, Fenakel G, Appelman Z et al. Nifedipine in the treatment of severe pre-eclampsia. *Obstet Gynecol* 1991; **77**: 331–7.

Forest MG, David M, Morel Y. Prenatal diagnosis and treatment of 21 hydroxylase deficiency. *J Steroid Biochem Molec Biol* 1993; **45**: 75–82.

Forest MG, Door HG. Prenatal treatment of congenital adrenal hyperplasia due to 21-hydroxylase deficiency. European experience in 233 pregnancies at risk. *Pediatrics* 1993; **33**: S3.

Frantz AG, Katz FH, Jailer JW. 6-Beta-hydrocortisol: high levels in human urine in pregnancy and toxaemia. *Proc Soc Exp Biol Med* 1960; **105**: 41–3.

Frenkel LM, Brown ZA, Bryson YJ et al. Pharmacokinetics of acyclovir in the term human pregnancy and neonate. *Am J Obstet Gynecol* 1991; **164**: 569–76.

Gardner DF, Cruishank DP, Hays PM, Cooper DS. Pharmacology of propylthiouracil (PTU) in pregnant hyperthyroid women: correlation of maternal PTU concentrations with cord serum and thyroid function tests. *J Clin Endocrinol Metab* 1986; **62**: 217–20.

Garland M, Szeto HH, Daniel SS et al. Zidovudine kinetics in the pregnant baboon. *J AIDS Human Retrovirol* 1996; **11**: 117–27.

Gembrach U, Hansman M, Bald R. Direct intrauterine fetal treatment of fetal tachyarrhythmia with severe hydrops fetalis by antiarrhythmic drugs. *Fetal Ther* 1988; **3**: 210.

Giacoia GP, Azubuike K, Taylor JR. Indomethacin and recurrent ileal perforations in a preterm. *J Perinatol* 1993; **13**: 297–9.

Goldberg HL, Nissim R. Psychotropic drugs in pregnancy and lactation. *Int J Psychiat Med* 1994; **24**: 129–49.

Gonik B, Feldman S, Pickering L. Pharmacokinetics of cefoperazone in the parturient. *Antimicrob Agents Chemother* 1986; **30**: 874–6.

Heikkila A, Erkkola R. The need for adjustment of dosage regimen for penicillin V during pregnancy. *Obstet Gynecol* 1993; **81**: 919–21.

Husemeyer RP, Davenport HT, Cummings AJ, Rosankiewicz JR. Comparison of epidural and intramuscular pethidine for analgesia in labour. *Br J Obstet Gynecol* 1981; **88**: 711–17.

Hytten FE, Leitch I. *The Physiology of Pregnancy* 1971; Oxford: Blackwell Scientific.

Hytten FE, Lind T. Indices of cardiovascular function. In Hytten FE, Lind T (eds) *Diagnostic Indices in Pregnancy* 1973, p 30; Basel: Documenta Geigy.

Ito S, Koren G, Harper PA, Silverman M. Energy dependent transport of digoxin across the renal tubular cell monolayers (LLC-PK1). *Can J Physiol Pharmacol* 1993; **71**: 40.

Kafetzis DA, Brater CD, Fanourgakis JE et al. Ceftriaxone distribution between maternal blood and fetal blood and tissues at parturition and between blood and milk. *Antimicrob Agents Chemother* 1983; **23**: 870–73.

Katz R, Karliner JS, Renik R. Effects of a natural volume overload state (pregnancy) on left ventricular performance in normal human subjects. *Circulation* 1978; **58**: 434.

Krauer B, Dayer P, Anner R. Changes in serum albumin and α_1 acid glycoprotein concentrations during pregnancy: an analysis of feto-maternal pairs. *Br J Obstet Gynaecol* 1984; **91**: 875–81.

Krauer B, Krauer F, Hytten F. Drug disposition and pharmacokinetics in the maternal–placental–fetal unit. *Pharmacol Therapeut* 1980; **10**: 301–28.

Krauer B, Krauer F, Hytten F. Pregnancy and its effects on drug handling. In Lind T (ed.) *Current Review in Obstetrics and Gynecology* 1984, pp 1–18; Edinburgh: Churchill Livingstone.

Krauer B, Krauer F. Drug kinetics and pregnancy. *Clin Pharmacokinet* 1977; **2**: 167–81.

Lander CM, Edwards VE, Eadie MJ, Tyrer JH. Plasma anticonvulsant concentration during pregnancy. *Neurology* (Minneapolis) 1977; **27**: 128–31.

Lander CM, Smith MT, Chalk B et al. Bioavailability and pharmacokinetics of phenytoin during pregnancy. *Eur J Clin Pharmacol* 1984; **27**: 105–10.

Lang R, Shalit I, Segal J. Maternal and fetal serum and tissue levels of ceftriazone in emergency cesarian section. *Chemotherapy* 1993; **39**: 77–8.

Lee MY, Smiley S, Kadkohodayan S et al. Developmental regulation of flavin-containing mono-oxygenase (FMO) isoforms 1 and 2 in pregnant rabbit. *Chem Biol Interact* 1995; **28**: 75–85.

Leighton BL, Norris ML, De Simone CL. Pre-eclampsia and healthy term pregnant patients have different chronotropic responses to isoproterenol. *Anesthesiology* 1990; **72**: 392–3.

Liebes L, Mendoza S, Wilson D, Dancis J. Transfer of zidovudine (AZT) by human placenta. *J Infect Dis* 1990; **161**: 203–7.

Lind T, Hytten FE. Blood glucose following oral loads of glucose, maltose and starch during pregnancy. *Proc Nutr Soc* 1969; **28**: 64A.

Lopez-Anaya A, Unadkat JD, Schuman LA, Smith AL. Pharmacokinetics of zidovudine: III. Effect of pregnancy. *J AIDS* 1991; **4**: 64–8.

Lotsham RR, Keegan JM, Gordon HM. Parenteral and oral acyclovir for the management of varicella pneumonia in pregnancy: a case report and review of the literature. *WV Med J* 1991; **87**: 204–6.

Lueke RH, Wosilat WD, Pearce BA. A physiologically based pharmacokinetics computer model of human pregnancy. *Teratology* 1994; **49**: 90–99.

Luxford AME, Kellaway GSM. Pharmacokinetics of digoxin in pregnancy. *Eur J Clin Pharmacol* 1983; **25**: 117–21.

McDonald-Gibson RG, Young M, Hytten FE. Changes in plasma nonesterified fatty acids and serum glycerol in pregnancy. *Br J Obstet Gynecol* 1975; **82**: 460–66.

Momotani N, Noh J, Oyanagi H et al. Antithyroid drug therapy for Grave's disease during pregnancy. Optimal regimen for fetal thyroid status. *N Engl J Med* 1986: **315**: 24–8.

Montella KR. Pulmonary pharmacology in pregnancy. *Clin Chest Med* 1992; **13**: 587–95.

Montgomery TL, Pincus IJ. A nutritional problem in pregnancy resulting from intensive resection of the small bowel. *Am J Obstet Gynecol* 1955; **69**: 865–7.

Mucklow JC. The fate of drugs in pregnancy. *Clin Obstet Gynecol* 1986; **13**: 161–75.

Nation RL. Drug kinetics in childbirth. *Clin Pharmacokinet* 1980; **5**: 340–64.

Nau H, Kuhnz W, Egger H-J et al. Research review: anticonvulsants during pregnancy and lactation—transplacental, maternal and neonatal pharmacokinetics. *Clin Pharmacokinet* 1982; **7**: 508-43.

Neuvonen PJ. Interaction with the absorption of tetracyclines. *Drugs* 1976; **11**: 45–54.

Nimmo WS, Wilson J, Prescott LF. Narcotic analgesics and delayed gastric emptying during labor. *Lancet* 1975; **i**: 890–93.

Notarianni LU. Plasma protein binding of drugs in pregnancy and neonates. *Clin Pharmacokinet* 1990; **18**: 20–36.

Nulman I, Rovet J, Stewart DE et al. Neurodevelopment of children exposed in utero to antidepressant drugs. *N Engl J Med* 1997; **336**: 258–62.

O'Sullivan MJ, Boyer PJJ, Scott GB et al. The pharmacokinetics and safety of zidovudine in the third trimester of pregnancy of women infected with human immunodeficiency virus and their infants. *Am Obstet Gynecol* 1993; **168**: 1510–16.

Olon B, Akesson BA, Dencker H et al. Pregnancy after jejunoileostomy because of obesity. *Acta Chir Scand* 1976; **142**: 82–3.

Ostesen M. Optimization of antirheumatic drug treatment in pregnancy. *Clin Pharmacokinet* 1994; **27**: 486–503.

Pacifi GM, Nottoli R. Placental transfer of drugs administered to the mother. *Clin Pharmacokinet* 1995; **28**: 235–69.

Parilla BV, Straburger JF, Socol ML. Fetal supraventricular tachycardia complicated by hydrops fetalis: a role for direct fetal intramuscular therapy. *Am J Perinatol* 1996; **13**: 483–6.

Parry E, Shields R, Turnbull AC. Transit time in the small intestine in pregnancy. *J Obstet Gynecol Br Commonw* 1970; **77**: 900–901.

Pereira CM, Nosbich C, Baughman WL, Unadkat JD. Effect of zidovudine on transplacental pharmacokinetics of ddI in the pigtail macaque. *Antimicrob Chemother* 1995; **39**: 343–5.

Perry JC, Ayres NA, Carpenter RJ. Fetal supraventricular tachycardia treated with flecainide acetate. *J Pediatr* 1991; **118**: 303.

Perucca E, Crema A. Plasma protein binding of drugs in pregnancy. *Clin Pharmacokinet* 1982; **7**: 336–52.

Philipson A. Pharmacokinetics of ampicillin during pregnancy. *J Infect Dis* 1977; **136**: 370–76.

Philipson A. Pharmacokinetics of antibiotics in pregnancy and labor. *Clin Pharmacokinet* 1979; **4**: 297–309.

Philipson A. Plasma levels of ampicillin in pregnant women following administration of ampicillin and pivampicillin. *Am J Obstet Gynecol* 1978; **130**: 674–83.

Pirani BBK, Campbell DM, MacGillivray I. Plasma volume in normal first pregnancy. *J Obstet Gynecol Br Commonw* 1973; **80**: 884–7.

Rayburn WF, Atkinson BD, Gilbert K, Turnbull GL. Short-term effects of inhaled albuterol on maternal and fetal circulations. *Am J Obstet Gynecol* 1994; **171**: 770–73.

Rebond P, Gronlade J, Groslambert PL, Colomb M. The influence of normal pregnancy and the post partum state on plasma proteins and lipids. *Am J Obstet Gynecol* 1963; **86**: 820–28.

Schou M, Amdisen A, Sheenstrap DR. Lithium and pregnancy—II. Hazards to women given lithium during pregnancy and delivery. *Br Med J* 1973; **ii**: 137–8.

Shoondermark-Van de Ven L, Galama J, Capmps W et al. Pharmacokinetics of spiramycin in the Rhesus monkey: transplacental passage and distribution in tissues in the fetus. *Antimicrob Agents Chemother* 1994; **38**: 1922–9.

Sibai BM. Treatment of hypertension in pregnant women. *N Engl J Med* 1996; **335**: 257–65.

Smego RA, Asperilla MD. Use of acyclovir for varicella pneumonia during pregnancy. *Am Coll Obstet Gynecol* 1991; **78**: 1112–16.

Smiley RM, Finster M. Do receptors get pregnant too? Adrenergic receptors alterations in human pregnancy. *J Matern Med* 1996; **5**: 106–14.

Smith CV, Rauburn W, Anderson NJ et al. Effect of a single dose of pseudoephedrine on uterine and fetal doppler blood flow. *Obstet Gynecol* 1990; **76**: 803–6.

Speiser PW, New MI. Prenatal diagnosis and management of congenital adrenal hyperplasia. *Clin Perinatol* 1994; **21**: 631–45.

de Swiet M. The cardiovascular system. In Hytten FE, Chamberlain GVP (eds) *Clinical Physiology in Obstetrics* 1980, p 31; Oxford: Blackwell Scientific Publications.

Wallace C, Couch R, Ginsburg J. Fetal thyrotoxicosis: a case report and recommendations for prediction, diagnosis and treatment. *Thyroid* 1995; **5**: 125–8.

Weinstein AJ, Gibbs RS, Gallagher M. Placental transfer of clindamycin and gentamicin in term pregnancy. *Am J Obstet Gynecol* 1976; **124**: 688–91.

Wendel PJ, Ramin SM, Barnett-Hamm C et al. Asthma treatment in pregnancy: a randomized controlled study. *Am J Obstet Gynecol* 1996; **175**: 150–54.

Wisner KL, Perel JM, Wheeler SB. Tricyclic dose requirements in pregnancy. *Am J Psychiatry* 1993; **150**: 1541–2.

Post-reproductive Years

Menopause

Brinda Wiita,[1] Michael Gast[2] and Veronica Ravnikar[3]

[1]Solvay Pharmaceuticals, Marietta, GA, [2]Wyeth-Ayerst Research, Philadelphia, PA,
and [3]University of Massachusetts Medical Center, Worcester, MA, USA

INTRODUCTION

Menopause, or the end of menstruation, usually occurs at about 50 years of age, with a range of 39–59 years (Treolar, 1981). Generations ago, menopause occurred near the end of a woman's life, and there was little time to experience the adverse consequences of estrogen deprivation. Now that the average lifespan has increased significantly, women live approximately one-third of their lives after menopause, and women over 50 are the most rapidly growing segment of the population. Women in the large segment of the US population born in the wake of World War II, known as 'baby boomers', are just entering this age range. Since the active health care and maintenance of these women will become such an important public health and fiscal issue in the next 20 years, the medical community has an important stake in optimizing, increasing and prolonging the use of postmenopausal estrogen therapy (ERT) and combined estrogen–progestin hormone replacement therapy (HRT).

Currently, although it is estimated that only 15% of eligible women take HRT, prescriptions for oral menopausal estrogens increased from 13.6 million in 1982 to 31.7 million in 1992, and prescriptions for the progestin medroxyprogesterone acetate (MPA) increased 4.9-fold (Wysowski, Golden & Burke, 1995). The majority of women discontinue treatment within a few months and refuse to continue using HRT chronically as recommended. There are many and complex reasons why women reject a therapy with obvious health benefits, which emphasizes replacement of lost hormones to restore the former physiological state, not treatment of a medical condition. Although rational assessments and statistical evaluations of the benefit–risk ratios of HRT conclude that the positive aspects of menopausal therapy far outweigh the negatives (Barrett-Connor, 1992; Grady et al, 1992; Harlap, 1992; Grodstein et al, 1997), personal reasons for rejecting HRT include fear of cancer, recurrence of menstrual-like bleeding, weight gain, cyclical mood changes and other HRT side-effects, as well as the well-intentioned, if sometimes inaccurate, advice of physicians, friends and family. Women are deluged with

Drug Development for Women. Edited by V.V. Ragavan. © 1998 John Wiley & Sons Ltd.

books, newspaper and magazine articles on the menopause which recommend alternative approaches to symptom relief, osteoporosis and heart disease prevention. Focus groups involving women aged 40–60 reveal that women know more about herbal medicines than estrogen, and that they receive more information on menopause from the lay press than from their physicians (Andrews, 1996). Faced with this information overload, it is often easier for women to do nothing at all than to see a physician and make an informed decision about HRT. This chapter will discuss the types and doses of natural and synthetic estrogens and progestins used in menopausal HRT regimens, both to treat symptoms and to prevent and treat osteoporosis and cardiovascular disease.

HISTORICAL PERSPECTIVE

Conjugated equine estrogens (CEE), the first estrogen preparation marketed for menopausal therapy in the USA, have been widely prescribed since 1950. In the last two decades, estrogens have been delivered in many additional formulations and by several different routes, and progestin addition has become the standard of care for women who have not undergone hysterectomy. Considerable epidemiological data are available on estrogens, and knowledge and understanding of the spectrum of benefits of estrogen therapy continue to grow as the extent and duration of usage expand. Until the 1970s, estrogens were most commonly used for symptomatic relief of hot flashes and preventing atrophy of the urogenital tract, but now their recognized therapeutic benefits include osteoporosis prevention and treatment (Lindsay et al, 1980; Lindsay, Hart & Clark, 1984; Ettinger, Genant & Cann, 1985; Lufkin et al, 1992), cardiovascular disease prevention and treatment (Stampfer et al, 1991; Wenger, Speroff & Packard, 1993; Grodstein et al, 1996), improvement of mood and quality of life (Siddle et al, 1990; Ditkoff et al, 1991), cognitive function and memory (Kampen & Sherwin 1994; Henderson et al, 1994; Paganini-Hill & Henderson, 1994) and retention of teeth (Krall et al, 1997).

ESTROGEN AND PROGESTERONE: PHYSIOLOGY AND PHARMACOLOGY

Estradiol is the signature hormone of the female reproductive cycle. Its sharp rises and falls are required to maintain reproductive cyclicity in the premenopausal woman and its absence in the postreproductive years leads to a variety of clinical problems including vasomotor instability, osteoporosis, cardiovascular disease and, most likely, diminished cognitive and physical function. In addition, the hormone is responsible for supporting skin, genito-urinary, muscular and other tissues.

The ovary ceases to secrete estradiol and progesterone at menopause, and declining ovarian hormone levels stimulate release of the gonadotropins follicle-stimulating hormone (FSH) and luteinizing hormone (LH) (Rossmansmith,

TABLE 11.1 Pharmacological properties of the progestins

Progestin class	Breast	Endometrium	Coag	Vascular	Lipids	CHO	Bone
19-nor testosterone	+/−	+	+/−	−	−	−	+
17-alpha-progesterone	+/−	−	+/−	−	−	−	+
Progesterone	+	−	+/−	+/−	+/−	+/−	+
Antiprogestins	+	+	+/−	+/−	+/−	+/−	+/−

Scherbaum & Lauritzen, 1991; Burger, 1996; McKinlay, 1996). Estrogen replacement therapy lowers gonadotropin levels significantly via the hypothalamic–pituitary neuro-endocrine feedback loop, but circulating levels of FSH and LH do not return to premenopausal levels. Ovarian stromal tissue remains functional in early menopause and continues to secrete testosterone under LH regulation (Adashi, 1994).

Interactions between estrogens and progestins occur at the cellular level and may modify estrogen actions on bone, vascular tissue, metabolic processes, and the central nervous system in postmenopausal women. Progestins appear to synergize with the positive actions of estrogens on bone to enhance the effects of low doses of estrogen on bone (Gallagher, Kable & Goldgar, 1990; Speroff et al, 1996). However, progestins may blunt the actions of estrogens on lipoprotein synthesis (Lobo et al, 1994; Miller et al, 1991) and antagonize estrogen-dependent coronary vasodilatation leading to vasoconstriction (Sullivan and Fowlkes, 1996). Identification of the best and safest progestins for use in HRT regimens, and selection of the doses required to avoid jeopardizing estrogen benefits, requires careful elucidation of both positive and negative consequences of progestin use during HRT regimens and characterization of estrogen–progestin interactions in appropriate clinical studies and animal models. Many currently available progestins for menopausal HRT were initially developed for use in contraceptives, and consequently they have been well characterized in contraceptive doses. Pharmacological characterization at the lower doses used in menopausal women is desirable, as well as elucidation of bone, breast and cardiovascular activity in combination with a specific estrogen used in HRT. Table 11.1, which shows the pharmacological properties of the various classes of progestins, is compiled from various animal models and clinical pharmacology studies.

Investigations of estrogen pharmacology have focused on estradiol, which acts in most tissues via its specific high-affinity receptors. Basic research related to the other estrogens used in HRT, such as estrone, equilin, equilenin and their derivatives, is less extensive and focused primarily on bone and the cardiovascular system. Study of concurrent estrogen and progestin effects in some cell types, particularly breast cancer cell lines, has received more extensive evaluation and review. The underlying molecular mechanisms and tools for defining cellular or molecular mechanisms of estrogen–progestin interactions and progestin selection to be combined with estrogen when a particular target organ is of concern have received less attention.

Recently, the identification of estrogen-responsive regions in the progesterone receptors of certain species and modification of non-receptor-mediated actions of estrogens by progestins have gained the attention of the basic science community. Nonetheless, significant work will be required to fill the gaps which separate clinical and basic knowledge about the consequences of progestins in HRT regimens. Recent developments have led to the targeted drug development of 'designer' estrogen analogs or selective estrogen receptor modulators with profiles of desired actions on specific tissues.

SELECTIVE ESTROGEN RECEPTOR MODULATORS (SERMS), 'ANTI-ESTROGENS' OR ESTROGEN ANALOGS

Approximately 15 years ago tamoxifen was developed as an 'anti-estrogen' designed to competitively inhibit the effects of low levels of endogenous estradiol and estrone in women who had been diagnosed with hormone-responsive adenocarcinoma of the breast. It is widely used as primary and maintenance therapy for estrogen-positive breast cancer. Over the last several years it has become apparent that tamoxifen is not a pure anti-estrogen, but rather a weak estrogen with an activity spectrum encompassing estrogenic actions on bone, lipoproteins and endometrium, and estrogen antagonist effects in breast (Daniel et al, 1996; Grey et al, 1995; Love et al, 1992). The absence of estrogenic stimulation in breast and the ability to bind to the estrogen receptor and prevent estrogen actions in breast tissue is what gives tamoxifen its positive clinical benefit in breast cancer patients. However, it is known to cause vasomotor symptoms, menstrual irregularities, endometrial polyps and vaginal bleeding or discharge.

Following several years of clinical use of tamoxifen, clinicians began to detect cases of adenocarcinoma of the endometrium which were similar but not identical to endometrial carcinomas seen earlier with long-term unopposed estrogen therapy in the 1970s (Rubin et al, 1990; Seoud, Johnson & Weed, 1993; van Leeuwen et al, 1994; Weiss et al, 1979). An increased incidence of uterine cancer was seen in large randomized trials and a case-control study in The Netherlands (van Leeuwen et al, 1994). These findings led to a careful re-evaluation of both the clinical and preclinical effects of tamoxifen and a requirement for routine gynecological care during treatment. It was determined that tamoxifen was indeed mildly estrogenic in its actions on the endometrium, and that over time it stimulated proliferation which may have contributed to the development of rare cases of endometrial carcinoma in breast cancer patients on long-term therapy. This spectrum of estrogenic activity makes tamoxifen a less than ideal substitute for estrogen in the healthy postmenopausal woman, although it would have some benefit in maintaining bone mineral density in women with a history of estradiol-responsive breast cancer. Careful endometrial surveillance would be needed in these patients (Daniel et al, 1996; Seoud, Johnson and Weed, 1993).

TABLE 11.2 SERMS in clinical development

Decreasing estrogen agonism ————————————————————————————→

System/agonist	Estradiol	Tamoxifen	Raloxifene	Droloxifene	ICI 182780
Bone	++++	++	++	++	–
Breast	+++	–	–	–	–
Cardiovascular	++++	+	+	+/–	–
CNS	++++	–	–	–	–
Endometrium	+	+	+/–	+	–

Compound	Company	Stage of development
Raloxifene	Lilly	Approved (USA) December 1997
Droloxifene	Pfizer	Phase III
Idoxifene	SmithKline Beecham	Phase III
Levonormeloxifene	Novo Nordisk	Phase III
TAT 59	Taiho-Synphar	Phase III
LY 353381	Lilly	Phase I
CP 336156	Pfizer	Phase I

The comparative estrogenic effects of a spectrum of estrogen receptor-active drugs on clinically significant outcomes in estrogen responsive tissues. These vary from tamoxifen to the 'pure' anti-estrogen ICI 182780. (+) implies a salutary or desired clinical change, such as anti-resorptive activity in bone. Estradiol is included as a standard against which the other agents may be compared.

Evaluation of tamoxifen's effect on the cardiovascular system and the bone metabolic cycle also produced some surprises. The most exciting of these was the positive effect that this 'anti-estrogen' had on bone. Tamoxifen was capable of producing 'anti-osteoporotic', anti-resorptive changes in bone biology not unlike those related to estrogen therapy (Kenny et al, 1995; Love et al, 1992).

In the early 1990s, after observing the positive effects of tamoxifen on bone, researchers began a concerted effort to identify new substances which would have desired clinical effects on bone, the cardiovascular system and the central nervous system and no proliferation-stimulating effects on the breast or uterus. The objective was to develop a variety of other estrogen mimetic substances in an effort to identify tissue selective agonists that would have an 'ideal' clinical profile for use either as HRT or as breast cancer treatment or prophylaxis.

The five tissues of primary interest in the HRT-treated patient are shown in Table 11.2. Of these, bone and cardiovascular system are of the greatest clinical import while breast and uterus address the oncologic aspects of the agents. Central nervous system effects reflect effects on mood, quality of life, cognitive function and development of Alzheimer's disease, and sexual function. The long-term effects of these compounds on cardiovascular risk and cognitive function remain to be elucidated.

The current spectrum of synthetic 'estrogen analogs' or 'modified estrogens' or 'selective estrogen receptor modulators or SERMs' include agents such as tamoxifen, raloxifene, idoxifene, droloxifene, centchroman, toremifene, levonormeloxifene

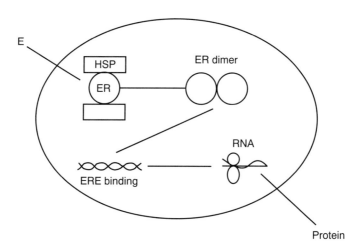

FIGURE 11.1 The classic model for estrogen receptor-mediated actions. Critical components include receptor dimerization and ERE binding. HSP = heat shock protein

and 'pure' estrogen antagonists like the compound ICI 182780 (Gradishar & Jordan, 1997). When considered as a group, these agents span a continuum of tissue selectivity from full agonist to almost complete antagonistic effects in estrogen-responsive tissues. Estrogen acts at the cellular level by binding to a specific receptor. This receptor then sheds its chaperoning heat shock proteins and dimerizes. The dimer translocates to nuclear DNA, where it acts on specific palindromic sequences known as estrogen response elements (ERE). These elements form part of a transcription initiation complex which ultimately leads to the synthesis of estrogen-responsive proteins (see Figure 11.1).

Tissue-specific estrogens can interfere with this process in a variety of ways. Classically, it is assumed that the tissue-specific estrogen interacts with the estrogen receptor and forms some type of sterically modified estrogen receptor dimer. According to classical theory, this abnormally configured estrogen receptor dimer interacts inappropriately with the ERE, blocking synthesis of estrogen-responsive proteins in the cell (Gast, 1997).

In fact, estrogen tissue selectivity is of significantly greater complexity. Most cells have more than one consensus ERE and often more than one non-consensus ERE. Thus, tissue selectivity may depend not only upon the configuration of estrogen receptor dimers but also on the number, position and structure of the EREs for a given estrogen-dependent protein. In this model, the tissue selectivity of estrogens can extend not just to whole cell types but to specific proteins within a cell. This model is probably more consistent with the in vivo findings and clinical realities of tissue selectivity. In addition, the existing cellular milieu, i.e. the available second messengers, interacting proteins and specific configuration of DNA within a given cell type is undoubtedly critical to tissue selectivity (Figure 11.2).

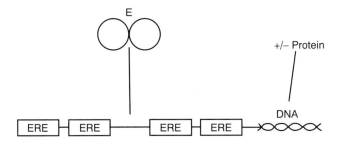

FIGURE 11.2 Tissue selectivity of steroids depends on the number, position and structure of the ERE for a given estrogen-dependent protein. The existing cellular milieu also influences the response to steroid hormones

Thus, a cell concurrently treated with a potent progestin might fail to exhibit or minimally exhibit a tissue selectivity where the same cell would have strong selective effects in the absence of concurrent therapy.

Finally, the recent elucidation of a second high-affinity estrogen receptor in the rat and the human has also changed our concepts of the process of tissue steroid specificity. This receptor, although highly conserved in its DNA binding region, has significant differences from the conventional estrogen receptor in the transcription activating factor (TAF) regions of the molecule (Kuiper et al, 1996; Mosselman, Polman & Dijkema, 1996). It may also be distributed preferentially in tissues such as ovary and testis. Because of differences in the human carboxyl terminus of the molecule, where primary conformational events of the estrogen receptor occur, it is possible that DNA interactions with the second receptor (designated ERβ) can occur in preference to, or as an alternative to, binding with conventional ERα. Additionally, workers evaluating the tissue-selective estrogen raloxifene have recently suggested that not only may the drug bind to estrogen receptor monomers as opposed to promoting dimerization, but may also exert some of its tissue activities by interacting with DNA at sites other than the traditional ERE (Yang et al, 1996).

Recent Phase II results and interim analyses of raloxifene Phase III data indicate that this new SERM may approach the desired profile for a modified estrogen or designer estrogen. Raloxifene prevents loss of bone mineral density, although to a lesser extent than conjugated equine estrogens (CEE) as assessed by measuring markers of bone metabolism and bone mineral density (Delmas et al, 1997). Preliminary information suggestive of a significant reduction in breast cancer risk during raloxifene treatment was also presented in June 1997, but longer-term data are needed to support any conclusions related to breast cancer risk. Endometrial stimulation was not evident after 2 years of treatment. The 60 mg daily dose of raloxifene, which was recently approved for osteoporosis prevention, does not relieve menopausal somatic symptoms. The incidence of vasomotor symptoms was increased by higher doses of raloxifene and the dose-related effects on the endometrium are unknown at this time.

HRT: CONSEQUENCES OF ESTROGEN AND ESTROGEN–PROGESTIN ADMINISTRATION

Clinical efforts to reduce the unfavorable impact of progestins on estrogens in HRT regimens have involved changes in the nature of the progestin component, the dose of progestin utilized, and the interval and duration of progestin administration. Recent studies have focused on the 'less than monthly' administration or 'extended cycle' progestin administration (Williams et al, 1994; Ettinger et al, 1994). Different progestins, including 'natural' progesterone, and synthetic progestins (medroxyprogesterone acetate (MPA), dydrogesterone, 17-α-acetoxyprogesterone derivatives, and 19-nortestosterone derivatives) and anti-progestins have been used. The metabolic consequences of these estrogen–progestin permutations and combinations and combined actions on bone mineral density appear to be small, but there is insufficient information on their impact on more enduring clinical outcomes for older women such as brain function, quality of life, breast cancer and cardiovascular disease.

Evaluation of the risks and benefits of HRT is an ongoing process; fortunately, the expected benefits of HRT continue to outweigh the potential risks (Grady et al, 1992; Harlap 1992; Grodstein et al, 1997). Clinicians continue to struggle to define the risks and areas in which concomitant progestin therapy moderates, eliminates or augments the use of estrogen in postmenopausal women. Careful clinical and laboratory research evaluation is required in order to avoid making rash judgments on these important clinical issues until adequate and accurate data have been obtained on all hormones under consideration. Data on the effects of HRT on cardiovascular disease and breast have been obtained from observational studies, which are inherently subject to bias and confounding factors. Prospective controlled trials of adequate size are needed to resolve questions about the effects of estrogens and progestins on these conditions.

New progestins in clinical development programs for HRT regimens have generally originated from oral contraceptive development programs in which they are combined with the synthetic estrogen, ethinyl estradiol. For use in postmenopausal women, these progestins are combined with natural estrogens such as estradiol or CEE and tested to determine the minimum effective dose for endometrial protection. This dose may be different from the target dose in an oral contraceptive, which has typically been characterized and developed for the task of blocking ovulation in women of reproductive age. Because of the convenience and generally favorable bleeding profiles associated with continuous combined HRT (Udoff, Langenberg & Adashi, 1995), relatively high monthly doses (70–140 mg) of MPA have become popular adjuncts to daily estrogen replacement. However, recent literature reports of clinical comparative trials cited by the American College of Obstetricians and Gynecologists (Andrews, 1996), challenge such regimens because they include more progestin in terms of dose, type and duration than the minimum exposure needed to achieve the primary objective, i.e. prevention of endometrial hyperplasia. Progestin doses of this magnitude produce undesirable changes in coagulation factors and serum lipoprotein-bound cholesterol, i.e. effects that dampen or reverse the effects of estrogens. Differences between the effects of progesterone and synthetic progestogen on HDL-cholesterol, an important predictor of cardiovascular risk, were seen in the PEPI study, a three-year trial in which the HDL increases caused by CEE were diminished to a greater extent by medroxyprogesterone acetate than by oral micronized progesterone (PEPI Writing Group, 1995, 1996).

Estrogen–Progestin Regimens

Progestins have been combined with estrogens in HRT since the early 1980s, principally to counteract prolonged estrogenic stimulation of the uterine endometrium leading to carcinoma and to induce endometrial sloughing or regression. Estrogen therapy given alone to women with intact uteri, even with a few hormone-free days per month, is associated in prospective clinical trials with unacceptably high rates of endometrial hyperplasia, which has been proposed as a marker for the later development of endometrial carcinoma (PEPI Writing Group, 1995; Woodruff et al, 1994). The undeniable association of postmenopausal estrogen therapy with a significantly increased risk of endometrial carcinoma was acknowledged at an FDA hearing in December 1975, which reviewed the findings of Smith et al (1975) and Ziel & Finkle (1975), who reported up to seven-fold increases in uterine cancer among postmenopausal women treated with estrogens to relieve symptoms. At that time, the FDA advisory committee recommended using the lowest possible dose of estrogen and discontinuing therapy occasionally to determine the need for continued use, and to evaluate lower doses. Subsequently, combining synthetic or natural progestins with estrogens (HRT) in women with intact uteri has become the standard of care in most countries, and several fixed combinations of estrogens and progestins are marketed or in clinical development. There are many forms of HRT used to prevent endometrial hyperplasia. Progestin can be administered at high or low doses, and duration may vary from a few days per month to daily or continuous dosing. Some HRT regimens utilize a medication-free interval at the end of every cycle, while others have advocated weekly interruption. The currently marketed CEE/MPA regimens are administered without a hormone-free interval, and several investigators have evaluated progestin interruption only every three months for 10–14 days (Williams et al, 1994; Ettinger et al, 1994). The cyclical form of HRT, in which estrogen is taken daily and progestin is taken for 12–15 days per month, is meant to resemble the menstrual cycle, and induces regular monthly vaginal bleeding. Continuous estrogen–progestin regimens, which eventually produce a high incidence of amenorrhea, administer the same doses of estrogen and progestin every day (Archer et al, 1994; Speroff et al, 1996). The daily dose of progestin given continuously may be lower than in the cyclical regimens, but the cumulative dose is often the same or higher. Bleeding may be initially experienced with a continuous regimen and usually lessens as treatment continues, but some women experience bleeding for a prolonged time and may decide to stop treatment for this reason.

Recent evidence that some progestins may diminish the positive effects of estrogens on lipoprotein-bound cholesterol and vasodilatation (Williams et al, 1992; Sullivan et al, 1995) have led some physicians to conclude that progestins added to estrogen therapy may diminish the long-term cardiovascular benefits of estrogens. The net effect of such pronouncements is to raise general alarm about HRT and to decrease the frequency and duration of HRT use beyond perimenopausal treatment for hot flashes and night sweats, when the greatest proportion of women choose to take HRT. Such long-term conclusions are probably fallacious, since they are based on the blunting and not the elimination of positive estrogenic shifts in predictors of cardiovascular risk, as consistently reported in clinical trials of estrogens combined with MPA or norethindrone acetate (Lobo et al, 1994: PEPI Writing Group, 1995; Speroff et al, 1996) instead of the more definitive cardio-vascular outcomes such as myocardial infarctions. Progesterone and dydrogester-one, which are non-androgenic progestins, tend to have little or no effect on the lipoprotein responses to estrogen (PEPI Writing Group, 1995; Gelfand et al, 1997).

Early efforts to determine the role of combined estrogen–progestin therapy in cardiovascular morbidity and mortality suggest no blunting of the estrogen-related sparing of myocardial infarctions and cardiovascular death (Falkeborn, Persson & Adami, 1992; Psaty et al, 1994; Grodstein et al, 1996) and long-term prospective studies focused on cardiovascular outcomes are ongoing. The time frame of clinical experience with estrogen–progestin regimens in postmenopausal women is much shorter than the experience with estrogen-only therapy, and the benefit–risk ratio of these regimens is not completely understood. Extensive mid- and long-term prospective randomized trials are being conducted in order to detect the multiple interactive effects of estrogens and progestins (discussed in detail in Chapter 12).

Breast Cancer

The breast, like the uterus, contains estrogen receptors and exhibits proliferative changes in response to estrogenic stimulation. In contrast to the uterus, however, breast tissue exhibits greater proliferative activity in the presence of both estrogen and progesterone than with estrogen alone (King, 1991). Female gender is the primary risk factor. The presence of estrogens in women under the age of 50 may contribute to the higher incidence of breast cancer in that age group (Barrett-Connor, 1994).

Breast cancer incidence in postmenopausal women receiving estrogens or HRT has been measured in several large epidemiological studies, but the evidence for no significant alteration in breast cancer risk lacks strength and consistency. The only conclusion that can be drawn at the present time is that there is neither a dramatic increase nor a decrease in breast cancer incidence with estrogen or estrogen–progestin replacement therapy. The Cancer and Sex Hormones (CASH) study conducted by the Centers for Disease Control and Prevention (CDC) did not detect an increase in the overall risk of breast cancer with postmenopausal estrogen replacement therapy (Wingo et al, 1987). A recent report from the Nurses' Health Study revealed that in this ongoing prospective observational study of more than 69 000 postmenopausal women, previous estrogen therapy had no influence on the risk of breast cancer, while current use for more than 5 years was associated with a slight but significant increase in the relative risk (RR) of breast cancer (RR = 1.46, 95% CI range = 1.20–1.76) (Colditz et al, 1995).

The long-term health benefits of estrogens have been unquestionably demonstrated in large long-term observational studies such as the Nurses' Health Study (Stampfer et al, 1991), and meaningful data on combined estrogen–progestin regimens are now being published (Grodstein et al, 1996). The Women's Health Initiative (WHI), sponsored by the National Institutes of Health, is evaluating the effects of no HRT, CEE therapy alone or combined with progestin, dietary modification, and calcium and vitamin D supplementation over a total observation period of approximately 12 years. Forty participating centers plan to enroll 160 000 women, and results will be available around 2006. The large size and long duration of studies of this type, which are necessary to properly evaluate the long-term effects of HRT, as well as the strong potential effects of diet and lifestyle, make it important to optimize estrogen–progestin therapy by using the lowest effective doses and treatment durations of estrogens and progestins. Such attempts will blunt criticism and maximize the acceptability of HRT usage.

US Development Guidelines for HRT Regimens

The postmenopausal estrogen–progestin drug development guidelines of the Food and Drug Administration (FDA) recommend studies designed to compare and evaluate the incidence of uterine endometrial hyperplasia in estrogen-only and estrogen–progestin treatment groups over a treatment duration of 1 year (FDA HRT Writing Group, 1995). While this treatment duration may be sufficient to assess endometrial stimulation by estrogen and its prevention by the concomitant administration of progestin, it does not support adequate investigations of positive and negative effects of these hormones on bone, breast and the cardiovascular system.

Guidelines for Prescribing Preventive HRT

Numerous treatment algorithms and guidelines for prescribing HRT for post-menopausal women have been created by professional societies, individuals, managed care organizations, and others. However, few if any of these have been implemented and validated in clinical practice. Guidelines issued by the American College of Physicians (1992) emphasize evaluation and risk assessment of the patient entering natural menopause, since this is the start of a period in life when risk for diseases such as coronary heart disease, stroke, cancer and osteoporosis become more prevalent. Ideally, each woman who is considering preventive HRT should be counseled on her risk for these various diseases and she should be able to judge the likely changes in her risk for disease and in life expectancy due to treatment. The decision should incorporate each woman's individual preferences concerning risks and benefits of therapy. Prior to initiating therapy, a pelvic examination should be done. An endometrial assessment should be conducted for non-hysterectomized women who will be prescribed estrogen-only treatment; no endometrial evaluation is required for women who will be prescribed combined estrogen–progestin therapy. Endometrial evaluation may be done by an office-based biopsy, but this procedure may be poorly tolerated by older women due to urogenital atrophy, decrease in size and compliance of the vaginal introitus, or stenotic cervical os. Transvaginal ultrasound has been used by some as an initial test to determine which women need endometrial sampling, on the theory that a biopsy will not be necessary if the endometrial thickness measured by ultrasound is between 0 and 4 mm (Holbert, 1997). This screening evaluation is, however, not universally accepted, and the validity of the test depends heavily on the available imaging equipment and the technical expertise of the examiner, as well as other factors. Older women, however, may also have difficulty with the ultrasound procedure. Annual mammograms and breast examinations should be conducted, and an annual endometrial evaluation should be considered in women on estrogen-only therapy. It is also important to evaluate heavy or unexpected vaginal bleeding in women on combined estrogen–progestin therapy.

Younger postmenopausal women are usually treated to relieve their vasomotor symptoms and disturbed sleep and to prevent osteoporosis and cardiovascular disease. The focus in older postmenopausal women shifts towards the prevention and/or treatment of osteoporosis, which affects approximately 25% of women over the age of 75 in the USA. Recent evidence suggests that ERT/HRT may play a significant role in the prevention of cardiovascular and neurodegenerative disease, as well as reducing the incidence of certain forms of cancer. Osteoporosis and cardiovascular disease are key causes of morbidity and mortality in the elderly, but the side-effects of vaginal bleeding and breast tenderness are often strong deterrents for the elderly woman deciding to begin or even continue HRT.

VASOMOTOR SYMPTOMS (HOT FLASHES OR FLUSHES)

Vasomotor symptoms or hot flashes are the classical sign of estrogen deficiency associated with the onset of menopause. Hot flashes are reported in population studies to affect about 75% of postmenopausal women, but only one in three will seek treatment for these symptoms. The hot flash is a sudden transient sensation of warmth or heat that spreads over the upper body, simultaneously with increased skin temperature and pulse rate (Molnar, 1975). Severe hot flashes may be accompanied by sweating and followed by a chill, and are more frequently experienced after oophorectomy (Kronenberg, 1990; Oldenhave et al, 1993; Oldenhave, 1994). Frequent and persistent hot flashes have a profound negative impact on quality of life, and they are often accompanied by psychosomatic complaints such as tension, fatigue, headaches, depression, and aches and pains (Oldenhave, 1994). Symptoms subside with time even if no HRT is taken, but approximately 25% of untreated women continue to have hot flashes for longer than 5 years (Hammond, 1996). Vasomotor symptoms respond rapidly to estrogen therapy, although complete relief often takes 6 weeks or longer to achieve (Haas et al, 1988). The mechanisms underlying the vasomotor instability which accompanies hot flashes is poorly understood; however, the efficacy of estrogens in producing symptomatic relief is undeniable. Estrogens are not unique in their ability to treat hot flashes. The effectiveness of progestins and androgens in modulating vasomotor instability indicates that the mechanism is not truly estrogen-specific. Although progestins in the doses used for HRT appear to have little influence on vasomotor symptoms, higher doses of progestins such as megestrol are capable of relieving hot flashes, and may be prescribed for symptomatic women with a history of breast cancer to lessen this estrogen deficiency-related symptom. Androgen replacement therapy in male doses has been shown to relieve hot flashes in hypogonadal men (DeFazio et al, 1984). The influence of other factors which may underly the varying incidence and severity of hot flashes between individual women is unknown.

OSTEOPOROSIS

Estrogen deficiency accelerates bone loss by causing an imbalance in normal bone cycle activity, which greatly favors resorption over formation, the net result being a decrease in bone mineral density and excessive fragility which leads to fractures.

Estrogen therapy alone or in combination with other agents effectively slows bone resorption, resulting in a net gain in axial and appendicular bone mineral density (BMD) and a significant decrease in the rate of fractures (Weiss et al, 1980; Kiel et al, 1987; Cauley et al, 1995). The impact of estrogen therapy on BMD is greatest in the first 5 years after menopause, when the rate of bone turnover is extremely high, but the desirable effects of resorption inhibition and fracture prevention by estrogen are also seen at ages from 30 years onwards in women. In the PEPI trial, the major factors influencing the actions of estrogen on bone mineral density (BMD) were age, baseline BMD, and previous HRT (PEPI Writing Group, 1996). Schneider, Barrett-Connor & Morton (1997) have demonstrated that women over 60 who begin estrogen therapy derive skeletal benefits which are nearly equal to benefits in younger women.

Since estrogens as a class conserve BMD and reduce the risk of vertebral and non-vertebral (femoral neck and distal radius) fractures, the relationship between their effects on BMD and fractures has been proven. Therefore, unlike new bone-active drugs, FDA does not require investigation of estrogens in clinical studies with fracture endpoints to obtain an osteoporosis indication. For an estrogen, the lowest effective dose which prevents osteoporosis (using BMD as a marker) must be identified in a 2-year double-blind controlled trial in women 1–3 years after menopause. BMD of the lumbar spine and proximal femur should be measured at intervals by dual-energy X-ray absorptiometry (DEXA). Markers of bone turnover should be measured, and endometrial biopsies should be done at 6–12 month intervals.

FDA guidelines for a clinical study investigating the efficacy and safety of a non-estrogen for the treatment of postmenopausal osteoporosis state that eligible women would be ambulatory outpatients at least 5 years following menopause, with one or more osteoporosis-related vertebral fractures and/or with a mean L2–L5 vertebral BMD at least 2 SD below the mean peak BMD for premenopausal women. The current FDA guidelines require a treatment duration of 5 years, with possible approval based on an interim analysis conducted at 3 years. Estrogen osteoporosis treatment studies are permitted to use BMD as a primary endpoint. Thus, these studies generally need to enroll a smaller number of patients than those aimed to demonstrate reduction in the incidence of new vertebral fractures, such as studies currently required for non-estrogens. European guidance for such programs differs modestly from FDA-directed programs.

The actions of estrogens on bone, unlike other tissues, are not blunted by progestins. In fact, androgenic progestins such as norethisterone acetate induce significantly higher increases in BMD than estrogen alone (Speroff et al, 1996). In the PEPI trial, although there were no significant differences in BMD between estrogen and estrogen–progestin groups at 1 and 3 years, the continuous MPA regimen, which contained the highest monthly dose of progestin, induced greater BMD increases than the other active treatment groups (PEPI Writing Group, 1996).

CARDIOVASCULAR

Cardiovascular disease is the most common cause of death in the USA, and epidemiological studies have demonstrated significant reductions in cardiovascular mortality and morbidity in women treated with long-term estrogen therapy (Stampfer et al, 1991). These observations may be subject to some bias because healthier women with better dietary and exercise habits may choose estrogen treatment, and consequently the apparent cardiovascular protection may be due to non-hormonal lifestyle factors. The long-term prospective controlled Women's Health Initiative Trial is expected to provide a definitive answer to whether younger healthy women are protected from cardiovascular problems by estrogen therapy added to good nutrition and exercise. Meanwhile, relatively short-term benefits in women with prior cardiovascular disease are being investigated in the Heart Estrogen/Progestin Replacement Study (HERS) and Women's Estrogen Stroke

Trial (WEST). The possible mechanisms for this cardiovascular protection include metabolic changes (e.g. lipids, homocysteine reduction), endothelial-mediated non-genomic responses (vasomotion or anti-atherogenic) or anti-oxidant activity.

Lipoprotein-bound cholesterol profiles are favorably influenced by estrogens, with oral administration having a greater impact than transdermal or topical administration (Walsh et al, 1991; Erenus et al, 1994). Elevated HDL-cholesterol and lowered LDL-cholesterol induced by oral estrogens reverse the shifts in lipoproteins which occur after menopause (Walsh et al, 1991). Transdermal estrogens decrease LDL but have little effect on HDL (Chetkowski et al, 1986). Estrogen also has a dramatic anti-atherosclerotic effect in arteries by augmenting vasodilatation (Williams et al, 1992; Herrington et al, 1994) and antagonizing platelet aggregation via the endothelium-dependent pathways of nitric oxide and prostacyclin. These activities have been demonstrated in both animal and clinical models. Data on the relationship between stroke incidence and estrogen replacement are still unclear, but the NHANES1 cohort study reported reduced relative risks for stroke mortality (RR = 0.86, CI 0.28–2.66) and stroke incidence (RR = 0.82, CI 0.46–1.47) (Finucane et al, 1993). No significant association was detected between stroke and use of HRT in a recent report from the Nurses' Health Study (multivariate adjusted RR, 1.09; 95% CI, 0.66–1.80) (Grodstein et al, 1996).

UROGENITAL ATROPHY

The normal vaginal mucosa consists of three distinct layers of cells, the lowest layer being composed of parabasal cells, which mature in the presence of estrogen, and succeeding layers being intermediate and superficial cells. The outermost superficial cells become 'cornified' during mid-cycle under the influence of high estradiol levels. During menopause, when there is a profound absence of estrogen, maturation of parabasal cells remains suppressed and the vaginal mucosa consists primarily of parabasal cells. The mucosa is then found to be thin and atrophic without protective superficial layers. The atrophic mucosa can become ulcerated and can easily become infected. In addition, the parabasal cells are not secretory in nature and the absence of secretions will lead to sensations of dryness and associated symptomatology. Estrogen treatment, given either systemically or locally, will convert the vaginal mucosa to intermediate and ultimately to superficial keratinized cells. This process is similar to the process found in the normal menstrual cycle, as keratinization typically occurs during the increase in estrogen in the follicular phase.

The urogenital estrogen deficiency syndrome, which affects most postmenopausal women, is composed of vaginal symptoms such as dyspareunia, vaginitis and vulvar itching, as well as symptoms involving the lower urinary tract, specifically involuntary urine leakage and lower urinary tract infections. Urge incontinence and to some extent stress incontinence have been linked to estrogen deficiency, but the effectiveness of estrogen therapy in relieving incontinence has not been conclusively demonstrated. Atrophic vaginitis can significantly impair quality of life due to sensations of dryness, dyspareunia, loss of libido, vaginal infections, bleeding and urological incompetence, as well as pathologic conditions such as chronic infections, discharge, ulcerations and bleeding.

Several estrogen-containing vaginal creams are available for the treatment of local symptoms and currently they provide better symptom relief than non-estrogen-containing products. Presently available products on the market are creams containing conjugated estrogens (Premarin®) and estradiol (Estrace®). Vaginally applied estrogen is well absorbed, and can relieve other menopausal symptoms such as hot flashes.

The vaginal effects of a wide range of estrogen doses have been studied. Mandel et al (1983) evaluated the histologic effects of different doses of conjugated estrogens for 4 weeks in postmenopausal women. Doses as low as 0.3 mg/day restored the vaginal mucosa to a premenopausal state. Even with the lowest doses, there was a significant increase in the estrogen index at week 1 and values remained above baseline until the end of the study. Dickerson et al (1979) observed relief of vaginal and vasomotor symptoms by vaginal creams containing either estradiol or conjugated estrogens.

In another study, Martin et al (1979) also studied the effects of Premarin® and Estrace® creams, given for 15 days, on vaginal mucosal cells. With both creams, there was a dramatic increase in superficial cells, from a baseline of 2% to 70% at 8 days, with no further change in 15 days. Luisi et al (1980) studied the effects of Ovestin® (0.5 mg estriol/day) and Premarin® (1.25 mg/day) for 2 weeks. A different measure of mucosal maturation (maturation value) showed a significant increase in maturation by day 8, without much further increase after that with estriol. Premarin® caused ferning and spinnbarkeit (tests on cervical mucus indicative of estrogen presence) while Ovestin® did not, probably due to the greater estrogenic potency of the conjugated estrogens preparation.

Smith et al (1993) evaluated the vaginal effect of a very low dose releasing vaginal ring. Even with small doses of estradiol, about $5-10$ μg/day, there was a significant increase in vaginal maturation, with parabasal cells decreasing from an initial value of 56% to 9% after 24 weeks. Corresponding shifts were seen in interstitial and superficial cells, and the percentage of superficial cells remained considerably lower (about 25%) than with higher oral doses. Patients also observed significant relief of symptoms.

Evaluation of efficacy of locally applied estrogens has involved the study of changes in both symptoms and maturation of vaginal cells. The former evaluation is a subjective one, especially in the open uncontrolled design commonly used for studes of topical estrogens, while the latter is an objective measure of estrogen's effect on the vaginal mucosa. Many studies have shown improvement in most if not all symptoms of atrophic vaginitis utilizing doses of estrogens mentioned above (Martin et al, 1979; Gordon et al, 1979; Carlstrom et al, 1982).

Vaginally administered estrogens are systemically absorbed, especially when given in amounts presently available in the marketplace, namely $0.1-0.2$ mg E_2 or

0.1–1.25 mg CEE. The efficacy of these ultralow doses of estrogens delivered by the vaginal route was recently reported by Naessen, Berglund & Ulmsten (1997), who observed that forearm bone density increased significantly in women over 60 years of age treated with vaginal estradiol rings, even though serum estradiol levels did not change perceptibly. They postulated that the end-organ effects of ultralow doses of estradiol were consistent with up-regulation of estrogen receptor sensitivity with advancing age and long-standing hypo-estrogenism. In particular, local safety of these products has been observed. Smith et al (1993) evaluated endometrial thickness by vaginal ultrasound after 90 days of vaginal administration delivering 5–10 μg of E_2 per day. Luisi et al (1980) evaluated the endometrium in women after 2 weeks of treatment with Premarin® or Ovestin® cream. The endometrium remained atrophic after Ovestin® treatment, but showed proliferative changes after treatment with Premarin®.

The mechanism of action of estrogen therapy on the urogenital tract is inadequately defined, but initial findings indicate that both receptor-mediated and non-receptor-mediated mechanisms are involved. Changes in connective tissue, glandular function, cell permeability, and improved vascular supply have all been implicated in urogenital symptom relief. Vaginal moisture, fluid volume, elasticity, epithelial integrity, and pH are indicators of vaginal health (Bachmann et al, 1991). Although only Premarin® and Estrace® creams, and more recently the vaginal ring, are available in the USA, several other products are available in Europe, such as Ovestin® (estriol cream) and Vagifem® (a vaginal tablet with 10 μg or 25 μg of estradiol). Vaginal rings made of silicone polymer (Silastic) containing estradiol, which deliver estradiol preferentially to the vaginal tract and minimize release into the systemic circulation, effectively relieve urogenital problems and may be more acceptable to patients because they eliminate messy applications.

QUALITY OF LIFE, PSYCHOLOGICAL STATUS AND SEXUAL FUNCTION

The climacteric spectrum of symptoms, encompassing perimenopausal and post-menopausal changes, includes emotional fluctuations, negative mood, cognitive impairment, and decreased sexual drive and enjoyment (Oldenhave, 1994). These events are related to hormonal deficiency, life events, and aging. Quality of life in postmenopausal women, and the impact of the climacteric on their lives, has been extensively studied in recent years. Evidence that quality of life is improved by HRT (Wiklund, Karlberg & Mattssen, 1993) influences patients' decisions to take such therapy and motivates them to continue treatment for the rest of their lives. Quality of life and mood improvement by HRT in controlled trials has been variable because of non-hormonal influences on these subjective parameters. Significant mood improvements were observed with HRT (Kupperman, 1953) and estrogen therapy may relieve depression (Klaiber et al, 1979). Surgically menopausal women, who may experience ovarian hormone withdrawal at a relatively young age, probably undergo greater psychological trauma and stress than naturally menopausal women (Johanssen et al, 1975). Androgen plays a critical role in the maintenance of sexual function in men and women, and androgen co-therapy with estrogen may improve sexual drive and enjoyment (Sherwin & Gelfand, 1985; Davis et al, 1995).

Cognitive Function

Although investigations of the effects of estrogen therapy on cognitive function in late and early menopause are still in their infancy, marked cognitive improvements have been reported after administering estrogens to women with Alzheimer's disease (Honjo et al, 1989; Ohkura et al, 1995), and cognitive improvements in normal menopausal women have been observed by Kampen & Sherwin (1994). Barrett-Connor & Kritz-Silverstein (1993) observed, in a longitudinal survey of older women in the Rancho Bernardo community, that estrogen-treated women did not exhibit better cognitive performance than untreated women, but Paganini-Hill & Henderson (1994) have observed a marked decrease in Alzheimer's disease-related deaths in estrogen-treated women that is dose- and duration-dependent. The sum total of available data is so promising that numerous researchers are currently studying cognitive function enhancement and prevention of senile dementia by estrogen therapy.

PRODUCTS FOR ESTROGEN REPLACEMENT AND ESTROGEN–PROGESTIN THERAPY

Types and doses of estrogen regimens prescribed for postmenopausal women have evolved since conjugated estrogens were first marketed 50 years ago. Estrogen tablets and vaginal creams were first marketed in the 1950s and 1960s, followed in the mid-1980s by transdermal twice-weekly estradiol reservoir-type patches containing ethanolic solutions of steroids. These systems tend to cause local skin irritation in a significant proportion of patients, particularly in hot and humid climates. The new matrix estradiol patches, which contain no organic solvents, and seldom cause local irritation, have been available in the US since 1995. A vaginal estradiol ring has been marketed in the USA since 1997, and a topical hydro-alcoholic estradiol gel is in late-stage clinical trials.

As the body of information on the long-term benefits and risks of estrogen replacement grows, utilization of the lowest effective estrogen dose is increasingly emphasized. Recommended oral dosages have seen steady decreases from 1.25 mg of conjugated or esterified estrogens or 2.0 mg estradiol to 0.625 mg or 1.0 mg, respectively, with a further trend towards 0.3 mg of conjugated or esterified estrogens or 0.5 mg of estradiol for osteoporosis prevention. Following initial

TABLE 11.3 Products for estrogen replacement and estrogen–progestin therapy

Brand name	Components	Daily dosage/route
Oral products		
Premarin® (conjugated estrogens, USP)	Equilin sulfate, estrone sulfate, 17-α-hydroxyequilin sulfate, δ 8,9 dehydroestrone, equilenin	0.3–2.5 mg/oral
Estrace® (micronized estradiol USP)	Estradiol 17-β	0.5–2.0 mg/oral
Ogen®	Piperazine estrone sulfate	0.3–2.5 mg/oral
Estratab® Menest® (esterified estrogens USP)	Estrone sulfate, equilin sulfate	0.3–2.5 mg/oral
Transdermals and topicals		
Estraderm®	Estradiol	0.05–0.1 mg/transdermal
Vivelle®	Estradiol	0.05–0.1 mg/transdermal
Climara®	Estradiol	0.035–0.1 mg/transdermal
Estring®	Estradiol	vaginal
Fempatch®	Estradiol	0.025–1.0 mg/transdermal
Premarin® vaginal cream	Conjugated equine estrogens (CEE)	
Estrace® vaginal cream	Estradiol-17-β	
Estrogen–progestin		
Premphase®	CEE + MPA	0.625 mg CEE + 5 mg MPA for 14 days/mouth
Prempro®	CEE + MPA	0.625 mg CEE + 2.5 or 5.0 mg MPA/day

introductions of conjugated and esterified estrogens and micronized estradiol in the 1950s, there were no additional products for HRT until 1987, when the first transdermal patch was introduced. The pace of new product introductions and clinical development activities has intensified significantly since 1995, when matrix estradiol patches and combined estrogen–progestin products were introduced on the US market (see Table 11.3 and Appendix).

Cyclical and Continuous Estrogen–Progestin Regimens

Combined estrogen–progestin products approved by the FDA are fixed regimens investigated in 1-year trials comparing the lowest effective dose of estrogen alone with combination regimens containing varying doses of progestin combined with the same dose of estrogen, in order to identify the regimen containing the lowest dose of progestin which prevents estrogen-induced endometrial hyperplasia.

Frequently used regimens administer a course of progestin once a month (cyclical or sequential regimen) or include a smaller dose of progestin given daily (continuous regimen). Combined estrogen–progestin regimens including conjugated estrogens and medroxyprogesterone acetate (MPA) (Premphase® and Prempro®) are available, and new drug applications (NDAs) have been submitted for regimens containing the estrogens ethinyl estradiol or estropipate combined with norethindrone acetate. Transdermal estrogen–progestin regimens with patches containing estradiol and norethindrone acetate are in Phase II and Phase III clinical trials.

The ultimate acceptance of these fixed combined regimens remains to be determined, since a flexible and customized approach is inherently important for hormone replacement, in order to restore the endogenous estrogenic balance of the individual being treated. Long-term compliance with estrogen–progestin regimens is significantly dependent on control of vaginal bleeding, which in turn depends on the patient's hormonal and endometrial status at initiation of therapy. Women in early menopause will have a greater incidence of irregular or breakthrough bleeding, and they are more likely to accept the regular bleeding of a cyclical regimen. Older women are less tolerant of vaginal bleeding and will do better on a continuous regimen, which should eliminate vaginal bleeding after being administered for 6–12 months. Patients must be informed about the nature and frequency of the anticipated bleeding patterns and reassured that such regimens significantly reduce the risk of developing endometrial cancer.

Due to concerns about the undesirable long-term effects of progestin and possible attenuation of estrogen benefits, particularly during long-term administration, there is a strong interest in reducing progestin doses as far as possible while still maintaining endometrial control. One solution was the development of regimens in which progestins were administered every 3 months (Ettinger et al, 1994). While success has been reported with these extended cycles, concern exists about the long-term endometrial safety and the amount of bleeding experienced during each 3-monthly bleeding episode.

Guidelines for development of combination estrogen–progestin hormone replacement therapy products were issued by the Food and Drug Administration in 1995. Unlike European requirements, these guidelines require an estrogen-only comparator group in order to follow the combination drug policy, which requires a combination drug to contain the lowest effective dosage of each of its active components for their respective labeled indications.

In order to obtain an indication for vasomotor symptoms, two double-blind placebo-controlled studies lasting 3 months or longer should be conducted in patients who experience at least 7 or 8 moderate to severe flashes per day (60+ hot flashes/week) at baseline, after HRT washout. The hot flashes are almost always documented by patient recording in daily diaries, although objective recording by thermography is preferred.

To obtain the endometrial protection indication for an estrogen–progestin combination, the lowest effective dose of estrogen which relieves vasomotor symptoms is investigated in combination with a range of progestin doses, in order to identify the lowest dose of progestin which prevents development of estrogen-induced endometrial hyperplasia or cancer. The dose of estrogen is studied alone and combined with at least two doses of progestin in a 12-month double-blind study. Endometrial assessments must be done by biopsies conducted at least at baseline and at the end of the study, although routine transvaginal ultrasonography is encouraged in order to support inadequate biopsy samples and to generate a prospective database correlating ultrasound and histological findings. Biopsy slides must be read by two independent pathologists using standardized criteria for diagnosis of endometrial hyperplasia, with a third independent blinded pathologist to adjudicate differences in interpretation.

Combining studies for prevention of endometrial hyperplasia and vasomotor relief is not advisable, since the highly symptomatic patients eligible for the hot flash indication will not be able to tolerate extended placebo treatment in a hyperplasia study. The retention of patients over 3 months of treatment and the preceding washout period is already problematic, since women with symptomatology which impairs quality of life may prefer to take an effective agent instead of possibly being assigned to treatment with placebo or an ineffective dose of estrogen.

NEW APPROACHES/OTHER THERAPY

Local Progestogen Application

Since endometrial hyperplasia may be inhibited by an agent acting solely within the uterine lumen, methods to deliver progestins selectively to the uterus have recently received marked attention as approaches which diminish the unwanted effects of systemic progestins. An intra-uterine device (IUD) releasing small amounts of levonorgestrel has been developed in Europe (Suhonen et al, 1995) and a vaginal gel containing progesterone has been approved by the FDA for relief of secondary amenorrhea and dysfunctional bleeding. Vaginal and intra-uterine delivery have the significant advantage of delivering lower amounts of progestin into the systemic circulation and perhaps avoiding attenuation of estrogen benefits (Archer et al, 1995). Also, vaginal delivery prevents the formation of progesterone metabolites, which have been implicated in the sedation-inducing side-effects of orally administered progesterone (Arafat et al, 1988).

Estrogen–Androgen Therapy

Postmenopausal women have been treated with androgens since the 1950s, but the usage of estrogen–androgen therapy is confined to a small fraction of patients. The ovaries produce approximately half of all endogenous androgen in women prior to menopause (Adashi 1994; Davis & Burger, 1996); levels decline immediately after surgical menopause and gradually after natural menopause (Vermeulen, 1976; Judd et al, 1974). Injectable androgen preparations and implants contain testosterone or its esters and oral preparations contain 17-alkylated testosterone or its derivatives. Clinical studies with androgen implants and low doses of oral androgen have demonstrated positive effects on sex drive, frequency and enjoyment, well-being, energy level and BMD (Davis et al, 1995; Sherwin & Gelfand, 1985; Watts et al, 1995). Side-effects of estrogen–androgen therapy include acne, hirsutism and voice changes, which are reversible if therapy is discontinued immediately after detection. Estrogen-induced increases in HDL are reduced by androgen (Barrett-Connor et al, 1996; Watts et al, 1995), but androgens have no negative effects on estrogen-induced coronary vasodilatation (Honore et al, 1996) and exert vaso-dilator actions in animal models (Yue et al, 1995; Chou et al, 1996). Although cardiovascular outcomes during long-term estrogen–androgen therapy have not been determined, market surveillance data suggest no dramatic increase in cardiovascular risk.

Tibolone, available in Europe, combines estrogenic, androgenic and progestogenic properties. This compound relieves climacteric symptoms, increases BMD and prevents endometrial stimulation (Milner et al, 1996; Bjarnason et al, 1996, 1997; Botsis et al, 1997); however, since it is a weak progestin, bleeding problems similar to those seen with continuous HRT may complicate therapy.

Estrogen Analogs

Estrogen analogs, also called tissue-selective estrogens or selective estrogen receptor modulators (SERMs), comprise a class of molecules with estrogenic activity which are designed to deliver the desired effects of estrogens at tissues and organs such as the bone and cardiovascular system and eliminate the undesired effects on the breast and uterus (described earlier). Pursuit of this new approach to menopausal therapy was initiated by the finding that tamoxifen, a breast cancer treatment which was characterized as an anti-estrogen, induced positive bone and lipoprotein changes in postmenopausal women. Long-term treatment with tamoxifen in a large breast cancer prevention trial conducted by the National Cancer Institute induced significant and atypical endometrial stimulation, and therefore tamoxifen cannot be used for postmenopausal HRT. Chemical derivatives of triphenylethylenes and other classes are in clinical development for the prevention and treatment of osteoporosis (Gradishar & Jordan, 1997).

One of the more promising SERMs in clinical development is raloxifene (Draper et al, 1995), which is in Phase II and III clinical trials for osteoporosis and other indications. Preliminary Phase III results demonstrate beneficial effects on bone and lipids. Classic dogma suggests that raloxifene, like tamoxifen and the other triphenylethylenes, binds to the estrogen receptor and blocks estrogen actions in breast and endometrial tissue, thus preventing growth and tumor development.

In other cell types, however, raloxifene activates the same genes as estradiol and displays the same pharmacological actions, e.g. bone and lipoprotein metabolism (Fuchs-Young et al, 1995). It has been suggested that some of the tissue-selective actions of raloxifene may be mediated by a polypurine sequence which does not require the DNA binding domain of the classical estrogen receptor (Yang et al, 1996). Unlike estrogen, raloxifene does not relieve vasomotor symptoms and tends to precipitate hot flashes at higher doses, which would limit its use in younger symptomatic women. The anti-estrogenic action of raloxifene in endometrium has the distinct advantage of eliminating the need to add progestin.

Phyto-estrogens

There is a rapidly growing interest in the use of natural plant-derived estrogens or phyto-estrogens for self-medication of menopausal complaints. Epidemiological studies show that menopausal symptoms are rare in countries where diets contain large amounts of soybeans and other phyto-estrogens. A phyto-estrogen-rich diet may contribute to relief of symptoms such as hot flashes and vaginal dryness (Brzezinski et al, 1997). Recent animal and clinical research investigations on the soy sterols genistein and daidzein have revealed that soy sterols have beneficial effects on lipoprotein-bound cholesterol (Anthony et al, 1996) with no accompanying vaginal stimulation (Cline et al, 1996). Clinical investigations of soy and other plant extracts are ongoing to determine the nature of their postulated tissue selectivity and the clinical applications of dietary factors which protect against cancer and heart disease.

Popular health food remedies for menopause-related complaints are ginseng, dong quai, black cohosh, primrose oil and licorice root. Long-term usage of such plant extracts without medical supervision should be avoided, since the minimum effective doses and side effects of these substances are unknown. A major concern is that endometrial growth induced by long-term use of these substances may not receive appropriate medical treatment, since women taking health food products may not see a physician regularly or even reveal that they are taking these substances. In addition, the phyto-estrogens are not as potent as estrogens or SERMs, and the long-term health benefits and risks (bone, cardiovascular, CNS) have not been determined.

POSTREPRODUCTIVE THERAPEUTICS IN THE FUTURE

When dealing with a therapy as global as HRT, it is perhaps difficult to imagine how it could change and broaden its scope to provide better health for women in their postreproductive years. Although current approaches to HRT are well accepted and used, such regimens are confined to approximately 15% of the eligible female population, and the duration of usage is far shorter than the ideal goal of lifetime hormone replacement therapy after menopause. Current and future efforts in this field are aimed at providing agents lacking the real or imagined disadvantages of estrogens and combined regimens and employing natural or non-hormonal approaches. Development goals for new tissue-selective estrogens are elimination of stimulation of the breast and endometrium while retaining positive effects on bone and the cardiovascular system. New estrogens with specific actions on the CNS, such as 17-α-estrogen derivatives, are also being sought. Concerns over acute and chronic metabolic events, dysphoria and vaginal bleeding have led to a search for new progestins, regimens and routes of delivery and to a closer look at natural progesterone. The goal of the search for new approaches in using progestins is to avoid modulating the benefits of estrogen-dominant HRT regimens. A wide variety of choices and flexible approaches which can be tailored to individual medical needs and personal preferences is essential to facilitate decision-making and patient compliance. Non-hormonal approaches such as non-steroidal entities and tissue- or disease-specific drugs are also needed in the therapeutic portfolio.

REFERENCES

Adashi EY. The climacteric ovary as a functional gonadotropin-driven androgen-producing gland. *Fertil Steril* 1994; **62**: 20–27.

American College of Physicians. Guidelines for counseling postmenopausal women about preventive hormone therapy. *Ann Intern Med* 1992; **117**: 1038–41.

Andrews WC. The transitional years and beyond. *Am J Obstet Gynecol* 1996; **85**: 1–5.

Anthony MS, Clarkson TB, Hughes CL Jr et al. Soybean isoflavones improve cardiovascular risk factors without affecting the reproductive system of peripubertal rhesus monkeys. *J Nutri* 1996; **126**: 43–50.

Arafat ES, Hargrove JT, Maxson WAS et al. Sedative and hypnotic effects of oral micronized progesterone may be mediated through its metabolites. *Am J Obstet Gynecol* 1988; **159**: 1203–9.

Archer DF, Fahy GE, Viniegra-Sibal A et al. Initial and steady-state pharmacokinetics of a vaginally administered formulation of progesterone. *Am J Obstet Gynecol* 1995; **173**: 471–8.

Archer DF, Pickar JH, Bottiglioni F for the Menopause Study Group. Bleeding patterns in postmenopausal women taking continuous combined or sequential regimens of conjugated estrogens with medroxyprogesterone acetate. *Obstet Gynecol* 1994; **83**: 686–92.

Bachman GA, Notelovitz M, Gonzalez SJ et al. Vaginal dryness in menopausal women; clinical characteristics and non-hormonal treatment. *Clin Pract Sexuality* 991; **7**: 25–32.

Barrett-Connor E. Risks and benefits of replacement estrogen. *Ann Rev Med* 1992; **43**: 239–51.

Barrett-Connor E, Kritz-Silverstein D. Estrogen replacement therapy and cognitive function in older women. *JAMA* 1993; **260**: 2637–41.

Barrett-Connor E. Postmenopausal estrogen and the risk of breast cancer. *Ann Epidemiol* 1994; **4**: 177–80.

Barrett-Connor E, Timmons C, Young R, Wiita B & The Estratest Working Group. Interim safety analysis of a two-year study comparing oral estrogen–androgen and conjugated estrogens in surgically menopausal women. *J Women's Health* 1996; **5**: 593–602.

Bjarnason N, Bjarnason K, Haarbo J, Christiansen C. Tibolone: prevention of bone loss in late postmenopausal women. *J Clin Endocrinol Metab* 1996; **81**: 2419–22.

Bjarnason N, Bjarnason K, Haarbo J et al. Tibolone: influence on markers of cardiovascular disease. *J Clin Endocrinol Metab* 1997; **82**: 1752–6.

Botsis D, Kassanos D, Kalogirou D et al. Vaginal ultrasound of the endometrium in postmenopausal women with symptoms of urogenital atrophy on low-dose estrogen or tibolone treatment: a comparison. *Maturitas* 1997; **26**: 57–6.

Brzezinski A, Adlercreutz H, Shaoul R et al. Short-term effects of phyto-estrogen-rich diet on postmenopausal women. *Menopause* 1997; **4**: 89–94.

Burger HG. The endocrinology of the menopause. *Maturitas* 1996; **23**: 129–36.

Cauley JA, Seeley DJ, Ensrud K et al. Estrogen replacement therapy and fractures in older women. *Ann Intern Med* 1995; **122**: 9–16.

Chetkowski RJ, Meldrum DR, Steingold KA et al. Biologic effects of transdermal estradiol. *N Engl J Med* 1986; **314**: 1615–20.

Chou TM, Krishnankutty S, Hutchison SJ et al. Testosterone induces dilation of canine coronary conductance and resistance arteries in vivo. *Circulation* 1996; **94**: 2614–19.

Cline JM, Paschold JC, Anthony MS et al. Effects of hormonal therapies and dietary soy phyto-estrogens on vaginal cytology in surgically postmenopausal macaques. *Fertil Steril* 1996; **65**: 1031–5.

Colditz GA, Hankinson SE, Hunter DJ et al. The use of estrogens and progestins and the risk of breast cancer in postmenopausal women. *N Engl J Med* 1995; **332**: 1589–93.

Daniel Y, Inbar M, Bar-Am A et al. The effects of tamoxifen treatment on the endometrium. *Fertil Steril* 1996; **65**: 1083–9.

Davis SR, McCloud P, Strauss BJG, Burger H. Testosterone enhances estradiol's effects on postmenopausal bone density and sexuality. *Maturitas* 1995; **21**: 227–36.

Davis SR, Burger HG. Androgens and the postmenopausal woman. *J Clin Endocrinol Metab* 1996; **81**: 2759–63.

DeFazio J, Meldrum DR, Winer JH, Judd HL. Direct action of androgen on hot flushes in the human male. *Maturitas* 1984; **6**: 3–8.

Delmas PD, Bjarnason NH, Mitlak B et al. Effects of raloxifene on bone mineral density, serum cholesterol concentrations, and uterine endometrium in postmenopausal women. *N Engl J Med* 1997; **337**: 1641–7.

Dickerson J, Bressler R, Christian CD, Hermann H. Efficacy of estradiol vaginal cream in postmenopausal women. *Clin Pharmacol Ther* 1979; **26**: 502–7.

Ditkoff EC, Crary WG, Cristo M, Lobo RA. Estrogen improves psychological function in asymptomatic postmenopausal women. *Obstet Gynecol* 1991; **78**: 991–5.

Draper MW, Flowers DE, Neild JA et al. Antiestrogenic properties of raloxifene. *Pharmacology* 1995; **50**: 209–17.

Erenus M, Kutlay K, Kutlay L, Pekin S. Comparison of the impact of oral versus transdermal estrogen on serum lipoproteins. *Fertil Steril* 1994; **61**: 300–302.

Ettinger B, Genant HK, Cann CE. Long-term estrogen replacement therapy prevents bone loss and fractures. *Ann Intern Med* 1985; **102**: 319–24.

Ettinger B, Selby J, Citron JT et al. Cyclic hormone replacement therapy using quarterly progestin. *Obstet Gynecol* 1994; **83**: 693–700.

Falkeborn M, Persson I, Adami HO. The risk of acute myocardial infarction after oestrogen and oestrogen–progestin replacement. *Br J Obstet Gynecol* 1992; **99**: 821–8.

FDA HRT Working Group. Guidance for clinical evaluation of combination estrogen/progestin-containing drug products used for hormone replacement therapy of postmenopausal women. *Menopause* 1995; **2**: 131–6.

Finucane FF, Madans JH, Bush TL et al. Decreased risk of stroke among postmenopausal estrogen users. Evidence from a national cohort. *Arch Intern Med* 1993; **153**: 73–9.

Fuchs-Young R, Glasebrook AL, Short LL et al. Raloxifene is a tissue-selective agonist/

antagonist that functions through the estrogen receptor. *Ann NY Acad Sci* 1995; **761**: 355–60.

Gallagher JC, Kable WT, Goldgar D. Effect of progestin therapy on cortical and trabecular bone: comparison with estrogen. *Am J Med* 1991; **90**: 171–8.

Gast M. The pharmacologic profile of conjugated equine estrogens. *Proceedings of the 2nd International Symposium on Women's Health and Menopause: Risk reduction strategies* 1997, in press.

Gelfand MM, Fugere P, Bissonnette F et al. Conjugated estrogens combined with sequential dydrogesterone or medroxyprogesterone acetate in postmenopausal women: effects on lipoproteins, glucose tolerance, endometrial histology, and bleeding. *Menopause* 1997: **4**: 10–18.

Gradishar WJ, Jordan VC. The clinical potential of new anti-estrogens. *J Clin Oncol* 1997; **15**: 840–52.

Grady D, Rubin SM, Petitti DB et al. Hormone therapy to prevent disease and prolong life in postmenopausal women. *Ann Intern Med* 1992; **117**: 1016–37.

Grodstein F, Stampfer MJ, Manson JE et al. Postmenopausal estrogen and progestin use and the risk of cardiovascular disease. *N Engl J Med* 1996; **335**: 435–61.

Grodstein F, Stampfer MJ, Colditz GA et al. Postmenopausal hormone therapy and mortality. *N Engl J Med* 1997; **336**: 1769–75.

Grey AB, Stapleton JP, Evans MC, Reid IR. The effect of the anti-estrogen tamoxifen on cardiovascular risk factors in normal postmenopausal women. *J Clin Endocrinol Metab* 1995; **80**: 3191–5.

Haas S, Walsh B, Evans S et al. The effect of transdermal estradiol on hormone and metabolic dynamics over a six-week period. *Obstet Gynecol* 1988; **71**: 671–6.

Hammond CB. Menopause and hormone replacement therapy: an overview. *Obstet Gynecol* 1996; **87**: 2–15S.

Harlap S. The benefits and risks of hormone replacement therapy: an epidemiologic overview. *Am J Obstet Gynecol* 1992; **166**: 1986–92.

Henderson VW, Paganini-Hill A, Emanuel CK et al. Estrogen replacement therapy in older women: comparisons between Alzheimer's disease cases and non-demented control subjects. *Arch Neurol* 1994; **51**: 896–900.

Herrington DM, Braden GA, Downes TR, Williams JK. Estrogen modulates coronary vasomotor responses in postmenopausal women with early atherosclerosis. *Am J Cardiol* 1994; **73**: 951–2.

Holbert TR. Transvaginal ultrasonographic measurement of endometrial thickness in postmenopausal women receiving estrogen replacement therapy. *Am J Obstet Gynecol* 1997; **176**: 1334–9.

Honjo H, Ogino Y, Naitoh K et al. In vivo effects by estrone sulfate on the central nervous system-senile dementia (Alzheimer's type). *J Steroid Biochem Mol Biol* 1989; **34**: 521–5.

Honore EK, Williams JK, Adams MR et al. Methyltestosterone does not diminish the beneficial effects of estrogen replacement therapy on coronary artery reactivity in cynomolgus monkeys. *Menopause* 1996; **3**: 20–26.

Jensen J, Riis BJ, Strom V et al. Long-term effects of percutaneous estrogens and oral progesterone on serum lipoproteins in postmenopausal women. *Am J Obstet Gynecol* 1987; **156**: 66–71.

Johanssen BW, Kaji L, Kullander S et al. On some effects of bilateral oophorectomy in the age range 15–30 years. *Acta Obstet Gynecol Scand* 1975; **54**: 449–61.

Judd HL, Judd GE, Lucas WE, Yen SSC. Endocrine function of the postmenopausal ovary: concentration of androgens and estrogens in ovarian and peripheral vein blood. *J Clin Endocrinol Metab* 1974; **39**: 1020–24.

Kampen DL, Sherwin BB. Estrogen use and verbal memory in healthy postmenopausal women. *Obstet Gynecol* 1994; **83**: 979–83.

Kenny AM, Prestwood KM, Pilbeam CC, Raisz LG. The short-term effects of tamoxifen on bone turnover in older women. *J Clin Endocrinol Metab* 1995; **80**: 3287–91.

Kiel DP, Felson DT, Anderson JJ et al. Hip fracture and the use of estrogens in postmenopausal women: the Framingham Study. *N Engl J Med* 1987; **317**: 1169–74.

King RJB. Biology of female sex hormone action in relation to contraceptive agents and neoplasia. *Contraception* 1991; **43**: 527–42.

Klaiber EL, Broverman DM, Vogel W, Kobayashi Y. Estrogen therapy for severe persistent depression in women. *Arch Gen Psychiat* 1979; **36**: 742–4.

Krall EA, Dawson-Hughes B, Hannan MT et al. Postmenopausal estrogen replacement and tooth retention. *Am J Med* 1997; **102**: 536–42.

Kronenberg F. Hot flashes: epidemiology and physiology. *Ann NY Acad Sci* 1990; **592**: 52–86.

Kuiper GGJM, Enmark E, Pelto-Huikko M et al. Cloning of a novel estrogen receptor expressed in rat prostate and ovary. *Proc Natl Acad Sci USA* 1996; **93**: 5925–30.

Kupperman HS. Comparative clinical evaluation of estrogenic preparations by the menopausal and amenorrheal indices. *J Endocrinol Metab* 1953; **13**: 688–703.

Lindsay R, Hart DM, Clark DM. The minimum effective dose of estrogen for prevention of postmenopausal bone loss. *Obstet Gynecol* 1984; **63**: 759–63.

Lindsay R, Hart DM, Forrest C, Baird C. Prevention of spinal osteoporosis in oophorectomised women. *Lancet* 1980; **2**: 1151–4.

Love RR, Mazess RB, Barden HS et al. Effects of tamoxifen on bone mineral density in postmenopausal women with breast cancer. *N Engl J Med* 1992; **326**: 852–6.

Lufkin EG, Wahner HW, O'Fallon WM et al. Treatment of postmenopausal osteoporosis with transdermal estrogen. *Ann Intern Med* 1992; **117**: 1–9.

Luisi M et al. A group-comparative study of effects of Ovestin cream vs Premarin cream in postmenopausal women with vaginal atrophy. *Maturitas* 1980; **2**: 311–19.

Lobo RA, Pickar JH, Wild RA et al for the Menopause Study Group. Metabolic impact of adding medroxyprogesterone acetate to conjugated estrogen therapy in postmenopausal women. *Obstet Gynecol* 1994; **84**: 987–95.

Mandel FP, Geola FL et al. Biological effects of various doses of vaginally administered conjugated equine estrogens in postmenopausal women. *J Clin Endocrinol Metab* 1983; **57**: 133.

Martin et al. Systemic absorption and sustained effects of vaginal estrogen creams. *JAMA* 1979; **242**: 2699–700.

McKinlay SM. The normal menopausal transition: an overview. *Maturitas* 1996; **23**: 137–45.

Miller VT, Muesing RA, LaRosa JC et al. Effects of conjugated equine estrogen with and without three different progestogens on lipoproteins, high-density lipoprotein subfractions and apolipoprotein A-1. *Obstet Gynecol* 1991; **77**: 235–40.

Milner MH, Sinnott MM, Cooke TM et al. A 2-year study of lipid and lipoprotein changes in postmenopausal women with tibolone and estrogen-progestin. *Obstet Gynecol* 1996; **87**: 593–9.

Molnar GW. Body temperatures during menopausal hot flushes. *J Appl Physiol* 1975; **38**: 499.

Mosselman S, Polman J, Dijkema R. ERβ: identification and characterization of a novel human estrogen receptor. *FEBS Lett* 1996; **392**: 49–53.

Naessen T, Berglund L, Ulmsten U. Bone loss in elderly women prevented by ultra-low doses of parenteral 17β-estradiol. *Am J Obstet Gynecol* 1997; **177**: 115–19.

Ohkura T, Isse K, Akazawa K et al. Long-term estrogen replacement therapy in female patients with dementia of the Alzheimer type: 7 case reports. *Dementia* 1995; **6**: 99–107.

Oldenhave A, Juszmann LJB, Everaerd WThAM. Hysterectomized women with ovarian conservation report more severe climacteric complaints than do normal climacteric women of similar age. *Am J Obstet Gynecol* 1993; **168**: 765–71.

Oldenhave A. Pathogenesis of climacteric complaints: ready for the change? *Lancet* 1994; **343**: 649–53.

Paganini-Hill A, Henderson VW. Estrogen deficiency and risk of Alzheimer's disease in women. *Am J Epidemiol* 1994; **140**: 256–61.

PEPI Writing Group. Effects of estrogen or estrogen/progestin regimens on heart disease risk factors in postmenopausal women. The postmenopausal estrogen/progestin interventions (PEPI) trial. *JAMA* 1995; **273**: 199–208.

PEPI Writing Group. Effects of hormone therapy on bone mineral density. Results from the postmenopausal estrogen/progestin interventions (PEPI) trial. *JAMA* 1996; **276**: 1389–96.

Psaty BM, Heckbert SR, Atkins D et al. The risk of myocardial infarction associated with the combined use of estrogens and progestins in postmenopausal women. *Arch Intern Med* 1994; **154**: 1333–9.

Rossmansmith WG, Scherbaum WA, Lauritzen C. Gonadotropin secretion during aging in postmenopausal women. *Neuroendocrinology* 1991; **54**: 211–18.

Rubin GL, Peterson HB, Lee NC et al. Estrogen replacement therapy and the risk of endometrial cancer: remaining controversies. *Am J Obstet Gynecol* 1990; **162**: 148–54.

Schneider DL, Barrett-Connor EL, Morton DJ. Timing of postmenopausal estrogen for optimal bone mineral density. The Rancho Bernardo study. *JAMA* 1997; **277**: 543–7.

Seoud MAF, Johnson J, Weed JC. Gynecologic tumors in tamoxifen-treated women with breast cancer. *Obstet Gynecol* 1993; **82**: 165–9.

Sherwin BB, Gelfand MM. Differential symptom response to parenteral estrogen and/or androgen administration in the surgical menopause. *Am J Obstet Gynecol* 1985; **151**: 153–60.

Siddle NC, Fraser D, Whitehead MI et al. Endometrial, physical and psychological effects of postmenopausal oestrogen therapy with added dehydroprogesterone. *Br J Obstet Gynaecol* 1990; **97**: 1101–7.

Smith DC, Prentice R, Thompson DJ, Herrmann WL. Association of exogenous estrogen and endometrial carcinoma. *N Engl J Med* 1975; **293**: 1164–7.

Smith P, Heimer G, Lindskog M, Ulmsten U. Oestradiol-releasing vaginal ring for treatment of postmenopausal urogenital atrophy. *Maturitas* 1993; **16**: 145–54.

Speroff L, Rowan J, Symons J et al for the CHART Study group. The comparative effect on bone density, endometrium, and lipids of continuous hormones as replacement therapy (CHART Study). A randomized controlled trial. *JAMA* 1996; **276**: 1397–403.

Stampfer MJ, Colditz GA, Willett WC et al. Postmenopausal estrogen therapy and cardiovascular disease. Ten-year follow-up from the Nurses' Health Study. *N Engl J Med* 1991; **325**: 756–62.

Suhonen SP, Holmstrom T, Allonen HO, Lahteenmaki P. Intrauterine and subdermal progestin administration in postmenopausal hormone replacement therapy. *Fertil Steril* 1995; **63**: 336–42.

Sullivan JM, Shala BA, Miller LA et al. Progestin enhances vasoconstrictor responses in postmenopausal women receiving estrogen replacement therapy. *Menopause* 1995; **2**: 193–9.

Sullivan JM, Fowlkes LP. The clinical aspects of estrogen and the cardiovascular system. *Obstet Gynecol* 1996; **87**: 36–43S.

Treolar AE. Menstrual cyclicity and the premenopause. *Maturitas* 1981; **3**: 249–64.

Udoff L, Langenberg P, Adashi EY. Combined continuous hormone replacement therapy: a critical review. *Obstet Gynecol* 1995; **86**: 306–16.

van Leeuwen FE, Benraadt J, Coebergh JWW et al. Risk of endometrial cancer after tamoxifen treatment of breast cancer. *Lancet* 1994; **343**: 448–52.

Vermeulen A. The hormonal activity of the postmenopausal ovary. *J Clin Endocrinol Metab* 1976; **42**: 247–53.

Walsh BW, Schiff I, Rosner B et al. Effects of postmenopausal estrogen replacement on the concentrations and metabolism of plasma lipoproteins. *N Engl J Med* 1991; **325**: 1196–204.

Watts NB, Notelovitz M, Timmons MC et al. Comparison of oral estrogens and estrogens plus androgen on bone mineral density, menopausal symptoms and lipoprotein profiles in surgical menopause. *Obstet Gynecol* 1995; **85**: 529–37.

Weiss NS, Szekeley DR, English DR, Schweid AL. Endometrial cancer in relation to patterns of menopausal estrogen use. *JAMA* 1979; **242**: 261–4.

Weiss NS, Ure CL, Ballard JH et al. Decreased risk of fractures of the hip and lower forearm with postmenopausal use of estrogen. *N Engl J Med* 1980; 1195–8.

Wenger NK, Speroff L, Packard B. Cardiovascular health and disease in women. *N Engl J Med* 1993; **329**: 247–56.

Wiklund I, Karlberg J, Mattsson LA. Quality of life of postmenopausal women on a regimen of transdermal estradiol therapy: a double-blind placebo-controlled study. *Am J Obstet Gynecol* 1993; **168**: 824–30.

Williams JK, Adams MR, Herrington DM, Clarkson TB. Short-term administration of estrogen and vascular responses of atherosclerotic coronary arteries. *J Am Coll Cardiol* 1992; **24**: 1757–61.

Williams DB, Voigt BJ, Fu YS et al. Assessment of less than monthly progestin therapy in postmenopausal women given estrogen replacement. *Obstet Gynecol* 1994; **84**: 787–93.

Wingo PA, Layde PM, Lee NC et al. The risk of breast cancer in postmenopausal women who have used estrogen replacement therapy. *JAMA* 1987; **257**: 209–15.

Woodruff DJ, Pickar JH for the Menopause Study Group. Incidence of endometrial hyperplasia in postmenopausal women taking conjugated estrogens (Premarin) with medroxyprogesterone acetate or conjugated estrogens alone. *Am J Obstet Gynecol* 1994; **170**: 1213–23.

Wysowski DK, Golden L, Burke L. Use of menopausal estrogens and medroxyprogesterone in the United States, 1982–1992. *Obstet Gynecol* 1995; **85**: 6–10.

Yang NN, Venugopalan M, Hardikar S, Glasebrook A. Identification of an estrogen response element activated by metabolites of 17β-estradiol and raloxifene. *Science* 1996; **273**: 1222–5.

Yue P, Chatterjee K, Beale C et al. Testosterone relaxes rabbit coronary arteries and aorta. *Circulation* 1995; **91**: 1154–60.

12

Cardiovascular Disease

Lian G. Ulrich

University Hospital of Copenhagen, Gentofte, Copenhagen, Denmark

HISTORICAL PERSPECTIVE

Often, today's contraindications become tomorrow's indications. One such example may be the use of estrogen replacement therapy (ERT) for cardiovascular disease.

Modern ERT therapy started almost six decades ago in the 1930s, and was initially used to treat women with severe menopausal symptoms. At that time, estrone and estradiol compounds were used. However, ERT did not become commonplace until the 1970s when it evolved from the 'feminine forever' concept of the 1960s (Bush & Barrett-Connor, 1985). Estrone was the first of the natural estrogenic hormones to be prepared in its crystalline form in 1929 and was initially extracted from the urine of pregnant women. This was followed by estriol, also in 1929, and estradiol extracted from porcine ovaries in 1935. The first commercial estrogen product used for the treatment of climacteric symptoms was Progynon (estrone benzoate) and was launched by Schering in Germany in 1929 (Frobenius, 1990; Schering AG, undated). Poor availability of natural estrogens led to the synthesis of ethinyl estradiol (EE), a synthetic, orally absorbed estrogen which was synthesized by Schering in 1937 but was not marketed until 1949 (Frobenius, 1990). Since the early 1970s, EE at first and, later, micronized natural estrogens have been the most commonly used agents used to treat menopausal symptoms in Europe, whereas Premarin, first marketed in the USA in 1942, is today the most widely used non-contraceptive estrogen worldwide with the USA remaining the primary market (Bush & Barrett-Connor, 1985).

The oral contraceptive pill (OC), which first became available in the early 1960s, is an estrogen–progestogen combination with EE or mestranol as the estrogenic component. Initial pills contained estrogens in high doses, viz. about 50–150 μg of EE in combination with various progestogens such as norethisterone and norgestrel. Initially, these estrogens and progestogens were used in OCs as well as for hormone replacement therapy (HRT). Because of the high potency of synthetic estrogens, side effects such as thromboembolic disease were found with these treatments.

Drug Development for Women. Edited by V.V. Ragavan. © 1998 John Wiley & Sons Ltd.

Changes in the formulation of natural estrogens, such as micronization, led to the use of natural estrogens for HRT, because smaller doses were needed for this indication. Presently, naturally occurring estrogens in physiological doses are primarily utilized in postmenopausal estrogen therapy, thus greatly reducing side effects related to the cardiovascular system more commonly seen with the more potent artificial estrogens used in OC preparations. As discussed later in this chapter, recent studies have actually found a beneficial effect of natural estrogens on cardiovascular disease in older women, which is in fact directly the opposite of earlier findings on OCs in younger women.

The findings in large OC studies remained a critical influence during the developmental phase of HRT investigations. The majority of studies investigating the relationship between fatal cardiovascular disease (CVD) and OCs were carried out in the UK (Thorogood & Vessey, 1990). The first studies, indicating an increased risk of CVD in OC users, were published in the late 1960s by Inman & Vessey. In 1968, two large-scale prospective cohort studies were started in the UK: the Royal College of General Practitioners Study, which followed 46 000 married women, half of whom used OCs at the time of recruitment, and the Oxford Family Planning Association (FPA) study on 17 000 married women, 10 000 of whom used the pill. Both studies have now run for more than 20 years and have resulted in well over 100 scientific publications. Both studies have demonstrated an increased risk of myocardial infarction as well as an increased risk of stroke (thrombotic as well as subarachnoid hemorrhage) in pill users. The Oxford Study has also shown an increased risk of pulmonary embolism. These studies, however, suffer from having started in the 1960s, when the use of high-dose synthetic estrogen-containing OCs (50–100 μg) was predominant. The studies also showed that the risk of myocardial infarction with OC use is markedly increased in the presence of other risk factors, particularly cigarette smoking and age. These studies and others still form the basis for present estrogen labeling, which states that OC use is contraindicated in women who smoke, especially after the age of 35 and in women with a history of cardiovascular disease. The latter caution is a relative contraindication for OC use. Because of the previously mentioned confusion between OCs and postmenopausal ERT, it is not unusual even today to find various forms of CVD listed as contraindications to postmenopausal therapy.

DEMOGRAPHIC/SOCIAL ISSUES

The Scope of the Problem

The male–female mortality ratios for coronary heart disease (CHD) vary from 3:1 to 6:1 in 27 countries (Lobo & Speroff, 1994). Despite these ratios favorable to women, CVD is the leading cause of death in women, claiming 500 000 women/ lives each year, or approximately one-fifth of the 2.5 million women hospitalized for this disease in the USA each year (Wenger, Speroff & Packard, 1993). Even so, for decades CVD has been considered a male disease, although in total, slightly more women than men succumb to CVD (Bush, 1990). Perhaps the reason is that very few women die of CVD before their 50s, whereas increased mortality and morbidity to this condition occurs in men much earlier, i.e., during their 40s. Data from the Framingham study indicate that the incidence of cardiac failure is higher in men than in women at any given age until the very late years of life (Kannel, Plehn & Cupples, 1988). Although overall more women than men die of CVD, this could be a reflection of women living longer than men and, in fact, cardiovascular mortality rates remain lower amongst women at every decade of life.

The Effect of the Menopause

The risk of dying from CHD increases with age, but women rarely die from CHD before their 50s. Since the average age of menopause is 51, and the incidence of CHD increases in women in their 50s, the menopause has been intensively discussed as a possible independent risk factor for CVD. Vital statistics, however, currently do not support the menopause per se as an important risk factor for CVD in women. The slope of the CVD mortality curve is no different for women aged 50–69 as compared to women aged 30–49 (Kannel et al, 1976). However, the menopause only occurs on average at age 51 and thus it may not be surprising that no abrupt change in the incidence is seen in the curve in this age group.

The effect of menopause in a population may actually be spread over two decades, between ages 35 and 55, as some women experience an early menopause while others start menopause much later. In the 20 year follow-up of the Framingham study, premenopausal status was compared to postmenopausal in all age groups less than 55 years. This data showed highly significant two-fold relative risk of occurrence of CVD in the postmenopausal group, although the groups were made up of small numbers (Kannel et al, 1976). Several confounding factors may influence the results; e.g. smokers tend to have an earlier menopause than non-smokers (Lindquist & Bengtsson, 1979). In the Nurses' Health Study cohort, where age and cigarette smoking were controlled, women who went through natural menopause were shown to have the same relative risk for CHD as premenopausal women (Colditz et al, 1987). In contrast, premenopausal women who had under-gone bilateral oophorectomy and who were not taking exogenous estrogens had a significantly increased risk of CHD compared to premenopausal women of the same age, and this increased risk was eliminated by estrogen use (Colditz et al, 1987). The weight of evidence supports the association of early surgical menopause with an increased risk of CVD and could be due to falling estrogen levels and/or some other yet to be determined factor (Bush, 1990; Stampfer, Colditz & Willett, 1990).

Another point of discussion, based on data from UK studies, is whether the apparently lower difference in mortality rates between men and women after their fiftieth year could be due to change in the mortality curves for men rather than in the corresponding curves for women (Heller & Jacobs, 1978). Death rates from ischemic heart disease (IHD) data from England and Wales (1970–1974) based on age seems to indicate that around their fiftieth year, the slope of the logarithmic curve decreased for men but not for women. There is speculation that women enjoy an apparent protection from CVD in their premenopausal years as compared to men—not because of their estrogen but because of an increased risk in the young male population due to as yet unknown factors, such as free testosterone or premature death in a high-risk group with congenital hyperlipidemias. Younger women could also be protected by estrogen, thus suggesting that a variety of factors, including hyperlipidemia with high LDL-cholesterol, may account for the difference in mortality, and with the loss of these differences in the 50s, men and women rapidly approach similar mortality and morbidity rates.

Hormone Replacement Therapy with Estrogen (and Progestogen?)

As discussed above, the data is still not clear as to whether menopause itself is a risk factor for CVD, but the overwhelming data has shown that ERT is associated with a decreased relative risk of CVD. A number of cohort studies have documented an association between decreased risk of various cardiovascular disease end points and ERT and/or estrogen/progestogen replacement therapy (HRT).

As can be seen from Table 12.1, the great majority of studies (Wilson et al, 1985, being the exception) indicate that ERT and HRT are associated with a decreased risk of CVD. It is important to note that, in spite of the overall conclusions, many of the studies included small numbers and, furthermore, not all studies reached statistical significance. The Framingham study (Wilson et al, 1985) has been intensely discussed, and it has been pointed out that the study group was small (302 out of 1234 women used ERT), and the increase in risk was primarily found in smokers. In addition, the authors chose to control for total cholesterol and HDL-cholesterol levels in their multivariate logistic regression. Surgical menopause occurred frequently among estrogen users and duration of estrogen treatment was not taken into account. Finally, morbidity but not mortality was found to be increased in estrogen users.

Several case-control studies have also been reported and well reviewed by Barrett-Connor & Bush (1991). Again, most of these studies included small numbers of women and yielded non-significant results, even though the trend was towards a decrease in risk with estrogen use. One notable exception is a study by Thompson, Meade & Greenberg (1989). This study, however, included women who were treated with progestogens only, and when this subgroup was removed from analysis, there was only a marginal increase in risk. Finally, a single clinical study of 168 women followed for over 10 years of therapy with HRT indicated a non-significant relative risk of 0.33 for myocardial infarction (MI) (Nachtigall et al, 1979).

TABLE 12.1 Studies on the association between ERT/HRT and risk of CVD

References	n	Follow-up years	Endpoint	RR	(Ever users)
Burch, Byrd & Vaughan, 1974	737	6–23 years	Fatal CHD	0.43	$p < 0.05$
		9 899 patient years			
Hammond et al, 1979	610	> 5 years	CVD	0.33	$p < 0.05$
Wilson, Garrison & Castelli, 1985	1 234	8 years	CHD	1.9	$p < 0.01$
Petitti, Perlman & Sidney, 1987	6 093	10–13 years	Acute MI	0.3	NS
Bush et al, 1987	2 270	8.5 years	Fatal IHD	0.34	(0.12–0.81)
Criqui et al, 1988	1 868	12 years	CVD	0.81	(0.61–1.08)
Hunt, Vessey & McPherson, 1990	4 544	11 years, average	Fatal CVD	0.41	(0.20–0.61)
Sullivan et al, 1990	2 268	10 years	Death	0.16	(0.04–0.66)
Avila, Walker & Jick, 1990	24 900	128 500 patient years	Non-fatal MI	0.7	(0.4–1.3)
Henderson, Paganini-Hill & Ross, 1991	8 853	7.5 years	Acute MI	0.6	$p < 0.001$
Wolf et al, 1991	1 944	16 years	Fatal CVD	0.66	(0.48–0.90)
Falkeborn et al, 1992	23 174	5.8 years	First MI	0.81	(0.71–0.92) ERT/ HRT
Lafferty & Fiske, 1994	157	25 years	MI	0.53	(0.3–0.87) HRT
				0.34	(0.09–1.34)
Grodstein et al, 1996b	59 337	16 years	CHD	0.6	(0.43–0.83) ERT
				0.39	(0.19–0.78) HRT

Evaluating the status today, there is good support in the literature that current use of non-contraceptive estrogen replacement therapy is associated with a decrease in the risk of CVD. The questions that presently remain unanswered relate to whether the addition of progestogens in any way changes the relative risk ratios. The available epidemiological evidence, although limited, supports HRT being as effective as ERT in the prevention of CHD. Other issues which need to be addressed are possible effects of dose, type of estrogen and route of administration. The latest and largest epidemiological study, the 16 year data from the Nurses' Health Study (Grodstein, 1996b) tries to answer some of these questions. Like with the Uppsala study (Falkeborn et al, 1992) this study indicates that HRT is as effective as ERT, low-dose estrogen being at least as good as high doses in the prevention of CHD. Biases can never be avoided in observational studies, and hence it is critical to determine whether secondary intervention is adequate or whether primary prevention is the preferred strategy for investigating the effect of HRT and its relationship to CVD in clinical studies. A couple of ongoing studies, the Wyeth-Ayerst HERS study (a secondary intervention trial) and the Women's Health Initiative (a prospective primary prevention trial) may provide some answers in the future.

CLINICAL EFFICACY CRITERIA

Although epidemiological studies indicate that the use of ERT and probably also HRT is associated with a decreased risk of CVD, it has often been stated that epidemiological, and especially case-control, studies can only generate hypotheses, whereas full-fledged clinical trials are needed to prove or disprove causal relationships.

Even though most epidemiological studies reported in the literature have attempted to correct for CVD risk factors, how to carry out these adjustments and how they affect outcomes still remains controversial. For example, low levels of HDL-cholesterol is a well recognized risk factor, but to adjust for this would be to affect one of the mechanisms by which ERT is said to act, as previously discussed in relation to the Framingham study. Randomized clinical trials overcome this problem. In fact, secondary interventions with lipid-lowering drugs have been studied. However, to be adequately powered, secondary intervention studies on HRT after myocardial infarction can easily require 3000 women per group, carried out for probably 2–5 years. Primary intervention trials are even more costly, increase the requirements for patient numbers by at least a factor of 10, and need to be carried out for close to a decade.

Because of these time frames, both academic research and pharmaceutical companies remain interested in surrogate end points, but such end points can create their own problems, too. Although certain surrogate end points, such as lipid levels, have been identified in epidemiological studies as important predictors, their relationship in particular to ERT remains questionable. Furthermore, dose relationships have rarely been investigated, raising questions about whether threshold levels exist and also, what kind of quantitative differences are important.

Lipids

Lipoprotein profiles have been widely used as surrogate end points in the assessment of the utility of drugs and their influence on the risk of cardiovascular diseases. Bush et al (1987) and Barrett-Connor & Bush (1991) estimated that approximately 20–50% of the beneficial effect of ERT in CVD could be accounted for by the effect on the lipid profile.

The relative importance of LDL-cholesterol decrease and HDL-cholesterol increase is still not settled. Intervention studies such the POSCH trial (Buchwald et al, 1992) have underlined the importance of lowering LDL, whereas the LRC studies (Bush et al, 1987) underlined the importance of increasing HDL in Premarin-treated women.

Another issue which has been raised is whether the same risk factors are equivalent in men and women and, in fact, whether studies conducted exclusively in men can be extrapolated to women. We know that several different subtypes may exist for all tested lipids, such as HDL2 and HDL3. It may very well be that sub-fractions resulting from ERT/HRT therapy may not be identical in ERT/HRT treated and untreated persons, a factor which epidemiological studies do not account for completely.

For instance, high triglyceride levels are known to increase the risk of CVD in the untreated subject, but are found to be elevated after unopposed estrogen treatment. The triglycerides which increase after estrogen treatment are considered to be of a more 'fluffy' variety than triglycerides found in untreated women. Furthermore, in the untreated, high triglyceride levels are most often linked to low levels of HDL-cholesterol, which is also a known risk factor, whereas in estrogen-treated women, HDL-cholesterol as well as triglycerides will increase, while progestogen added to the estrogen treatment tends to modify both HDL-cholesterol and triglyceride increases. A high HDL-cholesterol could be sufficiently protective to make LDL-cholesterol unimportant and, likewise, very low LDL-cholesterol levels may give sufficient protection to make HDL-cholesterol levels relatively unimportant. Data from the Framingham study provide some support for this concept. In this study, even a high level of total cholesterol was not related to a high incidence of CHD as long as HDL-cholesterol was also high, whereas the incidence of CHD was directly related to total cholesterol with lower levels of HDL-cholesterol (Castelli et al, 1986).

The effect of estrogen on lipids is to some extent dose-related. As an example, the study by Walsh et al (1991) on 0.625 mg vs. 1.25 mg conjugated equine estrogens (Premarin), as shown in Table 12.2, demonstrates that all lipids except HDL2-apo-A2 are significantly different between the two doses of CEE and placebo.

In the same study, 2 mg E2 (Estrace®) was compared to the 0.1 mg estradiol patch (Estraderm®TTS) given twice weekly (a small group), with the results shown

TABLE 12.2 Lipoprotein changes *vs.* placebo during treatment with different types, dosages and forms of administration of estrogen

Change from placebo	0.625 mg Conjugated equine estrogens (CEE)		1.25 mg CEE		2 mg Oral estradiol		0.1 mg TTS (transdermal estradiol, twice weekly)	
VLDL-T	+24%	$p = 0.003$	+42%	$p < 0.0001$	Large: +35% Small: +8%	$p = 0.05$ NS	Large: −4% Small: −3%	NS NS
VLDL-C	+16%	NS	+30%	$p = 0.008$	Large: +7% Small: −1%	NS NS	Large: −9% Small: +2%	NS NS
VLDL-apoB	+29%	$p = 0.02$	+22%	NS				
LDL-T	+20%	$p < 0.0001$	+30%	$p < 0.0001$	+30%	$p = 0.04$	+12%	NS
LDL-C	−15%	$p < 0.0001$	−19%	$p < 0.0001$	−14%	$p = 0.002$	−4%	NS
LDL-apoB	−10%	$p = 0.0009$	−9%	$p = 0.005$				
HDL-T	+32%	$p < 0.0001$	+43%	$p < 0.0001$	+26%	$p = 0.0001$	+10%	NS
HDL-C	+16%	$p < 0.0001$	+18%	$p < 0.0001$				
HDL2-C	+50%	$p < 0.0001$	+59%	$p < 0.0001$	+39%	$p = 0.0005$	+23%	$p = 0.015$
HDL2-apoAI	+46%	$p < 0.0001$	+39%	$p < 0.0001$				
HDL2-apoAII	−6%	NS	−3%	NS				
HDL3-C	+6%	$p = 0.0002$	+6%	$p = 0.0003$	+4%	NS	−5%	NS
HDL3-apoAI	+14%	$p < 0.001$	+22%	$p < 0.0001$				
HDL3-apoAII	+10%	$p < 0.0001$	+10%	$p < 0.0001$				

(Adapted from Walsh, 1991)

in Table 12.2. Transdermal administration showed no significant differences to placebo except those indicated in the table. Total triglycerides increased by 24%.

This study (Walsh et al, 1991) describes in detail the different lipid sub-fractions, while other studies have simply stated the effects on HDL, LDL, VLDL, total cholesterol and triglycerides. Dose relationship appears to be reflected primarily in VLDL and triglyceride fractions, whereas changes in HDL-cholesterol, LDL-cholesterol and apolipoproteins are only marginally improved with increasing doses. These findings would support the use of lower doses of Premarin for cardiovascular protection. Apo-A1, however, was directly related to Premarin dose in this study. The effect of oral E2 in the 2 mg dose on LDL-cholesterol was comparable to Premarin, whereas the effect on HDL-cholesterol and HDL2-cholesterol is somewhat lower. This study did not demonstrate major differences in dose effects, which is in agreement with previous findings by Henderson, Paganini-Hill & Ross (1991) in an epidemiological study. Data from the Nurses' Health Study do not indicate a positive dose–response curve either. On the contrary, higher doses may be less effective in the prevention of CHD (Grodstein, 1996b).

In addition, the study (Walsh et al, 1991) showed that the mechanism of hypertriglyceridemia induced by oral estrogens differs from that of familial hypertriglyceridemia. In the latter case, impaired lipolysis results in low HDL and high VLDL, whereas estrogen-induced hypertriglyceridemia is probably caused by increased production of triglycerides and apo-B. Estrogen increases LDL catabolism and levels of apo-A1. The latter is the most important sub-fraction involved in cardiovascular protection, partly because in vitro studies show that apo-A1 stimulates the efflux of cholesterol from cultured adipocytes loaded with LDL (Barbaras et al, 1987). This sub-fraction is low in men after puberty (Ohta et al, 1989) and it has been inversely related to coronary atherosclerosis in clinical studies (Puchois et al, 1987). Furthermore, although triglycerides have been shown to be an independent risk factor for CVD in women, this lipid fraction may be less important in estrogen-treated women.

Addition of progestogen to ERT in general reduces the estrogen-induced increase in HDL-cholesterol. This decrease is related to progestogen dose as well as to type and potency. The recently published PEPI trial (PEPI Writing Group, 1995) and the Nabulsi et al (1993) paper are the most widely cited papers on the effect of progestogen addition and CVD.

In the PEPI study, several regimens were compared: placebo; CEE (0.625 mg); CEE and MPA 10 mg for 12 days/month; CEE + MPA 2.5 mg continuous combined to CEE + MP (micronized progesterone) 200 mg 12 days/month. In this study, no substantial differences were found between the four actively treated groups with regard to LDL-cholesterol and triglycerides. With respect to HDL-cholesterol (mmol/l), however, a decrease of 0.03 was seen with the placebo, in contrast to an increase of 0.04 and 0.03 with CEE + MPA (cyclic and continuous) and increases of 0.14 and 0.11 with CEE and CEE + MP, respectively. The PEPI trial supported oral MP as a superior progestogen compared to MPA, as MP apparently does not influence the estrogen-induced changes in the lipoproteins.

This was also supported by the Darj & Nielsson (1992) study, which evaluated the lipid effects of E2 with different doses of progesterone (50–200 mg).

In contrast, the cross-sectional Nabulsi et al (1993) study found no major differences between users of estrogen and users of estrogen–progestogen (for all practical purposes, translating into Premarin and Provera) with respect to any of the lipid fractions, but it did find a non-statistical significant trend towards lower triglycerides with the use of combined therapy.

Claus Christiansen's group compared Trisequens Forte (4 mg micronized 17β-estradiol) for 22 days, with addition of 1 mg norethisterone acetate (NETA) on days 13–22, followed by 6 days of 1 mg E2), to Trisequens (the same as Trisequens Forte with 2 mg E2 instead of 4 mg), to half-dose Trisequens (1 mg E2), and placebo (Jensen & Christiansen, 1987). In this study, all of the active preparations also included estriol (E3) at half the dose of E2. Although the study stated that the effect on lipoproteins was dose-related, differences between the 1 and 2 mg doses is only apparent for total cholesterol, not for LDL-cholesterol and HDL-cholesterol.

Notelovitz et al's (1983) data further supported the findings noted above. This study compared oral micronized E2 at 1 mg and 2 mg, as well as CEE 0.625 mg and 1.25 mg given to subjects randomly for 3-month cycles (cyclic treatment for 3 out of 4 weeks), to baseline lipoprotein values. No major differences were found between treatment groups, but the groups were small and treatment time short in this study. There was, however, in this study a trend noted towards a more pronounced increase in HDL with E2 compared to CEE. This is in contrast to the finding in the earlier-quoted Walsh study (Ohta et al, 1989).

The effect of adding progestogens was also studied in a 2-year study comparing Trisequens (for composition, see above), Kliogest (continuous administration of 2 mg E2 and 1 mg NETA) and placebo (Munk-Jensen et al, 1994). Significant differences were noted between the two actively treated groups on total cholesterol, which decreased 1.01 mmol/l (Kliogest) and 0.58 mmol/l (Trisequens), and HDL2-cholesterol which decreased significantly (0.18 mmol/l) only in the Kliogest group. Expressed as percentage change from baseline, the following changes were noted. Kliogest: total cholesterol, −15%; LDL-cholesterol, −13%; HDL-cholesterol, −14%; Trisequens: total cholesterol, +8%; LDL-cholesterol, +10%; and total triglycerides, +18%. When these results are compared to the effects of CEE on lipids, the decreases in LDL-cholesterol are comparable, and the increase in triglyceride with Trisequens no more than that found with unopposed CEE. However, no increase was seen in HDL-cholesterol in this study and actually a decrease was found with Kliogest treatment.

The Framingham study, as well as the LRC study (Castelli, 1992; Bass et al, 1993) indicate that HDL-cholesterol as well as triglycerides are independent risk factors for CVD in women. Groups with low HDL-cholesterol (below 1.03 mmol/l) are particularly at risk when triglycerides are also found to be high, whereas women with high HDL-cholesterol (more than 1.30 mmol/l) apparently are not as influenced by high triglycerides.

Seen in this context, the lack of increase in HDL-cholesterol with some types of HRT may be worrisome. However, the lipoprotein profile seen with the Cyclo-progynova (2 mg estradiol valerate—E2V) for 21 days with the addition of 500 μg norgestrel (NG) or 250 μg levonorgestrel (LNG) may be interesting in this context (Vejtorp et al, 1986). The result of this study found that Cycloprogynova treatment (measured during the progestogen phase in the postmenopausal group) resulted in a 12% decrease in HDL-cholesterol, 19% decrease in LDL-cholesterol and 19% decrease in VLDL-cholesterol. Even so, Cycloprogynova is so far the only specific combination therapy that has been found to reduce the incidence of first myocardial infarction in an epidemiological study (Falkeborn et al, 1992). In this study, the protective effect of Cycloprogynova in prevention of myocardial infarction was at least comparable to the effect of unopposed estrogen therapy. The most recent data from the Nurses' Health Study (Grodstein, 1996b) also support the effect of HRT being at least as good as ERT in preventing CHD.

Based on the effect of the hormones alone or in combination on the lipo-proteins, the following can be concluded. It is likely that ERT as well as HRT in all the currently marketed formulations do indeed offer cardiac protection, even if some of the combined preparations do not increase or even decrease HDL-cholesterol. Even so, the best combination may be one that utilizes micronized progesterone with an estrogen. It probably does not matter much whether the estrogen is CEE or E2. Also, there may not be a significant dose effect as long as potent estrogens such as CEE and E2 are used in doses of at least 0.625 mg CEE or 1 mg E2.

Although some combined HRT products may lower HDL-cholesterol, this adverse effect may be overcome by other CVD-related effects, as demonstrated by the effect of Cycloprogynova on the lipoprotein profile. At this time, no clear evidence exists to distinguish one combination as being superior to any other. Furthermore, HRT may have a beneficial effect on triglycerides as compared to unopposed therapy, but since high triglycerides in studies of untreated populations are normally linked to low HDL-cholesterol, the importance of the triglyceride effect of estrogen remains unclear.

Other Surrogate Endpoints

Little is known about the dose-related effects of estrogens and progestogens on end points other than lipids which are normally related to CVD, and virtually nothing is known about the relative importance of these parameters compared to each other and to the lipids.

The effect of estrogen on coagulation factors has been investigated mainly in relation to ethinyl estradiol (EE). Gordon et al (1988) used 5, 10 and 20 μg of EE in combination with 0.5 or 1 mg NETA in postmenopausal women. Antithrombin III was significantly reduced only in the high estrogen dose group. Factor XII and partial thromboplastin time were slightly increased in all groups. The relationship between OCs and increased risk of thromboembolic disease has to a great extent been attributed to the estrogen effect on coagulation parameters. Not only does EE have an effect on these parameters, so do natural estrogens. However, since most of the effects of unopposed estrogens on these parameters are of an adverse nature, a lowering of the estrogen dose for the protection against CVD is likely to be advantageous. Recent epidemiological studies investigating the effect of OCs as well as ERT and HRT on the risk of venous thrombosis, especially related to coagulation, will be further discussed in the section on safety issues.

Nabulsi et al (1993) investigated CEE vs. CEE + MPA users and found significant differences in factor VII and protein C activity between the two actively treated groups. Lower values for both factors were found in the combined CEE–MPA group as compared to the CEE group. These differences reflect an increase in these factors for the unopposed estrogen group, with no apparent difference between the HRT and non-treated/previously treated groups. Unfortunately, the study does not differentiate between the two actively treated groups, only comparing users to non-users. High factor VII and low protein-C increase the risk of thrombosis.

No differences were observed between the opposed and unopposed groups with respect to insulin and glucose levels—both were lower than in the untreated groups. Blood pressure was not different in any of the groups.

Fasting glucose was significantly decreased in all treatment groups in the PEPI trial (PEPI Writing Group, 1995). Fasting insulin levels as well as levels 2 h postprandial did not change significantly in any of the groups, neither did any treatment group experience any clinically significant change in blood pressure. In addition, a significant increase in fibrinogen was found in the placebo treatment group, with no change in any of the treated groups.

Recently, a Finnish group has published the results from a non-randomized cross-sectional trial investigating the extent of atherosclerotic plaques in untreated women vs. treated women (Punnonen et al, 1995). These women were treated for approximately 10 years on average with combinations similar to Progynova and Cyclopro-gynova: E2V and E2V/LNG 2 mg estrogen dose (40 women per group). The total number of atherosclerotic plaques did not differ between actively treated groups and was significantly lower in these groups as compared to the untreated group.

Liebermann et al (1994) found improved endothelium-dependent flow-mediated dilatation in the brachial artery after 9 weeks of treatment with 1 or 2 mg estradiol. No dose-related effects were found.

Gilligan et al (1995), however, demonstrated that although acute intra-arterial infusion of estradiol potentiated forearm vasodilatation induced by acetylcholine, this effect could not be maintained during a subsequent 3 week treatment with 0.1 mg E2 patch. Estradiol levels during acute infusion were 345 pg/ml compared to the 120 pg/ml levels obtained with the patch. He concluded that E2 levels obtained with the patch were too low to have an effect. Another possible explanation is that the treatment time with the patch was relatively too short. Gangar et al (1991) only found an effect of transdermal estradiol on pulsativity index after 9 weeks or more of treatment, implying a time dependency for endothelial response. Since acute perfusion results in the higher blood levels, this method of administration may work directly on the myocytes of the damaged vessel, whereas an endothelial effect may take a longer time. The beneficial effect of ERT and HRT with no difference between the two is also supported by animal studies, showing reduced size of atherosclerotic plaques in monkeys (Adams et al, 1990) and rabbits (Haarbo et al, 1991) treated with ERT or HRT while on a high cholesterol diet as compared to controls.

Clinical Efficacy Parameters: Conclusion

There is now a significant body of evidence describing the effect of different estrogen–progestogen combinations on various cardiac surrogate end points, such as lipoprotein profile, coagulation, blood pressure and glucose insulin metabolism. Ultrasound measurement of atherosclerotic plaques has also been studied, as have flow measurements in different arteries, radiographic studies of stenosis and vascular diameters. Different combination therapies seem to have given different results, but very little is known about the relative importance of these various parameters.

Epidemiological studies have indicated a significant relationship between estrogen treatment and decreased risk of CVD. Most of these studies have primarily included women treated with unopposed estrogen, but the few studies which have included women treated with combined estrogen and progestogen have shown no difference in effect between ERT and HRT with respect to the hard end points in CVD, such as onset of angina or myocardial infarction, despite differences in surrogate end points.

Many hypotheses have been discussed with respect to the mechanism by which estrogens influence cardiovascular risk. But there appears to be no uniform conclusion in the published literature. Most likely the observed effects are multifaceted. The importance of the lipoproteins has probably been overestimated in the past, and the acute effects underestimated in view of recent findings indicating that the cardio-protective effect is related to current rather than past use of ERT (Grodstein, 1996b). It is also not known whether a true dose relationship and/or thresholds exist for these effects.

At present, further research is needed into the mechanism of action of estrogen and progestogens, including dose relationship. Clinical studies are needed on primary and secondary prevention of heart disease and acute myocardial infarction. Such studies have been started and will be described in more detail in the section on 'Ongoing Clinical Research'. The two most important studies are the NIH-sponsored 'Women's Health Initiative' (WHI) on primary prevention of CVD and the Wyeth-Ayerst-sponsored HERS study on secondary prevention of CVD by estrogens. Furthermore, studies are much needed to evaluate the dose effect of various ERT/EPRT regimens to determine threshold effects. These are potentially expensive but critical studies.

SAFETY ISSUES

The most important safety issue with regard to hormonal treatment is the influence on the risk, albeit small, of breast cancer. Another important safety issue is the increased risk of endometrial cancer with unopposed estrogen therapy. Although most of the data with regard to the effect of ERT on cardiovascular disease have been conducted in women who were given unopposed estrogen, current consensus states that a progestogen should be added to ERT for at least 10 days per 28 day cycle in order to protect the endometrium against estrogen-induced hyperplasia. Only limited data on the effect of combined regimens are available at present. Possible adverse effects of progestogen on estrogen's positive effect on CVD has been discussed previously.

As previously described, progestogens attenuate some of the positive estrogen-induced changes in the lipid profile, which have been thought to account for the major part of the cardioprotective effects of estrogens. Some authors have estimated that the cardioprotective effects of HRT are somewhat less than those of ERT, but the magnitude is not known (Daly et al, 1992). Others have argued that adding progestogens, notably MPA, may even improve the protective effect (Nabulsi et al, 1993) because of favorable effects on coagulation factors and triglycerides. Some have argued that 17-hydroxyprogesterone derivatives such as MPA may be less harmful on the cardiovascular system than are the 19-nortestosterone derivatives, but this discussion has been based on comparisons using non-equivalent doses. One of the most often cited papers (Hirvonen, Malkonen & Manninen, 1981) used 10 mg MPA, 10 mg NET and 0.5 mg LNG, whereas appropriate comparative doses would have actually been in the order of 5–10 mg MPA to 0.35–1 mg NET and 0.075–0.15 mg LNG. In a later study, the effects of different progestogens on the lipid profile were not shown to be very different from each other (Ottesen et al, 1985).

Whether progestogens in reality change estrogen's cardioprotective effect is still not entirely clear. However, two epidemiological studies are now available with sufficient numbers of women treated with HRT to make it feasible to analyze this group separately: the Uppsala study from Sweden (Falkeborn et al, 1992) and the latest update of the Nurses' Health Study (Grodstein, 1996b). In the Swedish study, prescriptions were collected from approximately 23 000 women who took estrogens in the period 1977–1980. Approximately 21% of the women in the study belonged to a cohort who took one single fixed brand, Cyclabil (2 mg estradiol valerate for 21/28 days, with the addition of 0.5 mg norgestrel for at least 10 days). This combination was previously found to have lowered HDL-cholesterol, HDL2-cholesterol and LDL-cholesterol, but triglycerides remained relatively unchanged (Vejtorp, 1986). Since HDL-cholesterol was also lowered, this could be seen to be a disadvantage, but in fact, the relative risk of first-time myocardial infarction in this cohort was 0.53 (0.30–0.87) for women less than 60 years of age at entry and 0.5 (0.28–0.8) in the whole group of women taking this fixed combined brand.

In the Nurses' Health Study the majority continue to use unopposed estrogen, but in the latest update, there were enough women on combination use to analyze the users of estrogen alone and those using combinations with progestogens (Grodstein, 1996b). The relative risk of major coronary disease multivariate adjusted was found to be 0.60 (0.43–0.83) for users of unopposed estrogen and 0.39 (0.19–0.78) for users of combined estrogen and progestogen. The number of cases in the combined group is small (8 cases in 27 161 person/years), but when observed in relation to the Swedish study, the two major epidemiological studies both indicate that the protection against CVD with HRT is at least comparable with that obtained with ERT alone. Furthermore, the women in the Swedish study primarily used estradiol in combination with 19-nortestosterone derivatives (levonorgestrel), whereas the Nurses' subjects primarily used conjugated equine estrogens combined with medroxyprogesterone acetate. The fact that both studies showed similar levels of protection against CVD may indicate no major differences between the various estrogens and progestogens with respect to their cardiovascular effects.

The Nurses' Health Study indicates a significantly reduced risk of major CVD with the dose of 0.625 mg of conjugated estrogens, with no significant trend. However, the groups using other estrogen doses were small in number and the only safe conclusion from this information is the lack of a dose relationship curve in relation to coronary disease.

However, a significant trend was found in this study towards an increased risk of stroke with higher estrogen doses. The overall risk of stroke was not significantly increased but a significantly increased risk of ischemic stroke was found in current estrogen users. This finding should, however, be treated with caution as other studies have found a decreased risk of stroke with ERT/HRT (Falkeborn et al, 1993; Paganini-Hill, Ross & Henderson, 1985). Previously, venous thromboembolism (VTE) has not been considered a safety issue with postmenopausal ERT/HRT, although the increased risk of VTE has been well recognized with oral contraceptives. Studies, although small, had not shown any increased risk with the use of natural estrogens, but the recent publications may change this (Daly et al, 1996; Jick et al, 1996; Grodstein, 1996a).

In the Oxford Regional Health Study, which is a case-control study ($n = 39$), the relative risk of venous thromboembolism (VTE), including deep venous thrombosis (DVT) and pulmonary embolism (PE), was found to be 3.5 (1.8–7.0) in current HRT users compared to non-users (Daly et al, 1996). There was no association between past ERT/HRT use and VTE, and the risk appeared to be higher for short-term users than for long-term users. There was an increased risk of VTE associated with use of higher doses of estrogen as compared to lower doses, whereas no difference was found between users of ERT and HRT. At the request of the UK researchers, investigators of the Puget Sound Study conducted a similar case-control investigation (Jick et al, 1996). Based on 42 cases of VTE (31 DVT and 11 PE) matched to 168 controls, current estrogen users were found to have a relative risk of VTE of 3.6 (1.6–7.8). This study indicated an increased risk with increasing estrogen dose, but the number of cases on estrogen doses other than 0.625 mg was extremely small. A relatively high risk of VTE was found in women who had used estrogen for less than 1 year, but the numbers were small and the relationship between treatment time and risk less clear compared to the British data. Furthermore, the cases included may be rather selective as 43 potential cases were not included, based on discharge summaries. Finally the latest update of the Nurses' Health Study seems to support the two case-control studies in that current users of postmenopausal replacement therapy had an increased risk of primary PE (Grodstein, 1996). The relative risk of PE adjusted for multiple risk factors in these women was 2.1 (1.2–3.8). In this study no association was found between estrogen dose and relative risk, but women who had used estrogen for less than 5 years tended to have an increased risk compared to longer-term users. The numbers in all of these sub-analyses were, however, small. Thus, based on the most recent evidence, VTE may potentially be a safety issue with ERT/HRT. The increased risk in short-term users may indicate acute effects and/or multifactorial pathogenesis.

Epidemiological data gathered thus far do not support any difference between HRT and ERT with respect to cardiovascular protection, so it is possible, although not yet proven, that progestogens may not cause any major safety concern from a cardiovascular point of view, despite the adverse effect of progestogens on HDL-cholesterol levels. Likewise, there seem to be no major differences between ERT and HRT with regard to VTE.

Based on surrogate end points, HRT may appear to be preferable to ERT with respect to the effect on coagulation (Nabulsi et al, 1993). ERT tends to decrease antithrombin III (ATIII), which in theory increases the risk of thrombosis. However, the changes that occur naturally at menopause also include an increase in ATIII and Factor VII. These changes are reversed by HRT, which also tends to decrease factor VII. Furthermore, the changes which take place remain within the normal range and thus most thinkers have favored the view that these changes are probably of little clinical significance.

Based on the recent epidemiological evidence, this view may change, but it should be kept in mind that earlier studies have not shown any relationship between VTE and use of postmenopausal estrogens, although the present studies are larger, many of the conclusions are still based on small numbers, and the absolute increased risk is probably in the order of one case of VTE in 5000 current estrogen users.

The effect of ERT and HRT on other surrogate end points may theoretically also be a safety issue. Diabetes has previously been considered a relative contraindication for HRT therapy, but some evidence suggests that diabetics may in fact benefit from estrogen replacement therapy (Luotola, Pyorala & Loikkanen, 1986). Hypertension is another contraindication which has been inherited from oral contraceptives, but with HRT, the trend is actually towards normalization of BP, and controlled hypertension should not be considered a contraindication to HRT (Hassager et al, 1987).

Treatment with HRT tends to provoke fluid retention. In a state of poorly compensated heart disease, this could, in theory, pose a potential clinical problem. No data exists to actually determine whether congestive heart failure is worsened with HRT treatment.

Based on present evidence, however, it seems safe to conclude that no major safety concerns apply with HRT with regard to cardiovascular issues. Ongoing research should help clarify some of the above-mentioned issues.

Risk/Benefit

Evaluating the status of risk/benefit from a patient's point of view, at this time HRT appears to provide primarily benefits. However, an important risk factor is related to the risk of breast and endometrial cancer, and perhaps an increased risk of gallstones, and based on recent reports of increased risk of venous thrombo-embolism. Unless an individual woman carries a higher than usual risk of breast cancer, or has already suffered from the disease, the cardiovascular and bone benefits outweigh the risk of breast cancer.

The real question is not whether or not HRT is beneficial to the bone and heart, but rather, when and for how long it should be taken. Some investigators have suggested that a major benefit to bone is derived only if women are treated immediately after the menopause and continue for at least 7–10 years or maybe for the rest of life or, alternatively, that some benefit may be obtained by treatment some 10–20 years after the menopause (Felson et al, 1993).

Furthermore, the question of whether HRT should be given for prevention of cardiovascular disease or for secondary prevention, and which approach is most cost-effective, still remains to be answered. No studies are yet available to make this determination. Radiographic studies have indicated that the largest effects occur in women with the most advanced atherosclerosis (Sullivan et al, 1990). If HRT is primarily given to high-risk women, such as women with previous or manifest coronary disease or perhaps to diabetics or women with hyperlipidemia, and further disease can be prevented, this could be a cost-effective approach to therapy. HRT is definitely effective in correcting some forms of hyperlipidemia (Tonstad et al, 1995) and high-risk women are easily identified on the basis of previous myocardial infarction, hyperlipidemia, diabetes or perhaps even early surgical menopause.

With regard to developing drugs for cardiovascular indications, there continues to be a level of disagreement between industry and regulatory agencies. Regulatory agencies have insisted on prospective studies providing hard clinical end points, claiming that surrogate end points are not adequate and, furthermore, have often rejected epidemiological studies, claiming that these studies in the published literature contain serious biases. The present status of the use of ERT and HRT for the prevention of cardiovascular disease is that while practicing clinicians prescribe estrogens, regulatory agencies have not provided approval of the indication, per se. If the regulatory agencies require studies with clinical end points, the costs to industry can be prohibitive for both obtaining the indication for old drugs and for development of new drugs. If a drug is already on the market, it is hard for a company to justify a large clinical study as being cost-effective. In addition, there is very little to distinguish one HRT regimen from another, and hence, they could be viewed as generic treatments. It is unlikely that many companies will find this kind of investment appropriate, without patent protection. Even so, some of the large companies, such as Wyeth-Ayerst, are conducting secondary prevention studies, while other companies are apparently taking a more passive approach and continue to investigate short-term surrogate end points, possibly hoping to benefit from competitor products.

Studies under way on secondary intervention, such as the Wyeth-Ayerst HERS study, will only provide the specific indication of secondary prevention. However, from a public health standpoint, the major impact will in fact be on primary prevention. Since such studies are extremely costly, it is unlikely that industry will sponsor primary prevention studies. We must rely on governmental funding agencies to complete these types of studies.

In the meantime, doctors will continue to prescribe HRT for its possible benefits, even if the pharmaceutical industry cannot promote such an indication. Unfortunately, patients will be placed on HRT without the assistance of well grounded clinical studies.

Ongoing Clinical Research

Current efforts in the industry are focused on obtaining cardiovascular indications with drugs already registered for the prevention of osteoporosis and/or treatment of the menopausal symptoms. Studies are also ongoing on the class of drugs called estrogen antagonists, or selective estrogen receptor modulators (SERMs) such as tamoxifen derivatives. However, most studies on cardiovascular effects are in early stages and are only investigating surrogate end points, such as lipids, glucose tolerance, coagulation and the direct effect on vessel walls. A few major studies, however, deserve special attention.

In the USA, the 3-year results from the PEPI study were published in 1995 (PEPI Writing Group, 1995). A total of 875 women were randomly assigned to five treatment groups: placebo; CEE 0.625 mg; CEE + cyclic MPA, 10 mg/daily; CEE + MPA 2.5 mg, given continuously; or CEE + MP 200 mg/day, given cyclically. Primary end points were: HDL-cholesterol, systolic BP, serum insulin and fibrinogen. Based on the lipid results, this study concluded that, from a cardiovascular protection perspective, CEE alone is the best regimen, but for women with an intact uterus, CEE + MP was the preferred treatment to prevent an increased risk of endometrial cancer with unopposed estrogen. This study cannot be seen as definitive with respect to preferred HRT regimen, as it is based on surrogate end points only, but based on the favorable results with estrogen and natural progesterone, companies may find development of such combinations attractive.

Given the importance of this area of endeavor and the many missing pieces of critical information, the National Institutes of Health (NIH) in the USA is presently funding a very large study to evaluate prospectively the benefits of HRT on cardiovascular outcomes in women, amongst other clinical end points. This study is called the Women's Health Initiative (WHI) (Marshall, 1993). In the WHI, 57 000 postmenopausal women will be recruited and studied from 45 centers at a cost in excess of $600 million. The effect of low fat diet, HRT, vitamin D and calcium on heart disease, cancer and osteoporosis will be investigated. A further 100 000 women will be recruited in an observational study to collect baseline data on the incidence of disease through the menopause. These women will be followed for 9 years and 25 000 of them are to take HRT, either estrogen alone or estrogen in combination with progestogen. It is hoped that this study may provide the basis for obtaining a cardiovascular indication for the products being studied. What is not known is whether such an indication will result in class labeling for a range of similar products or for only the studied products. In the UK a large primary prevention study called WISDOM, funded by the British Medical Research Council, is also about to start.

The Heart and Estrogen–Progestin Replacement Study (HERS) is a secondary prevention study in 2340 women. Recruitment started in January of 1993 and 15 clinical sites are involved in this randomized placebo-controlled double-blind trial. This is the first true secondary prevention trial. However, one problem with this study is the lack of an estrogen-alone trial group, which would have provided invaluable data on the effect of estrogen by itself in secondary prevention. The women are randomized to two trial groups: continuous combination of CEE 0.625 mg + MPA 2.5 mg, or placebo. Women in the study must be postmeno-pausal and have had a heart attack, angioplasty, bypass surgery or a serious blockage of the coronary arteries as shown by angiography. In addition, they must be less than 76 years old and have an intact uterus. The study is planned to run for 5.5 years. The final aim of the study is to obtain the indication of secondary prevention of heart disease in women.

There are other secondary prevention studies in the planning stages. A Swedish group has been attempting to get a study started on secondary prevention and progestogen, called the Women's Oestrogen Myocardial Infarction North European Secondary Prevention Study (WOEMINS). So far, the group has not been successful in obtaining sponsorship and financial back-up for such a study. A couple of angiographic studies are under way: the ERA trial is a three-arm double-blind angiographic trial measuring the effect of conjugated equine estrogen, with and without blind continuous low-dose progestin, on the progression of coronary atherosclerosis. The WELL-HART study is of similar design, using estradiol with and without cyclic MPA in women already on lipid lowering therapy. The ATW and EAGAR are even newer angiographic trials investigating the joint and independent effects of estrogen and anti-oxidant therapy and the effect of estrogen on progression of graft atherosclerosis. Finally, the CARMEN study, planned in France, will investigate the effect of different estrogen and progestogen therapies in women already suffering from coronary atherosclerosis.

In conclusion, at the present time, it appears that only a few HRT combinations are likely to obtain registration for prevention of coronary heart disease in this century based on well controlled studies.

Status of Basic Research

An area of intense and interesting research is the mechanisms involved in the action of HRT drugs on prevention of heart disease. In fact, many investigations are focusing on several broad categories of mechanisms. Present thinking tends towards attributing about 10–30% of the protective effects of estrogens via their action on lipids. Other mechanisms currently suggested include a direct effect on the vessel wall, effects on glucose metabolism/insulin resistance, or anti-oxidant effects. A recent finding which could result in development of therapeutics is the finding that estrogen treatment circumvents the lack of endothelial factor in atherosclerotic vessels and causes dilatation in response to acetylcholine in women, but not in men (Collins et al, 1995). This finding suggests a specific role of estrogen in women, which may possibly be receptor-mediated, but not via the classic steroid receptor complex, since the effect of estrogen in this model is seen within minutes.

Another area of investigation involves the study of partial estrogen agonists on cardiovascular effects, in the hopes that these products will not need the addition of full doses of progestogen, because they would avoid the endometrial effects of estrogen itself. Products already marketed are mixed-action estrogens such as Livial (Organon) and tamoxifen (Zeneca). Both products have estrogen-like effects as well as other effects such as androgen/progestogen (Livial) and anti-estrogen effects (tamoxifen). Other such products are also being studied, such as raloxifene, levomeloxifene and other partial estrogen agonists. The cardiovascular effects of this group of drugs is not known, but recent findings of endometrial cancer in women treated with tamoxifen for prevention of breast cancer are not encouraging (van Leeuwen et al, 1968; Ismail, 1996).

Combinatorial chemistry and designer drugs are also being investigated for their effect on cardiovascular disease. These techniques utilize concepts relating to differences in steroid receptors found in specific organs, such as bone, breast, endometrium, etc., to develop drugs which show the desired profile from a basic design point of view. Hopefully, a combination of chemistry and molecular biology will yield drugs with the ability to target specific organs positively, while successfully circumventing undesired effects. Whether these products will successfully reach the market place remains to be seen, many years from now.

Conclusion

With respect to CVD, the male:female ratio remains favorable to women in any age group until very old age, but in absolute numbers, slightly more women than men succumb to CVD. Even so, there continues to be a presumption amongst the health professionals that CVD is a male disease. Consequently, in many countries, women are not screened for CVD or treated to the same extent as men with lipid-lowering drugs and/or low-dose aspirin.

Recent data from a number of epidemiological trials indicating that ERT/HRT have positive effects in the prevention of CVD have been published and become more widely known to general practitioners and other non-specialist doctors. This has resulted in a rise in prescriptions for ERT/HRT for the prevention of CVD although, strictly speaking, no clinical trials have yet definitively proven a causal relationship between ERT/HRT and decreased risk of CVD.

Significantly more data are available for a single estrogen product, Premarin, given as monotherapy, than any other estrogen, primarily because the majority of the studies have been conducted in the USA, where Premarin is the leading prescribed estrogen. In Europe, however, physicians seem to extrapolate the results derived from US epidemiological studies to other estrogens and to combination therapy with progestogens. Thus, in Europe, it is not uncommon to see estradiol in combination with various progestogens prescribed to women at risk for CVD.

Historically, the medical community has often prescribed drugs for diseases or even for prevention without official regulatory approval, but based on published data. When such therapy becomes established, clinical trials on these conditions often are considered unethical by physicians, even if the therapy has not been conclusively established with controlled clinical trials. The situation with ERT/HRT therapy may be at this stage now, with such therapy considered critical to prevent CVD in women, based on observational studies only. Even if, in the absence of a formal indication, the pharmaceutical industry cannot promote and market products for this indication, treatment may become established without such promotion. One of the problems, then, remains the lack of knowledge of critical dose–response relationships and the effects of different types of estrogens and progestogens on CVD. We will see the random use of various combinations without substantial scientific evidence.

In spite of the presence of the clinical situation, it is important for the pharmaceutical industry to persevere to obtain data in collaboration with national and international health authorities and possibly regulatory agencies. It is critical, in the very near future, to obtain data from clinical trials on the effect of ERT/HRT on the critical clinical end points, based on various types and doses of estrogens, with and without progestogens. This information at this time may be even more important than the development of new types of estrogen agonists and antagonists.

REFERENCES

Adams MR, Kaplan JR, Manuck SB et al. Inhibition of coronary artery atherosclerosis by 17-beta-estradiol in ovariectomized monkeys. *Arteriosclerosis* 1990; **10**: 1051–7.

Avila MH, Walker AM, Jick H. Use of replacement estrogens and the risk of myocardial infarction. *Epidemiology* 1990; **1**: 128–33.

Barbaras R, Puchois P, Fruchart JC, Ailhaud G. Cholesterol efflux from cultured adipose cells is mediated by LpA1 particles but not by LpA1:AII particles. *Biochem Biophys Res Commun* 1987; **142**: 63–9.

Barrett-Connor E, Bush T. Estrogen and coronary heart disease in women. *JAMA* 1991; **265**: 1861–7.

Bass KM, Newschaffer CJ, Klag MJ, Bush TL. Plasma lipoprotein levels as predictors of cardiovascular death in women. *Arch Intern Med* 1993; **153**: 2209–16.

Buchwald H, Compos CT, Matts JP and the POSCH Group. Women in the POSCH trial. *Ann Surg* 1992; **216**: 389–97.

Burch JC, Byrd BF Jr, Vaughn WK. The effects of long-term estrogen on hysterectomized women. *Am J Obstet Gynecol* 1974; **118**: 778–82.

Bush TL, Barrett-Connor E. Noncontraceptive estrogen use and cardiovascular disease. *Epidemiol Rev* 1985; **7**: 80–104.

Bush TL, Barrett-Connor E, Cowan LD et al. Cardiovascular mortality and non-contraceptive use of estrogen in women: results from the Lipid Research Clinics Program follow-up study. *Circulation* 1987; **75**(6): 1102–9.

Bush TL. The epidemiology of cardiovascular disease in postmenopausal women. *Ann NY Acad Sci* 1990; **592** (part V): 263–71.

Castelli WP, Garrison RJ, Wilson PWF et al. Incidence of coronary heart disease and lipoprotein cholesterol levels. *JAMA* 1986; **256**: 2835–8.

Castelli WP. Epidemiology of triglycerides: a view from Framingham. *Am J Cardiol* 1992; **70**: 3–9H.

Colditz GA, Willett WC, Stampfer MJ et al. Menopause and the risk of coronary heart disease in women. *N Engl J Med* 1987; **316**: 1105–10.

Collins P, Rosano GMC, Sarrel PM et al. 17-Beta-estradiol attenuates acetylcholine-induced coronary arterial constriction in women not men with coronary heart disease. *Circulation* 1995; **92**: 24–30.

Criqui MH, Suarez L, Barrett-Connor E et al. Postmenopausal estrogen use and mortality. *Am J Epidemiol* 1988; **128**: 606–13.

Daly E, Roche M, Barlow D et al. HRT: an analysis of benefits, risks and costs. *Br Med Bull* 1992; **48**: 368–400.

Daly E, Vessey MP, Hawkins MM et al. *Lancet* 1996; **348**: 977–80.

Darj E, Crona N, Nilsson S. Effects on lipids and lipoproteins in women treated with estradiol and progesterone. *Maturitas* 1992; **15**: 209–15.

Falkeborn M, Persson I, Adami HO et al. The risk of acute myocardial infarction after estrogen and estrogen–progestogen replacement. *Br J Obstet Gynaecol* 1992; **99**: 821–8.

Falkeborn M, Persson I, Terent A et al. Hormone replacement therapy and the risk of stroke. *Arch Intern Med* 1993; **153**: 1202–9.

Felson DT, Shang Y, Hannan MT et al. The effect of postmenopausal estrogen therapy on bone density in elderly women. *N Engl J Med* 1993; **329**: 1141–6.

Frobenius WA. *A Triumph of Scientific Research* 1990. Carnforth, Lancs: Parthenon Publishing Group.

Gangar KF, Vyas S, Whitehead M et al. Pulsatility index in the internal carotid artery in relation to transdermal estradiol and time since menopause. *Lancet* 1991; **338**: 839–42.

Gilligan DM, Badar DM, Panza JA et al. Effects of estrogen replacement therapy on peripheral vasomotor function in postmenopausal women. *Am J Cardiol* 1995; **75**: 264–8.

Gordon EM, Williams SR, Frenchek B et al. Dose dependent effects of postmenopausal estrogen and progestin on antithrombin III and factor XII. *J Lab Clin Med* 1988; **111**: 52–6.

Grodstein F, Stampfer MJ, Goldhaber SZ et al. Prospective study of exogenous hormones and risk of pulmonary embolism in women. *Lancet* 1996a; **348**: 983–7.

Grodstein F, Stampfer MJ, Manson JAE et al. Postmenopausal estrogen and progestin use and the risk of cardiovascular disease. *N Engl J Med* 1996b; **335**: 453–61.

Hammond CB, Jelovsek FR, Lee KL et al. Effects of long term estrogen replacement therapy. *Am J Obstet Gynecol* 1979; **133**: 525–36.

Haarbo J, Leth-Espensen P, Stender S, Christiansen C. Estrogen monotherapy and combined estrogen-progestogen replacement therapy attenuate aortic accumulation of cholesterol in ovariectomized cholesterol-fed rabbits. *J Clin Invest* 1991; **87**: 1274–9.

Hassager C, Riis BJ, Strom V et al. The long term effect of oral and percutaneous estradiol in plasma and renin substrate and blood pressure. *Circulation* 1987; **76**: 753–8.

Heller RF, Jacobs HS. Coronary heart disease in relation to age, sex and the menopause. *Br Med J* 1978; **1**: 472–4.

Henderson BE, Paganini-Hill A, Ross RK. Decreased mortality in users of estrogen replacement therapy. *Arch Intern Med* 1991; **151**: 75–8.

Hirvonen E, Malkonen M, Manninen V. Effect of different progestogens on lipoproteins during postmenopausal replacement therapy. *N Engl J Med* 1981; **304**: 560–63.

Hunt K, Vessey M, McPherson K. Mortality in a cohort of long-term users of hormone replacement therapy: an updated analysis. *Br J Obstet Gynecol* 1990; **97**: 1080–6.

Ismail SM. Endometrial pathology associated with prolonged tamoxifen therapy: a review. *Adv Anat Pathol* 1996; **3**(4): 266–71.

Jensen J, Christiansen C. Dose–response effects on serum lipids and lipoproteins following combined estrogen-progestogen therapy in postmenopausal women. *Maturitas* 1987; **9**: 259–66.

Jick H, Derby LE, Myers MW. Risk of hospital admission for idiopathic venous thromboembolism among users of postmenopausal estrogens. *Lancet* 1996; **348**: 981–3.

Kannel WB, Hjortland MC, McNamara PM, Gordon T. Menopause and risk of cardiovascular disease. *Ann Int Med* 1976; **85**: 447–52.

Kannel WB, Plehn JF, Cupples LA. Cardiac failure and sudden death in the Framingham Study. *Am Heart J* 1988; **115**(4): 869–75.

Lafferty FW, Fiske ME. Postmenopausal estrogen replacement replacement: A Long Term Cohort Study. *Am J Med* 1994; **97**: 66–77.

Liebermann EH, Gerhard MD, Uehata A et al. Estrogen improves endothelium-dependent, flow-mediated vasodilatation in postmenopausal women. *Ann Intern Med* 1994; **121**: 936–41.

Lindquist O, Bengtsson C. Menopausal age in relation to smoking. *Acta Med Scand* 1979; **205**: 73–7.

Lobo R, Speroff L. International consensus conference on postmenopausal hormone therapy and the cardiovascular system. *Fertil Steril* 1994; **61**(4): 592–5.

Luotola H, Pyorala T, Loikkanen M. Effects of natural estrogen/progestogen substitution therapy on carbohydrate and lipid metabolism in postmenopausal women. *Maturitas* 1986; **8**: 245–53.

Marshall E. Big Science enters the clinic. *Science* 1993; **260**: 744–7.

Munk-Jensen N, Ulrich LG, Obel EB et al. Continuous combined and sequential estradiol and norethindrone acetate treatment of postmenopausal women: effect on plasma lipoproteins in a two-year placebo-controlled trial. *Am J Obstet Gynecol* 1994; **171**: 132–8.

Nabulsi AA, Folsom AR, White A et al. Association of hormone replacement therapy with cardiovascular risk factors in postmenopausal women. *N Engl J Med* 1993; **328**: 1069–75.

Nachtigall LE, Nachtigall RH, Nachtigall RD, Beckman EM. Estrogen replacement therapy. II. A prospective study in the relationship to carcinoma and cardiovascular and metabolic problems. *Obstet Gynecol* 1979; **54**: 74–9.

Notelovitz M, Gudat JC, Ware MD, Dougherty MC. Lipids and lipoproteins in women after oopherectomy and the response to estrogen therapy. *Br J Obstet Gynaecol* 1983; **90**: 171–7.

Ohta T, Hattori S, Murakami M et al. Age and sex related differences in lipoproteins containing apoprotein A-1. *Arteriosclerosis* 1989; **9**: 90–95.

Ottesen UB, Johansson BG, Von Schoultz B. Subfractions of high-density lipoprotein cholesterol during estrogen replacement therapy: A comparison between progestogens and natural progesterone. *Am J Obstet Gynecol* 1985; **151**: 746–50.

Paganini-Hill A, Ross RK, Henderson BE. Postmenopausal estrogen treatment and stroke: a prospective study. *Br Med J* 1988; **297**: 519–22.

PEPI Writing Group (for the PEPI trial). Effects of estrogen or estrogen/progestin regimens on heart disease risk factors in postmenopausal women. *JAMA* 1995; **273**: 199–208.

Petitti DB, Perlman JA, Sidney S. Noncontraceptive estrogens and mortality: long-term follow-up of women in the Walnut Creek Study. *Obstet Gynecol* 1987; **70**: 289–93.

Puchois P, Kandoussi A, Fievel P et al. Apolipoprotein A-1 containing lipoproteins in coronary artery disease. *Atherosclerosis* 1987; **68**: 35–40.

Punnonen RH, Jokela HA, Dastidar PS et al. Combined estrogen–progestin replacement therapy prevents atherosclerosis in postmenopausal women. *Maturitas* 1995; **21**: 179–87.

Schering AG, West Germany. *From a Chemist's Shop to Multinational Enterprise*, undated. Sheringianum: Press and Public Affairs Dept.

Stampfer MJ, Colditz GA, Willett WC. Menopause and heart disease. *Ann NY Acad Sci* 1990; **592**(IV): 193–203. In Flint M, Kronenberg F, Utian W (eds) *Multidisciplinary Perspectives on Menopause*.

Sullivan JM, Swaag RV, Hughes JP. Estrogen replacement and coronary artery disease. *Arch Intern Med* 1990; **150**: 2557–62.

Thompson SG, Meade TW, Greenberg GJ. The use of hormonal replacement therapy and the risk of stroke and myocardial infarction in women. *J Epidemiol Commun Health* 1989; **43**: 173–8.

Thorogood M, Vessey MP. An epidemiological survey of cardiovascular disease in women taking oral contraceptives. *Am J Obstet Gynecol* 1990; **163**: 274–81.

Tonstad S, Ose L, Gorbitz C. Efficacy of sequential hormone replacement therapy in the treatment of hypercholesterolemia among postmenopausal women. *J Intern Med* 1995; **238**: 39–47.

van Leeuwen FE, Benraadt J, Coebergh JWW. Risk of endometrial cancer after tamoxifen treatment of breast cancer. *Lancet* 1994; **343**: 448–52.

Vejtorp M, Christensen MS, Vejtorp L, Larsen JF. Serum lipoprotein changes in climacteric women induced by sequential therapy with natural estrogens and medroxyprogesterone acetate or norgestrel. *Acta Obstet Gynecol Scand* 1986; **65**: 391–5.

Walsh BW, Schiff I, Rosner B et al. Effects of postmenopausal estrogen replacement therapy on the concentrations and metabolism of plasma lipoproteins. *N Engl J Med* 1991; **325**: 1196–204.

Wenger NK, Speroff L, Packard B. Cardiovascular health and disease in women. *N Engl J Med* 1993; **329**: 247–72.

Wilson PWF, Garrison RJ, Castelli WP. Postmenopausal estrogen use, cigarette smoking and cardiovascular morbidity in women over 50. *N Engl J Med* 1985; **313**: 1038–43.

Wolf PH, Madans JH, Finucane FF et al. Reduction of cardiovascular disease-related mortality among postmenopausal women who use hormones: evidence from a national cohort. *Am J Obstet Gynecol* 1991; **164**: 489–94.

13

Osteoporosis

Pirow J. Bekker[1], David Juan[2], Russell T. Burge[2], Samarendra N. Dutta[3]* and Michael Gast[4]

[1]*Amgen Inc., Thousand Oaks, CA,* [2]*Proctor and Gamble Co., Cincinatti, OH,* [3]*Food and Drug Administration, Rockville, MD, and* [4]*Wyeth-Ayerst Research, Philadelphia, PA, USA*

BACKGROUND

Osteoporosis is one of the most poorly understood health problems confronting an older patient population. People who suffer from the disorder, or are at great risk, are often unaware of the nature of osteoporosis or of its consequences. Patients and physicians are often unfamiliar with the techniques designed to diagnose, prevent and treat this potentially crippling disorder. New understanding of biology of osteoporosis as well as new diagnostic and therapeutical modalities in the last 5 years have made the field of bone health a very exciting one recently.

As the population ages, osteoporosis, a disorder common to both men and women, is likely to increase in its prevalence. Although commonly associated with the postmenopausal woman, it is not exclusively a disease of women. As men live longer, osteoporosis will be seen more and more frequently in men in their 70s and 80s. The signs and symptoms of the disease are identical in both sexes. A decrease in stature with a bowing of the thoracic spine (known as Dowager's hump in the female) are the most visible physical manifestations of osteoporosis. This bowing, caused by spinal compression fractures, can cause severe physical pain and lead to varying degrees of immobilization. Other significant clinical problems associated with osteoporosis include fractures of the hip (proximal femur), wrist (Colles' fracture or distal radial or ulnar fractures) and silent spinal compression fractures (see Figure 13.1) (Melton, 1995).

Perhaps the most serious short- and long-term consequences of osteoporosis are fractures of the proximal femur (i.e. hip). In the USA there are an estimated 300 000 hip fractures annually for the over-50 population (US Congress, Office of Technology Assessment, 1994), and the annual incidence is predicted to exceed 840 000 by the year 2040 (Schneider & Guralnik, 1990). The long-term outcome of hip fractures is poor because most of these fractures occur in relatively frail

---

* Comments made in this report do not necessarily represent the decisions or the stated policy of the US Food and Drug Administration.

Drug Development for Women. Edited by V.V. Ragavan. © 1998 John Wiley & Sons Ltd.

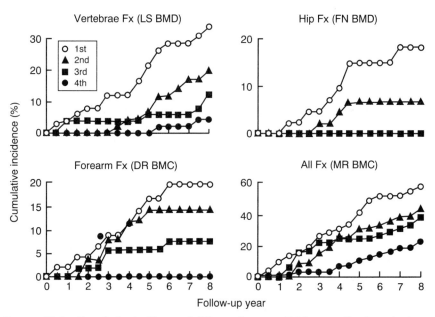

FIGURE 13.1 Cumulative incidence of different fractures (Fx) by quartiles from the lowest (1st) to the highest (4th) of baseline bone mineral density (BMD) of the lumbar spine (LS) and femoral neck (FN) and bone mineral content (BMC) of the distal radius (DK) and mid-radius (MR) among an age-stratified sample of Rochester (Minnesota, USA) women. Reprinted from Melton et al (1993), *Journal of Bone and Mineral Research*, **8**: 1227–1228, Figure 2, with permission of the American Society for Bone and Mineral Research

elderly patients and result in prolonged immobilization, therefore the incidence of fracture-related illnesses such as thrombo-embolism and other emboli is quite high. In addition, immobilization can lead to ulceration of aging skin and muscle tissue, with resulting superinfection. The incidence of other sorts of medical problems, e.g. metabolic imbalances, malnutrition and cardiovascular events, is also high in the postfracture, postoperative period in this group of individuals.

Short-term consequences of hip fracture are far more serious, including high rates of mortality and disability. Approximately 18–28% of patients over age 65 suffering hip fractures die within one year of their fracture (Magaziner et al, 1989; Kenzora et al, 1984; Ahmad, Eckhoff & Kramer, 1994). Upon discharge from an acute care hospital, about 41% of hip fracture patients over age 50 are admitted to a nursing home, and after one year two-thirds are discharged to home or will die, while one-third are still in the nursing home (US Congress, Office of Technology Assessment, 1994). About 12% of patients are discharged to a rehabilitation hospital or other short-stay facility following their acute care hospital stay (US Congress, Office of Technology Assessment, 1994). Among those patients discharged from the acute care hospital to their homes, about one-third of these receive paid home health care services and most others receive non-medical home

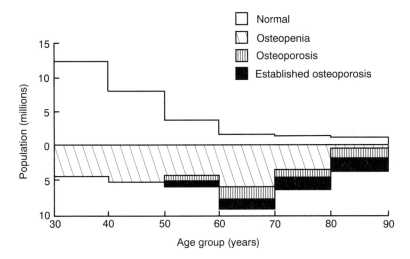

FIGURE 13.2 Estimated skeletal status: US white women (1990), based on WHO definitions. Adapted from Melton (1995)

care services from either friends, family or through paid or volunteer groups or individuals (US Congress, Office of Technology Assessment, 1994).

The total economic cost of osteoporotic fractures worldwide is staggering. In the USA alone the cost of osteoporosis is estimated to be at least $13.8 billion per year (Ray et al, 1997). Among the various types of osteoporotic fractures (hip, vertebral, distal forearm), the costs of hip fractures account for the greatest share, with estimates of $5.4–$8.7 billion per year (US Congress, Office of Technology Assessment, 1994; Praemer, Furner & Rice, 1992). It appears likely that the costs of osteoporosis will continue rising over the next century, as the over-55 age group will be the largest growing age group in our world population.

INCIDENCE AND PREVALENCE

Loss of bone from the skeleton or osteoporosis is a universal event associated most particularly with the loss of sex steroid hormone support for metabolic bone activity. Other factors, however, such as growth hormone and its downstream cascade and adrenal steroid production may affect bone maintenance as these endocrine and paracrine processes decrease with aging. As seen in Figure 13.2 (Melton et al, 1993), the percentage of women with osteoporosis and osteopenia (form of disease prior to symptomatology) (not clinically apparent form of the disease) increases throughout the decades of life. In women, by the 8th decade of life, the incidence of severely decreased mineralization of bone approaches 100%. Notably, osteoporosis and its complications in both men and women is now probably 100% preventable.

There are limited data available to assess the difference in prevalence of osteoporosis by racial groups or regions. However, the best data for making such comparisons relate to hip fractures (WHO, 1994). There were an estimated 1.7 million hip fractures worldwide in 1990 (Cooper, Campion & Melton, 1992), with higher incidence rates for women and for Caucasians (compared to Asians and Africans). Among Caucasian populations, age- and sex-adjusted incidence rates are higher in Scandinavian countries compared to countries in southern Europe, North America or Oceania (Melton, 1991; Johnell et al, 1992). The prevalence of osteoporosis in a region depends on the ethnic composition, the size of the population and the age distribution. In 1990 there were an estimated 380 million people age 35 and over in Europe, North America and Oceania, and 920 million in Asia. However, nearly one-half of the hip fractures occurred in the former regions— despite the lower population total—due to the older average age and greater Caucasian composition. About one-third of the world's total number of hip fractures occur in Asia, even though, because of the large population base, the incidence rate is much lower (Melton, 1988; Kanis & Pitt, 1992).

Possible explanations for the differences in hip fractures by sex and race include greater bone mass in men vs. women and in people of African heritage; and differences in physical activity, balance, stature, strength and diet by region and culture (Melton, 1991; Kanis & Passmore, 1989; Ross et al, 1991). For example, calcium intake may have an important effect on bone mass (Dawson-Hughes et al, 1990; Chevalley et al, 1992). Greater physical activity or exercise among women of Asian or African heritage may partly explain their lower prevalence of osteoporosis (Melton, 1991).

BONE BIOLOGY

Basic Biology

The extracellular compartment of bone consists of inorganic and organic components. The inorganic component is mostly hydroxyapatite and the organic component mostly type I collagen; other organic components are proteoglycans and proteins such as osteocalcin, and osteopontin and bone sialoprotein (BSP). In general, bone consists of two components: compact, dense, cortical bone, and sponge-like, less dense, trabecular bone. The former is found mostly in the diaphyses of long bones and provides strength to bones which are weight-bearing, such as the femur and tibia. The latter is found in epiphyses of long bones, as well as in the vertebrae and ribs. Trabecular bone contains hematopoietic bone marrow.

Bone is a dynamic organ, with constant renewal. This is accomplished by basic multicellular units (BMUs). These are teams of cells named osteoclasts (bone-resorbing cells) and osteoblasts (bone-forming cells). Turnover of bone is higher in the trabecular bone (25% per year) compared to cortical bone (3% per year) (Dempster, 1997), because the surface area of trabecular bone is higher than that of cortical bone. Therefore, there are more BMUs in a unit of trabecular bone compared to cortical bone.

Osteoclasts

Differentiated osteoclasts are large, multinucleated cells (see Figure 13.1), which originate from bone marrow precursors, most likely the colony-forming units—monocytes (CFU-M) line (Jotereau & LeDouarin, 1978; Kahn & Simmons, 1975; Nijweide, Burger & Feyen, 1986; Scheven, Visser & Nijweide, 1986; Udagawa et al, 1990). The main function of these cells is bone resorption: the peripheral part of the osteoclast's cell membrane attaches to the bone surface through podosomes (Marchisio et al, 1984, 1987) and forms a sealing zone (Schenk, Spiro & Wiener, 1967). Podosomes are short membranous protrusions with cores of microfilaments linked to the plasma membrane by talin, vinculin and α-actinin (Marchisio et al, 1984, 1987). A specific β_3 integrin of the RGD (arginine–glycine–aspartate) superfamily of matrix receptors ($\alpha_v\beta_3$ integrin) is expressed on the podosome surfaces and plays a role in substrate recognition, which is an early step in osteoclastic bone resorption (Davies et al, 1989; Zambonin-Zallone et al, 1989). Several matric adhesion proteins are involved in this process, e.g. vitronectins and RGD-containing proteins such as osteopontin, collagen I and BSP (Reinholt et al, 1990; Teti, Marchisio & Zambonin-Zallone, 1991). Binding of the RGD-containing proteins to the osteoclast integrin receptor results in decrease in osteoclastic intracellular Ca++ (Hruska et al, 1993) and tyrosine phosphorylation (Neff et al, 1992) which activate bone resorption (Miyauchi et al, 1991).

Through a microtubular assembly–disassembly process, cytoplasmic vacuoles migrate to the plasma membrane included within the sealing zone, and merge with the membrane to increase its surface area. This leads to extensive folding of the plasma membrane to form the so-called ruffled border membrane. This membrane has a high density of a H^+-ATPase, which acts as a proton pump (Bekker & Gay, 1990b; Blair et al, 1989; Vaananen et al, 1990). The proton pump extrudes protons, generated by the action of carbonic anhydrase II (CAII) (Gay & Mueller, 1974), into the resorption lacuna, which is formed between the osteoclast ruffled border and the bone surface. Defective Ca^{++} leads to osteopetrosis (Sly et al, 1983). A Na^+/K^+-ATPase (Baron et al, 1986) and HCO_3^-/Cl^- and Na^+/H^+ exchangers (Chakraborty et al, 1991; Hall & Chambers, 1989; Horne et al, 1991; Teti et al, 1989) in the osteoclast basolateral plasma membrane reverse the alkalinity and hyperpolarization created by proton pumping. The pH in the resorption lacuna decreases and the acidic environment results in degradation of the inorganic component of bone. It also creates an environment for secreted enzymes such as cysteine-proteases to be activated, which results in degradation of the organic component of bone. Procollagenase is activated to collagenase by cysteine-proteases (Eeckhout & Vaes, 1977). Since collagenase is active at neutral pH, degradation of collagen probably occurs after the osteoclast dislodges from the bone surface, resulting in pH return to neutral (Baron et al, 1993).

Enzymes which are instrumental in organic degradation are lysosomal enzymes such as cysteine-proteases (cathepsin B, C, and L) (Baron et al, 1993; Delaisse

& Vaes, 1992; Delaisse, Ledent & Vaes, 1991) β-glucuronidase, arylsulfatase and β-glycerophosphatase (Andersson et al, 1986; Baron et al, 1985, 1988; Doty & Schoefield, 1972; Lucht, 1971; Reinholt et al, 1990) and non-lysosomal enzymes such as stromelysin (Delaisse & Vaes, 1992), tissue plasminogen activator (Grills et al, 1990) and lysozyme (Hilliard, Meadows & Kahn, 1990). Transport of these enzymes to the ruffled border domain of the osteoclast is accomplished by association with the mannose-6-phosphate (M-6-P) receptor (Baron et al, 1988) in the Golgi apparatus. The newly synthesized enzymes are bound to M-6-P, which binds to the M-6-P receptors in the Golgi membranes (Creek & Sly, 1984). These enzymes are then channeled to the ruffled membrane where, under acidic conditions, the enzymes are released from the receptor (Baron et al, 1988, 1990).

The osteoclast also secretes tartrate-resistant acid phosphatase (TRAP), the function of which is unclear. Osteoclasts also have a plasma membrane Ca^{++}-ATPase which extrudes calcium from the cells (Bekker & Gay, 1990a). The presence of a calcium sensor on the osteoclast plasma membrane regulates osteoclast attachment to bone: the higher the calcium concentration in the resorption lacuna, the less attached the osteoclast is. This allows release of calcium and degradation products to the interstitial fluid and plasma (Hruska et al, 1993).

Osteoclasts generate oxygen-derived free radicals (Garrett et al, 1990; Key et al, 1990) which are involved in bone resorption. Their exact physiological role is unclear.

There is continual osteoclastic bone resorption. One reason for this is to renew bone. Since bone is continually under stress, microdamage may occur over time. Osteoclasts remove damaged bone and prepare the way for osteoblasts to form new bone. Another reason for bone resorption is to supply the body with calcium and phosphorus. In times of low dietary calcium and/or phosphorus intake, osteoclasts supply the body with calcium and phosphorus for vital cellular functions in nerve, muscle and other tissues. Under certain conditions, bone resorption is increased; examples include estrogen deficiency during the menopause, during periods of low calcium intake, immobilization, hyperparathyroidism, or malignant conditions such as multiple myeloma.

Osteoclasts create lacunae on the bone surface. These lacunae may result in weakening of bones if their numbers are large and/or they are situated at critical sites, e.g. if two lacunae occur at opposing sides on a trabecula. Therefore, under normal conditions, the lacunae are rapidly filled with new bone through the action of osteoblasts.

Many cytokines affect osteoclasts in different ways. Interleukin-1 (IL-1), for example, is widely accepted as a stimulator of bone resorption (Gowen, Meikle & Reynolds, 1983). It acts through its receptor, IL-1R (Garrett, Black & Mundy, 1990). High IL-1 production by peripheral blood monocytes has been linked to a form of high-turnover osteoporosis (Pacifici et al, 1987, 1989). Several other cytokines have bone effects: IL-4, IL-6, colony-stimulating factor (CSF), tumor necrosis factor (TNF), lymphotoxin, leukemia inhibitory factor, interferon-γ, and osteoclastpoietic factor. Contradictory results have been found for many of these cytokines. IL-6 is an example: in bone, IL-6 is produced by osteoblasts (Feyen et al, 1989). Even though osteoblasts have IL-6 receptors, the IL-6 effect on bone formation is unclear. IL-6 was shown to stimulate bone resorption in certain models (Black, Garrett & Mundy, 1991; Klein et al, 1991), but not in another (Al-Humidan et al, 1991).

Macrophage-colony-stimulating factor (M-CSF) plays an important role in osteoclast formation. This was demonstrated by studying the osteopetrosis op/op mouse model. These mice have a coding defect in the M-CSF region (Yoshida et al, 1990); M-CSF administration resolves the bone abnormalities (Felix, Cecchini & Fleisch, 1990; Kodama et al, 1991).

Osteoblasts

Osteoblasts are derived from mesenchymal cells. They are basophylic, cuboidal, polar cells, which are alkaline phosphatase-positive and have parathyroid hormone (PTH) receptors (see Figure 13.2). Alkaline phosphatase is an ectoenzyme (located on outside of plasma membrane), which could be shed in matrix vesicles (Ali, Sajdera & Anderson, 1970). Even though it may be involved in bone mineralization, its precise function is unclear. An obvious role may be to increase the local concentration of phosphate by degrading pyrophosphate, dephosphorylating matrix proteins, or by acting as an ion transporter (Wuthier & Register, 1985). The phosphate then binds with calcium as part of hydroxyapatite crystallization. Its importance in mineralization is demonstrated by the severe osteomalacia caused by its absence in congenital hypophosphatasia (Whyte, 1989).

During proliferation, osteoblasts produce type I collagen, fibronectin, and tissue growth factor β (TGF-β). Fibronectin contains the prototypical GRGDS (glycine–arginine–glycine–aspartate–cysteine) cell adhesion sequence. Osteoblasts produce many substances which will be described briefly below.

TGF-β appears to be important in extracellular matrix biosynthesis (Joyce et al, 1990; Sporn et al, 1983). During matrix maturation, AP transcription reaches a peak. Osteopontin, bone sialoprotein and osteocalcin are secreted during the subsequent mineralization phase. Studies suggest that these proteins are assembled in packets which mineralize shortly after secretion (Bianco, 1993; McKee et al, 1993).

Osteopontin is an RGDS (arginine–glycine–aspartate–cysteine)-containing protein, which is sialic acid-rich and binds calcium (Oldberg, Frauzen & Heinegard, 1986). It is highly phosphorylated and sulfated (Nagata et al, 1989). Osteopontin's exact role is unknown, but it is postulated to play a role in cell adhesion (Reinholt et al, 1990) and bone mineralization (Addadi et al, 1987; Glimcher, 1989). Osteopontin is produced earlier in bone formation than osteocalcin (Mark et al, 1987). Osteopontin mRNA has been found in osteoclasts (Merry et al, 1993; Shiraga et al, 1992), which suggests that these cells may form their own adhesion protein.

BSP is similar to osteopontin and is also found at sites of new bone formation (Weinreb, Shinar & Rodan, 1990). Osteopontin and BSP are likely candidates to act as initiation sites for bone mineralization, especially BSP, which is found only in bone.

Osteocalcin is a 5.7 kDa vitamin K-dependent, calcium-binding protein. Its expression peaks with mineralization of the extracellular matrix. It may be an inhibitor of mineral nucleation (Boskey, Wians & Hauschka, 1985) and it may also be an osteoclast activator (Glowacki & Lian, 1987). It was shown to be chemotactic for osteoclast and osteoblast precursors (Lucas, Price & Caplan, 1988; Malone et al, 1982; Mundy & Poser, 1983).

Osteonectin is a phosphoglycoprotein found at sites of new bone formation. As its name indicates, it has an affinity for calcium and can bind up to 12 calcium ions per molecule at low affinity binding sites (Termine et al, 1981a, b). Its function is related to bone remodeling, regulation of proliferation (Funk & Sage, 1991, 1993), and cell–matrix interactions (Everitt & Sage, 1992; Lane & Sage, 1990; Sage & Bornstein, 1991).

Thrombospondin is synthesized by osteoblasts and found in bone matrix. This complex class of molecules mediates bone–cell adhesion (Gehron Robey et al, 1989). More work is needed to define its exact role.

A large chondroitin sulfate proteoglycan (CSPG) is formed in the interstitial mesenchyme early in bone formation. It is thought to occupy the space which is about to be mineralized (Le Baron, Zimmermann & Ruoslahti, 1992). As bone formation progresses, CSRG is degraded and replaced by biglycan and decorin, two smaller proteoglycans (Bianco et al, 1990). Decorin may play a role in regulation of collagen formation (Vogel & Trotter, 1987). Biglycan's function is unclear. Cell-surface associated proteoglycans, such as β-glycan, may mediate cell responses to certain growth factors, such as transforming growth factor β (TGF-β) (Lopez-Casillas et al, 1993).

TGF-β has a proliferative effect on osteoblasts (Roberts et al, 1981). It was found to increase transcription of collagen (Centrella, Massague & Canalis, 1986; Centrella, McCarty & Canalis, 1987; Centrella & McCarty, 1988). It also stimulates its own production, suggesting an autocrine effect. It appears to enhance the formation of extracellular matrix and its own stabilization by inhibition of degradation; the latter is achieved by an increase in secretion of protease inhibitors and also by a decrease in protease secretion (Chiang & Nilsen-Hamilton, 1986; Laiho et al, 1986; Overall, Wrana & Soldek, 1989). TGF-β is found at active bone formation sites (Heine et al, 1987). It has also been implicated as a coupling factor between bone resorption and formation, since it is stored in bone and can be activated by low pH conditions such as with bone resorption (Oreffo et al, 1989). Osteoclast formation and bone resorption are inhibited by TGF-β (Chenu et al, 1988; Pfeilschrifter, Seyedin & Mundy, 1988).

Recombinant bone morphogenic proteins (BMPs) have been demonstrated to initiate de novo cartilage and subsequent bone formation when injected into soft tissue (Wang et al, 1990). This indicates that these molecules are important early regulators of bone formation. BMPs were shown to stimulate osteoblastic lineage

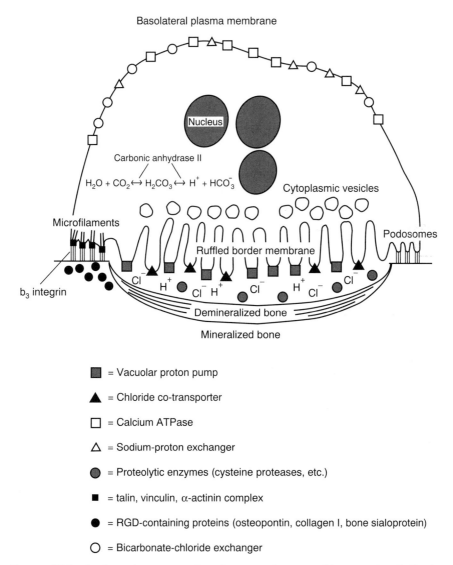

Basolateral plasma membrane

Nucleus

Carbonic anhydrase II

$$H_2O + CO_2 \leftrightarrow H_2CO_3 \leftrightarrow H^+ + HCO_3^-$$

Cytoplasmic vesicles

Microfilaments

Podosomes

Ruffled border membrane

b_3 integrin

Cl^- H^+ Cl^- H^+ Cl^- H^+ Cl^- Cl^-

Demineralized bone

Mineralized bone

▪ = Vacuolar proton pump

▲ = Chloride co-transporter

□ = Calcium ATPase

△ = Sodium-proton exchanger

⬤ = Proteolytic enzymes (cysteine proteases, etc.)

■ = talin, vinculin, α-actinin complex

● = RGD-containing proteins (osteopontin, collagen I, bone sialoprotein)

○ = Bicarbonate-chloride exchanger

FIGURE 13.3 A schematic representation of a mature bone resorbing osteoclast, indicating key structural and functional aspects of these cells

proliferation (Chen et al, 1991; Maliakal, Hauschka & Sampath, 1991). There is also evidence that it promotes osteoblastic differentiation (Yamaguchi & Kahn, 1991) and chemotaxis (Padley et al, 1991).

IL-1 plays a role in proliferation and differentiation of osteoblasts (Keeting et al, 1991; Lorenzo et al, 1990). This effect may be secondary to its stimulatory effect on bone resorption (Boyce et al, 1989).

After osteoid is laid down, it is mineralized through hydroxyapatite crystallization. Through a process called modeling, bone is constantly laid down in response to stress, resulting from weight bearing and/or muscle action. This action has primarily an osteoblastic component. On the other hand, remodeling is the process by which bone is resorbed by osteoclasts and then regenerated by osteoblasts.

Bone volume peaks in the second decade of life (Kimmel, 1990) and decreases thereafter, faster in women than in men, which is mostly related to the menopause. The age-related decline in bone volume is thought to be related to decreased bone formation by the osteoblasts. However, it was also found that the osteoclastic resorption depth decreases with age; therefore, the lower bone formation rate may be compensatory (Parfitt, 1992). Trabecular thinning and perforation postmenopause results in increasing bone fragility. Even though the diameter of long bones increases with age because of slight positive bone balance, the cortical bone thickness decreases, because of a negative bone balance endocortically.

Osteocytes

Osteocytes originate from osteoblasts buried in bone. They have long cytoplasmic projections (similar to dendrites) which extend deep into bone. There are gap junctions between osteocytes by which these cells may communicate (Miller, Bowman & Smith, 1980). It is thought that osteocytes are important stress detectors, which transduce signals to other cells. If, for example, bone is under high stress, these cells detect it and signal other cells such as osteoblasts or periosteal lining cells to respond by increased bone formation (Aarden, Burger & Nijweide, 1994; Yeh & Rodan, 1984).

Bone Lining Cells

In adults, flat bone lining cells cover bone surfaces. These cells originate from osteoblasts. Their function is unclear. There are gap junctions between these cells and osteocytes, suggesting intercellular communication.

DIAGNOSIS OF OSTEOPOROSIS AND MEASUREMENT TECHNIQUES

The definition of osteoporosis has been agreed to by a consensus panel (Consensus Development Conference, 1993). It is defined as 'a progressive systemic skeletal disease characterized by low bone mass and micro-architectural deterioration of bone tissues, with a consequent increase in bone fragility and susceptibility to fracture'. The inverse relationship between bone mineral density and fracture risk

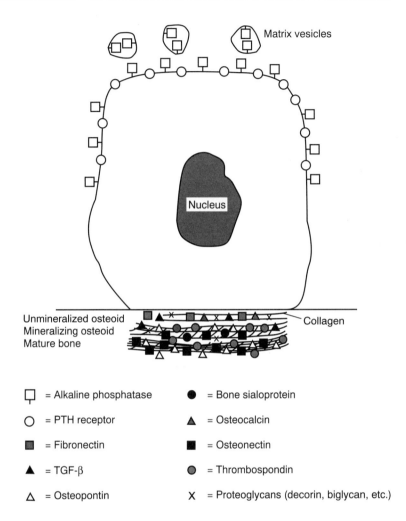

Matrix vesicles

Nucleus

Unmineralized osteoid
Mineralizing osteoid
Mature bone

Collagen

☐ = Alkaline phosphatase   ● = Bone sialoprotein

○ = PTH receptor   ▲ = Osteocalcin

■ = Fibronectin   ■ = Osteonectin

▲ = TGF-β   ● = Thrombospondin

△ = Osteopontin   X = Proteoglycans (decorin, biglycan, etc.)

FIGURE 13.4 A schematic representation of a typical mature osteoblast which forms new bone

has been demonstrated by several studies (Ross et al, 1990, 1991; Seeley et al, 1991). It is generally accepted that 1 SD reduction in bone mineral density (BMD) from the age-specific mean population value confers a two- to threefold increase in fracture risk. Even though there are other risk factors for fractures, it is only BMD that can be measured with high precision and accuracy. The measurement of BMD forms the basis for the diagnosis of osteopenia and osteoporosis. It is well appreciated that a mass-based diagnostic approach does not give the complete information on bone quality, since fracture risk is higher in the elderly than in the young with the same BMD. The ideal measurement is one which gives accurate information, not only about bone mass but also about bone quality, which involves alterations in bone composition, loss of trabecular connectivity, cement line accumulation, increased cortical porosity and bone fatigue damage.

In 1994, the WHO published guidelines (WHO, 1994) for the diagnosis of osteopenia and osteoporosis using dual energy X-ray absorptometry (DXA) for BMD determination, as follows:

1. *Normal.* BMD or bone mineral content (BMC) within 1 SD of the young adult reference mean.
2. *Osteopenia.* BMD or bone mineral content (BMC) greater than 1 SD below the young adult mean but less than 2.5 SD below this value.
3. *Osteoporosis.* BMD or BMC 2.5 SD or more below the young adult mean.
4. *Severe osteoporosis* (established osteoporosis). BMD or BMC 2.5 SD or more below the young adult mean in the presence of one or more fragility fractures.

There are several sources of diagnostic inaccuracies in the measurement of bone mineral density by DXA: inadequate machine calibration, inadequate reference ranges, vertebral deformities due to osteoarthrosis, Scheuermann's disease, severe scoliosis, previous fracture, contrast media (spine), overlying metal objects, vascular calcifications (especially in the spine) and osteomalacia.

Other investigative techniques in the diagnosis of osteoporosis include: quantitative computed tomography (QCT), ultrasound, various radiographic techniques (analysis of Moiré patterns from plain X-rays of trabecular bone), and magnetic resonance imaging (MRI). It is unknown at present whether these newer techniques are better in providing a more accurate assessment of bone quality than the DXA. A recent review critically examines the non-invasive bone mineral measurements as diagnostic tools (Grampp et al, 1997).

There is intensive research in the development of biochemical markers of bone formation and resorption. Recently, data were presented to show that biochemical markers, especially the bone resorption markers, may have predictive value for subsequent fractures or BMD responses to drug therapy (Melton et al, 1997; Gonnelli et al, 1997; Christiansen, 1994).

TREATMENT

Targets for Therapeutic Intervention

Osteoclasts

Since osteoclasts remove bone, therapeutic intervention targeting these cells should result in an increase in bone volume and therefore an increase in protection against fractures. With estrogen depletion after menopause, bone turnover is increased

(Fogelman et al, 1984). Therefore, therapies aimed at reducing turnover have been shown to be effective.

The number of osteoclasts could theoretically be reduced by reducing the number of precursors of osteoclasts. Therapeutic intervention could occur at different stages of differentiation, starting at the CFU-M stem cells and ending at the mature osteoclastic level. *Bisphosphonates* may reduce osteoclast recruitment (Boonekamp et al, 1986; Hughes et al, 1989; Lowik et al, 1988). The exact mechanism of action is unclear. *Etidronate* was shown to decrease activation frequency of BMUs and increase cancellous bone volume and trabecular thickness by decreasing the osteoclastic resorption depth (Parfitt, 1991).

For osteoclasts to be active, they need to migrate to bone surfaces (Chambers, 1980; Parfitt et al, 1996; Skjodt & Russell, 1992). The mechanism involved in osteoclast chemotaxis is unclear. As mentioned above, matrix proteins may play a role. Nevertheless, once understood, therapeutic intervention may be targeted to the process which delivers osteoclasts to bone surfaces.

Osteoclasts need to adhere to bone surfaces before they can start the resorption process. Therapeutic intervention may target this adhesion process, either by blocking the RGD-binding sites in bone matrix or by blocking the osteoclast integrin receptor. Therapeutic intervention could also be targeted at reversal of the adherence process, i.e. cause osteoclasts to detach from the bone surface after adherence has already occurred. This could be mediated by an agonist for the plasma membrane calcium sensor. *Bisphosphonate* exposure has been shown to result in osteoclast detachment (Flanagan & Chambers, 1989; Rowe & Hausmann, 1976, 1980; Rowe & Hays, 1983).

Calcitonin also results in contraction of osteoclasts (Chambers et al, 1986). It acts through a G-protein-linked plasma membrane receptor on osteoclasts (Lin et al, 1991). Calcitonin was shown to increase BMD (Overgaard et al, 1992) most likely through its inhibitory effect on osteoclasts.

The mechanism resulting in vacuolar incorporation into the osteoclast plasma membrane, which forms the ruffled border, presents a potential therapeutic target. It is known that intracellular microtubular assembly and disassembly is involved in this process. Inhibition of microtubular assembly interferes with osteoclast function (Baron et al, 1990; Hunter, Schraer & Gay, 1989). The intracellular actin network is involved in osteoclast motility. Agents which interfere with this actin network would decrease osteoclast motility and would inhibit function.

IL-1 receptor antagonists block the effect of IL-1 receptors to stimulate bone resorption. However, this occurs at high doses and the therapeutic potential needs to be demonstrated (Garrett et al, 1990).

Carbonic anhydrase II and the plasma membrane proton pump of the osteoclast are other putative entities for therapeutic intervention. Although the proton pump is similar to the vacuolar proton pump in many regards, it may have unique subunits which present unique targets. For example, two isoforms of the B-subunit of the H^+-ATPase have been demonstrated (Nelson et al, 1992; Puopolo et al, 1992). A certain *bisphosphonate (tiludronate)*, but not another (*alendronate*), was shown to inhibit the function of this pump (David et al, 1996). Other putative targets for intervention include the Na^+/K^+-ATPase, HCO_3^-/Cl^- exchanger or the Na^+/H^+ exchanger, present on the osteoclast basolateral plasma membrane.

Osteoclastic secretory enzymes such as collagenases and cysteine proteases are susceptible to inhibitors. These inhibitors could be aimed directly at osteoclasts (interfere with transcription, translation or post-translational processing) or to bone surfaces where osteoclastic resorption may release the inhibitor to act on the enzymes.

By increasing the body's ability to retain *calcium*, osteoclastic function could be controlled to some extent. Adequate calcium intake has been shown definitively to be effective in this regard (Aloia et al, 1994; Reid et al, 1993).

Even though calcium intake may be sufficient, intestinal malabsorption may occur with aging. *Vitamin D* and analogs increase calcium absorption and prevent excessive renal calcium loss (Gallagher et al, 1980). Bone cells have *1,25(OH)₂* *vitamin D* receptors, but its function here is unclear. *Vitamin D + calcium* has been demonstrated to be effective in reducing the risk for hip fracture in the elderly (Chapuy et al, 1992).

Estrogen deficiency, such as seen in the postmenopausal state, results in bone loss. Estrogen replacement prevents this bone loss mostly by reducing the activation frequency of BMUs (Steiniche et al, 1989). Estrogen binds to cytoplasmic steroid receptors; the estrogen–receptor complex is transported to the nucleus where it binds to DNA at an estrogen receptor-binding domain and influences transcription. Osteoblastic (Eriksen et al, 1988; Komm et al, 1988) and osteoclastic estrogen receptors have been demonstrated (Oursler et al, 1991). Estrogen was shown to have a direct suppressive effect on osteoclasts (Oursler et al, 1994). In vitro, estrogen was shown to downregulate IL-6 production (Girasole et al, 1992), which increases osteoclasts (Black, Garrett & Mundy 1991; Klein et al, 1991). IL-6-deficient mice, however, had normal trabecular bone and ovariectomy did not result in bone loss (Poli et al, 1994).

Selective estrogen receptor modulators, such as *raloxifene*, have estrogenic effects on bone and cardiovascular systems (Black et al, 1994; Draper et al, 1996), but appear to be devoid of the side effects of estrogen, e.g. breast tenderness and effects associated with endometrial hyperplasia (Black, Jones & Falcone, 1983).

The life-span of osteoclasts could be shortened by inducing early apoptosis. *Bisphoshonates* may be agents which cause accelerated apoptosis (Hughes et al, 1995; Rogers et al, 1996).

Knockout of *c-src* proto-oncogene results in osteopetrosis, indicating the importance of this gene in bone resorption (Soriaho et al, 1991). There are high levels of the protein product of *c-src*, $pp60^{c-src}$, in osteoclasts (Horne et al, 1992), where it may play a role in membrane fusion and vesicle targeting (Baron et al, 1993). Interference with *c-src* or $pp60^{c-src}$, resulting in inhibition of bone resorption, may be beneficial in treating osteoporosis.

A novel secreted glycoprotein, *osteoprotegerin*, which was identified recently, was shown to regulate bone resorption (Simonet et al, 1997). Osteoprotegerin is a member of the TNF receptor superfamily. It blocks the later stages of osteoclast differentiation and may potentially be used in treatment of osteoporosis.

Osteoblasts

Since osteoblasts are essential for the generation of new bone, therapeutic interventions aimed at these cells is being pursued actively. Bone formation is a complex process involving osteoblastic proliferation, matrix formation and maturation, and bone mineralization. One goal of therapeutic intervention is to stimulate proliferation of osteoblasts or their precursors. However, this may not have the desired outcome if the osteoblasts fail to differentiate. Another approach is to stimulate bone matrix formation. Matrix mineralization could also potentially be enhanced.

Mitogenic agents increase the number of osteoblasts. The therapeutic target could be any cell along the differentiation pathway from the early mesenchymal stem cell to the osteoblast. The earlier one could intervene in the differentiation pathway, the greater the potential gain. *Fluoride* has a mitogenic effect on osteoblasts (Kassem et al, 1991). The mechanism is unclear. It was postulated that it inhibits acid phosphatase, which leads to an increase in tyrosine-phosphorylated proteins and therefore affects signal transduction (Lau et al, 1989). Fluoride stimulates bone formation, without affecting bone resorption. It causes an increase in wall thickness, with no effect on resorption depth and resulting positive bone balance (Eriksen, Mosekilde & Melsen, 1985). However, because mineralization of new bone matrix is lagging, mineralization defects may form, especially with high doses. Fluoride is also directly incorporated into bone to form fluorohydroxyapatite. This may weaken bone. Lower doses of fluoride may prevent fluorosis.

Agents aimed at accelerating osteoblastic differentiation may also be an effective route of intervention. *Glucocorticoid* excess results in bone loss. However, in lower concentrations, these hormones (and the synthetic form, *dexamethasone*) appear to stimulate bone formation (Bellows, Aubin & Heersche, 1987). These effects may result from stimulation of osteoprogenitor cells to differentiate (Bellows, Heersche & Aubin, 1990). *Retinoic acid* was also found to stimulate differentiation of immature osteoprogenitor cells in vitro (Heath et al, 1989; Ng et al, 1988). Retinoic acid stimulates BMP-2 expression in bone-derived cells (Ghosh-Choudry et al, 1992). Whether retinoic acid will have beneficial effects in vivo, is not known. Acute administration of *vitamin D* downregulates proliferation of osteoblasts in vitro whereas differentiation is promoted. In contrast, chronic administration blocks differentiation (Majeska & Rodan, 1982).

Since osteoblasts have *parathyroid hormone* (PTH) receptors, they may have an anabolic effect on bone. This was indeed observed in rats and humans (Dempster et al, 1993). The effect may be caused by positive bone balance because of shallower resorption cavities, as seen in patients with mild hyperparathyroidism (Eriksen, 1986). It was also shown that PTH increases the number of new BMUs, but decreases the bone formation rate (Eriksen, 1986; Melsen, Mosekilde & Christensen,

1977; Meunier et al, 1981). However, since osteoclasts are also activated with PTH stimulation (Holtrop & Raisz, 1979; Holtrop, Raisz & Simmons, 1974; Miller, 1978), the increase in bone formation at certain sites may be accompanied by increased bone resorption at other sites. The mechanism for the anabolic effect of PTH is unknown. It causes increase in *IGF-1* and *TGF-β-1* production in osteoblasts. PTH acts on plasma membrane receptors which, through their intracytoplasmic domains, interact with GTP-binding proteins and affect adenylate cyclase, phospholipases and ion channels (Juppner et al, 1991). The PTH-signal-generating complex also has an effect on increasing cytosolic calcium from intracellular stores as well as extracellular calcium entry through calcium channels (Bidwell et al, 1991; Kruska et al, 1987). PTH has been shown to increase GM-CSF production by osteoblasts (Horowitz et al, 1989). PTH also stimulates IL-6 production, which affects osteoclastic activity.

Osteoblasts respond to *prostaglandin E_1* and *E_2* (PGE$_1$ and PGE$_2$), many interleukins and growth factors and such as *insulin-like growth factor I* and *II* (IGF-I and -II), *transforming growth factor β* (TGF-β), *epidermal growth factor* (EGF), *fibroblast growth factor* (FGF), *platelet-derived growth factor* (PDGF), and *interleukin-1* (IL-1). However, many of these molecules have been shown to produce different and often opposite responses in different systems. PGE$_1$ and PGE$_2$ stimulate periosteal and endosteal bone formation (Jee, Ke & Li, 1991). Whether any of these factors would be beneficial in managing bone disease is unknown.

Growth hormone is important in skeletal growth. It has plasma membrane receptors on osteoblasts and has been shown to stimulate collagen I and II, alkaline phosphatase and osteocalcin synthesis (Kassem et al, 1993). It stimulates IGF-I production in the liver but also in osteoblasts. IGF-I stimulates cartilage growth in the growth plates (Daughaday et al, 1972). Growth hormone and IGF-I increase bone turnover in humans (Johanssen, Lindh & Ljunghall, 1992). Both IGF-I and IGF-II stimulate osteoblast proliferation and differentiation (Canalis et al, 1989; Weinreb, Shinar & Rodan, 1990). This action is mediated through IGF binding proteins. IGF-I plus IGF binding protein 3 increase trabecular thickness in rats (Bagi et al, 1994).

Osteoblasts could potentially be stimulated to secrete more procollagen. Estrogen has been shown to stimulate procollagen synthesis in vitro. Since estrogen stimulates IGF-I synthesis in the liver, it may exert a positive skeletal effect through IGF-I.

Therapeutic intervention may also be targeted at increasing the life-span of osteoblasts. This would allow each osteoblast to form more matrix during its lifetime.

Osteocytes

Exercise stimulates the stress receptors in osteocytes, which results in an anabolic effect. Because of their location, these cells are not easily accessible to pharmacologic intervention. It is theoretically conceivable that agents which act on stress receptors may induce an anabolic effect.

Frost postulated that a mechanostat regulates the bone balance in an individual (Frost, 1992). For example, someone with high bone volume has a lower setpoint than someone with a low volume. This implies that bones in the individual with a lower setpoint respond at a lower stress level than in an individual with a higher setpoint. It is reasonable to postulate that the osteocyte is the site of the mechanostat. It may be possible in future to reset an individual's mechanostat.

Bone Lining Cells

By affecting these cells, periosteal bone formation may be enhanced. This is interesting because periosteal bone formation is more important biomechanically than the endosteal bone formation.

In summary, osteoclasts, osteoblasts, osteocytes and bone lining cells work in concert to maintain bone health. Detailed understanding of their function, as well as an understanding of the bone matrix, will lead to new paths of intervention. This will undoubtedly contribute to the treatment and prevention of osteoporosis and other bone diseases.

CLINICAL TRIALS: STUDY DESIGNS AND RELATED ISSUES

INTRODUCTION

Albright defined osteoporosis as a condition characterized by 'low bone mass and fractures' over 50 years ago. Since then, there have been multiple clinical trials conducted in postmenopausal osteoporotic women with a variety of bone-active agents such as calcium, vitamin D, fluoride, estrogen, bisphosphates and parathyroid hormone. The following discussion will focus primarily on selected randomized clinical trials for the prevention and/or treatment of postmenopausal osteoporosis.

Randomized Clinical Trials in Postmenopausal Osteoporosis

All randomized clinical trials, if properly designed and executed, have several important features as follows:

1.   Use of a proper control group.
2.   Randomized treatment assignment.
3.   Equalization of interference by means of double-blind.
4.   Low dropout.

5. Adequate statistical power.
6. Prospectiveness.

It is generally not appreciated that in clinical trials, the placebo effect may dampen the response range of the pharmacological agent. In osteoporosis trials, the response range may be further constricted by co-administration of either calcium and/or vitamin D supplementation, since both agents are known to exert some positive effect on bone (Aloia et al, 1994; Chevalley et al, 1994). Moreover, other confounding factors include exercise and socialization.

In osteoporosis trials, a dropout rate of 10% during the entire 2–3 years' duration of the trial is considered unusually good. However, the reality is that most often than not, the dropout rate approaches 20% or more. Why? The reasons include: (a) long duration of trial; (b) co-existent medical illnesses which make patients less willing to participate; (c) elderly studies; and (d) more intolerance to adverse effects. This high dropout rate tends to erode randomization, since it is not a random process resulting in substantial widening of the confidence intervals for both the active agent and the control groups. Most trials usually enroll more patients than needed, so that in the end there is enough power to draw conclusions about the treatment effect. However, even a small dropout rate has a profound effect on the outcome measure. Thus, it is important to try to track down those patients who drop out of the trials to obtain the key outcome measure(s) whenever possible.

In a recent review, Heaney discussed five unique design features for conducting osteoporosis trials (Heaney, 1996). The following summarizes some of his viewpoints.

1. *Long response time of bone.* Treatment should ideally be carried out for 4–5 years or until the targeted bone mass increase has been achieved before studying the effect on fracture rate.

2. *Bone remodeling transient.* Bone formation and bone resorption are coupled processes. Most bone-active drugs alter either the former or latter process, which will produce transient changes in BMD and is often misinterpreted. When an antiresorptive drug interferes with osteoclast function, there will be less bone resorbed per unit time. However, bone formation proceeds normally. Therefore, more bone is formed than resorbed, leading to measurable increase in bone mass. For example, a 50% reduction in activation in a normal skeleton will result in a one-time increase in spine BMD of approximately 3% over a period of 7–9 months. If drug treatment is continued, there will be no further change after the first remodeling cycle. However, if drug treatment is withdrawn, the remodeling space expands again, and the measurable increase in BMD is lost, thus the term 'transient' is used to describe this phenomenon. All activation suppressors will produce a positive remodeling transient, i.e. bisphosphonates, calcitonin, estrogen or calcium. But it is unclear which ones, if any, will alter the steady-state remodeling balance.

3. *Timing for bone mass measurement.* For a 2-year study, double measurements in the beginning and at the end (four in all) would yield a distribution of slopes with a variance only half as large as would be produced by five measurements performed every 6 months, thus saving 20% of work and money.

4. *Weighting data by duration of observation.* Since measurement uncertainty for BMD is greater than the treatment-induced short-term change, Heaney recommends weighting the observations by the duration of observation. He estimates that a 4-year slope has a precision that is approximately 5 times better than a 1-year estimate and approximately 2.5 times better than a 2-year estimate.

5. *What should be measured?* Bone mass could be determined by a variety of techniques: single photon absorptiometry (SPA), dual photon absorptiometry (DPA) and dual energy X-ray absorptiometry (DXA). Bone density is not the ultimate endpoint for the study of bone, since it does not tell us anything about skeletal micro-architecture. In fact, for the same micro-architecture, the bone strength is a function of its mass (BMC) whereas the relation to bone density is quite complex and at times the opposite is seen (fluoride, for example). Originally, SPA determinations of BMC and area were independent, with BMC being more precise than BMD since it has a smaller coefficient of variation for repeat measurements. However, with the improved technology, DPA and DXA, the measurements of area and BMC are included in the same software. For most short-term treatment trials in adults, BMD and BMC will vary in parallel. DXA is preferable to use in BMD determination because of its superior precision. Thus, BMC and BMD do not measure the same thing.

Clinical Trials in the Treatment and Prevention of Postmenopausal Osteoporosis

In the recent GREES guidelines, the various components which go into the study design of prevention and treatment trials are outlined (Recommendations, 1995). Table 13.1 summarizes the recommendations.

SPECIFIC APPROVED DRUGS FOR THE PREVENTION OR TREATMENT OF POSTMENOPAUSAL OSTEOPOROSIS

Currently, in the USA, estrogen and alendronate are the only drugs approved for the prevention indication, and calcitonin (subcutaneous or nasal), estrogen and alendronate for the treatment of postmenopausal osteoporosis. The following discussion of Estraderm and alendronate is derived from either transcripts of the Advisory Board meeting minutes or the Summary Basis of Approval (SBA) (Endocrinologic and Metabolic Drugs Advisory Board, 1985, 1995).

TABLE 13.1   Recommendations for study design of prevention and treatment trials

Component	Treatment trial	Prevention trial
Primary endpoint	Reduction in new vertebral/hip fracture	BMD (spine)
Secondary endpoint	BMDs (hip, spine); bone markers; non-vertebral fracture rate; worsening of previous fracture; quality of life	BMDs (hip, etc.); bone markers
Design	Double-blind, prospective randomized, placebo-controlled	Double-blind, prospective randomized, placebo-controlled *or* active agent vs. estrogen
Population	T score < −2 spine/hip; 1 vertebral fracture and T score < −2; at least 2 vertebral fracture	Spinal BMD T score −1 to −2 within 5 years of menopause
Duration	At least 2 years	At least 2 years
Statistical analyses	Intention-to-treat; valid completer analyses, Kaplan Meier analysis alpha = 0.05; beta = < 20%	Intention-to-treat; valid completer analyses, Kaplan Meier analysis alpha = 0.05; beta = < 20%
Diet supplements	0.5–1.0 g Calcium/day; 400–800 IU vitamin D/day	0.5–1.0 g Calcium/day
Fracture	X-ray yearly, central reader with validated criteria	
Bone safety	Paired biopsy, read centrally	

Etidronate

Etidronate was the first of the bisphosphonates to be introduced into clinical practice for the treatment of metabolic bone diseases characterized by excessive bone resorption, i.e. Paget's disease and postmenopausal osteoporosis. Even though it was not approved for use in the USA for the treatment of postmenopausal osteoporosis, it had been approved in most countries in Europe and Japan for this indication. Recently, it was approved in the UK for the prevention of post-menopausal and corticosteroid-induced osteoporosis. Table 13.2 summarizes the key clinical trial-related parameters.

In the US multicenter trial, the proportion of patients completing the 3-year blinded period was: placebo 90/105 (86%), phosphate 88/106 (83%), etidronate 92/105 (88%) and etidronate + phosphate 93/107 (87%). The second pivotal trial was conducted in Europe, specifically in Denmark. Three years of placebo and etidronate treatments were completed by 21/33 (64%) and 20/33 (61%) of patients, respectively. Watts et al (1990) published the results on the US trials and Storm et al (1990) published the European trials.

The vertebral compression fractures were identified with lateral spinal radiographs and read by a single expert radiologist, Dr Harry K. Genant, blinded

TABLE 13.2 Parameters for key clinical trials of etidronate in USA (sample size 429) and Europe (sample size 66)

Parameter	Trial measures
Primary endpoints	Lumbar spine BMD
Secondary endpoints	Urine OHP, Uca, PTH femoral neck and greater trochanter BMD, radius BMD
Design	Double-blind, randomized parallel group, placebo-controlled, 24 months*
Inclusion criteria	45–75 Years ≥ 12 months postmenopausal lumbar spine BMD > 1–4 vertebral fracture plus osteopenia
Exclusion criteria	Treatment with estrogen, glucocorticoids, androgens, anabolic steroids, phosphates; Ca < 1.0 g/day; vitamin D < 1000 IU/day previous 6 months or thiazide previous 2 months treatment with fluoride, any bisphosphonate or calcitonin; < 40 kg or > 80 kg; secondary osteoporosis; confounding conditions (active RA, GI or liver chronic alcoholism, renal impairment)
Doses**	400 mg × 14 days every 3 months
Safety	Bone biopsy in subset of patients
Diet supplement	500 mg Ca × 74 days every 3 months

*   The original study design was a 3 year blinded study followed by 2 years of open label.
** Patients were treated with phosphate 2 g or corresponding placebo for 3 days, followed by etidronate 400 mg (Didronel) or placebo daily for 14 days (2 h before meals with water, black coffee, tea or juice, but not with milk or other dairy products) and then elemental calcium for eight cycles over 24 months.

to the treatment. Vertebral Deformity Score (VDS) was used to assess the deformity of each vertebral body from T4 to L4, as shown in Table 13.3.

Fracture definitions used in these trials include:

1. *Vertebral Deformity Index* (VDI) is defined as the sum of the VDSs for an individual patient divided by the number of vertebrae assessed. Increases in VDI include: those with new fractures, those with worsening of previous fractures and those with both.

2. *Vertebral fracture* is defined as occurring when the VDS of an individual vertebra increases compared with the assigned score from the previous radiograph, with increments of 0.5 used to reflect interval changes.

Fracture assessments used in the etidronate clinical trials are shown in Table 13.4.

In the US multicenter trial, the bone mass of the lumbar spine, hip and radius was measured at baseline and every 6 months. Dual-photon absorptiometry was used to determine the BMD with a LunarDP3 densitometer, Norland 2600 densitometer and a modified Ohio Nuclear Series 84 γ-camera. Comparability of BMD measurements between centers was ensured with cross-calibration of instruments with a standard phantom (Hologic X-Caliber) which was measured twice yearly at each study site. All these instruments measured BMC within 5% of the nominal value, but BMD (calculated as BMC divided by area) varied more because of differences in edge-detection algorithms. Since the treatment response

TABLE 13.3 Assessment of deformity in vertebral bodies T4–L4 (Vertebral Deformity Score)

Grade 0 = Normal vertebra	
Grade 1 = Mild fracture	20–25% Reduction in any (anterior, middle, posterior) vertebral height or 10–20% reduction in vertebral area
Grade 2 = Moderate fracture	25–40% Reduction in any vertebral height or 20–40% reduction in vertebral area
Grade 3 = Maximum severe fracture	> 40% Reduction in any vertebral height or > 40% reduction in vertebral area

Increments of 0.5 were used as necessary to reflect intermediate changes between grades.

TABLE 13.4 Vertebral fracture assessments used in USA/Europe etidronate clinical trials

Assessment	Definition
Vertebral fracture incidence	The number of patients experiencing a fracture divided by total number of patients, expressed as a percentage
Vertebral fracture rate	The number of vertebral fractures per 1000 patient-years of exposure
Change in VDI	Change in the index of total vertebral deformity (higher numbers signify greater deformity); accounts for both the number of vertebral fractures and their severity
Life-table estimates of vertebral fracture incidence	Survival curves of the percentage of patients remaining free of fracture

was calculated as the percentage change from baseline, the absolute differences in BMD had a minimal effect on the final analyses. Single-photon absorptiometry with a ^{125}iodine source was used to determine the BMC (expressed in g/cm) of the radius of the non-dominant arm or the right arm, using Lunar SP2 densitometers, Nuclear Data 1100 densitometers, Norland Bone Mineral Analyzer Model 178 or 278 and Osteoanalyzer SPSHA110.

In the European trials, BMC of the lumbar spine was measured by dual-photon absorptiometry using the Novo Diagnostic Systems. The regional BMC of the distal nondominant forearm was measured with the single-photon absorptiometry with ^{125}iodine using the NovoGT 35 from Novo Diagnostic Systems.

The etidronate IND (Investigational New Drug notification) for the treatment indication was submitted to the FDA in 1992. An NDA was initially submitted in 1990 and it was felt by the Advisory Committee meeting (1991) that longer-term data were needed. Therefore, the NDA was resubmitted in August 1992.

Estraderm

Estraderm (estradiol transdermal system) was approved in 1991 for both the prevention and treatment of postmenopausal osteoporosis. Table 13.5 summarizes the key features of the two placebo-controlled pivotal trials.

TABLE 13.5 Key features of two placebo-controlled trials of Estraderm

Parameter	Trial 1	Trial 2
Primary endpoint	Lumbar spine BMD; radial BMD	Lumbar spine BMD
Secondary endpoint	Bone markers (osteocalcin, bone) specific alkaline phosphatase, vitamin D metabolite, urine OHP, Ca, E, E2, Lh, FSH, PTH)	Bone markers (osteocalcin, bone-specific alkaline phosphatase, urine OHP), Ca height, vaginal/cervical cytology, BMD proximal femur, BMC mid-radius and iliac crest
Design	Double-blind, randomized parallel group, placebo-controlled; 24 months	Double-blind, randomized placebo-controlled; 12 months; stratum I $\leq$ 10 years; stratum II > 10 years
Inclusion criteria	> 40 years old, hysterectomized 2 weeks–2 years prior to study	45–75 years old, with FSH > 30 mIU/ml; 1 non-traumatic vertebral fracture; BMD < 1.14 g/cm^2
Exclusion criteria	No HRT within 2 months; severe hot flushes on diuretics	No HRT within 2 months; severe hot flushes on diuretics
Estradiol dose	0.025, 0.05, 0.1 mg/day every 3.5 days	0.1 mg/day every 3.5 days, days 1–22
Progesterone dose	None	MPA 10 mg/day (days 13–22)
Safety	Mammogram every 6 months, vaginal bleed assessment	Mammogram every 6 months, vaginal bleed assessment
Diet supplement	No calcium	700 mg calcium/day
Sample size	127 Enrolled; 93 completed	76 Enrolled; 67 completed

The protocol in Trial 1 was started in April 1985 and completed in July 1989. During the trial, there were eight amendments: (a) exclusion of patients with active systemic granulomatous disease; (b) standard calcium preparation; (c) vaginal smear examinations; (d) analyses of vitamin D metabolites and bone-specific alkaline phosphatase; (e) reduction in minimum age from 45 to 40 years; (f) inclusion of patients who had hysterectomy/oophorectomy 6 weeks to 2 months prior to study entry but had not gone without estrogen replacement therapy for more than 6 months; (g) no ERT within 2 months prior to study; (h) yearly mammogram for those over age 50 and every other year for those < 49 years. In Trial 2, there were three amendments: (a) DPA at 6-month visit; (b) endometrial biopsy in women with abnormal bleeding and if endometrial hyperplasia found, patient was withdrawn; (c) bone biopsy parameter to be evaluated (bone formation rate/bone volume, bone balance, activation frequency, resorption rate per bone volume).

The power calculations for these two trials are of interest. In Trial 1, a sample size of 20 per group (completed 24 months) was estimated to detect mean difference in lumbar spine BMD at least 2.5% of placebo treatment difference with 95%

TABLE 13.6   Parameters for treatment indication in key clinical trial of alendronate

Parameter	Pivotal trials
Primary endpoint	Lumbar spine BMD
Secondary endpoints	Hip BMD; total body BMD; vertebral fractures; Spine Deformity Index; height; non-vertebral fractures; bone markers (urine deoxypyridinoline, pyridinoline, osteocalcin)
Design	Double-blind, randomized, placebo-controlled, 36 months*
Inclusion criteria	45–80 years ≥ 5 years postmenopausal lumbar spine BMD < 2.5 SD below the mean of premenopausal women
Exclusion criteria	Other causes of osteoporosis, e.g. glucocorticoids; other metabolic bone diseases; hyper- or hypothyroidism; active peptic ulcer disease; any recent or current treatment with the potential to cause gastro-intestinal irritation; health problems that could affect participation or interpretation of data; abnormal renal function (serum creatinine > 1.5mg/dl); abnormal hepatic function; abnormalities of lumbar spine precluding BMD assessment (min. 3); history of hip fracture; prior treatment with bisphosphonates; treatment within 12 months with estrogen, progestin, calcitonin, fluoride or anabolic steroids
Doses	5, 10, 20 mg (at 24 months, the 20 mg group switched to 5 mg)**
Safety	Bone biopsy in subset of patients
Diet supplement	500 mg Calcium
Sample size	994 Enrolled, 909 completed 12 months; 881 with paired spine films

*   The original study design was a 2-year blinded trial followed by 1 year open label which was later modified to include 3 years of double-blind treatment.

**   The switch was done because another study suggested that 20 mg was not needed for the BMD change.

power. In Trial 2, a sample size of 60 was estimated to detect a mean difference in lumbar spine BMD at least 2% in 12 months with 90% power.

Alendronate

Alendronate was the first bisphosphonate to be approved by the FDA for the prevention and treatment of postmenopausal osteoporosis. Table 13.6 summarizes the key clinical trial-related parameters for treatment indication.

The US multicenter trial randomized 478 patients (192 placebo, 98 alendronate 5 mg, 94 alendronate 10 mg, 94 alendronate 20 mg). Four hundred and six patients completed the 3-year trial. The second pivotal trial was conducted outside the USA in 19 centers (Australia, Austria, Belgium, Canada, France, Germany, Israel, Mexico, New Zealand, Argentina, Brazil, Chile, Colombia, Switzerland and the UK). These 19 centers randomized 516 patients (205 placebo, 104 alendronate 5 mg, 102 alendronate 10 mg, 105 alendronate 20 mg) and 418 patients completed 3 years of treatment. The results of the two pivotal trials were published in 1995 by Liberman et al (1995) and the ex-USA trial was published in 1996 by Devogelaer et al.

The techniques used in the efficacy endpoints deserve comment. The BMD of the lumbar spine, femoral neck, trochanter, forearm and total body were measured by DXA with Hologic QDR-1000/W, Lunar DPX-L or Norland XR-26 densitometers. All DXA scans were reviewed at a central facility by people who had no knowledge of the treatment assignment. All lateral spine films were sent to the radiology center, where vertebral heights were determined by observers blinded to the treatment assignment or film sequence. All films were digitized. Whether or not a vertebral fracture was present at baseline was determined by comparing the woman's baseline vertebral height ratios with those of a reference group. These ratios were calculated as follows: the anterior and middle heights were compared with the posterior height of the same vertebra, and the posterior height was compared with the posterior height of an adjacent vertebra. A vertebral height ratio more than 3 SD below the corresponding reference ratio was considered to be a previous vertebral fracture. A new fracture was defined as a reduction of at least 20% with an absolute decrease of at least 4 mm in the height of any vertebral body between baseline and follow-up observations. The SDI was used to determine vertebral deformities. SDI was developed as a continuous measure of vertebral deformities in patients with a history of vertebral fractures (Sauer et al 1991). Height was measured with a Harpenden stadiometer, which measures height to the nearest mm. During the trial, three measurements were obtained from each woman and two additional measurements were made if any two values differed by more than 4 mm.

In terms of statistical analyses, it was predetermined that data from the two pivotal studies from the three alendronate groups would be pooled, since neither trial alone, nor any one dose group, was sufficiently large to permit the detection of a significant effect of alendronate on the incidence of new fractures. For the analyses of the proportion of females with one or more new vertebral fractures, the Breslow–Day test was used to determine whether or not there was any interaction between the treatment group and the trial, since there were no trials. If no interaction, then the Cochran–Mantel–Haenzel test was applied to the pooled data to compare the placebo group with the alendronate group. The chi-squared test was used to compare the proportions of women with progressive vertebral deformities (i.e. those with increased SDI) in both the placebo and the alendronate group. ANOVA was used to analyze changes in height from baseline. Non-vertebral fractures were analyzed with Cox proportional-hazards models, with each of the two trials as a stratification factor. All analyses of the drug efficacy were based on the intention-to-treat principle. The power analyses were set to show a 3% difference between any of the alendronate treatment groups and placebo with 80–90% power.

The alendronate IND for the treatment indication was submitted to the FDA on August 30, 1988 and the drug was finally approved in September 1995. During this time, there were at least 12 meetings between Merck and the FDA on various aspects of drug development for the treatment indication. There were a total of 17 phase I studies. There was one phase IIa, an early dose-ranging bone marker study in 65 early postmenopausal women randomized to a 6-week trial with either placebo, 5, 20 or 40 mg alendronate per day. Dose-dependent reductions in urinary deoxypyridinoline (less with serum osteocalcin) ranged from 28–48%, a value comparable to the response seen in hormone replacement treatment. Based on this study, it was felt that 5–40 mg was a reasonable dose range to explore in the phase IIb dose-ranging study, and later the 5–20 mg into phase III trials. In addition to the two phase III pivotal efficacy studies, there were three other efficacy studies: one phase IIb study (188 patients, 2 years), one salmon calcitonin comparative study (286 patients) (Adami et al, 1995) and one elderly patient study (359 patients, 2 years).

Merck also conducted two pivotal trials (Vertebral Deformity Trial, Clinical Fracture Trial) for the fracture prevention indication. The various features of the study design were published (Black et al, 1993). Table 13.7 summarizes key characteristics of these studies. The patients were recruited from population-based mailing lists at 11 clinical center across the USA. This model of 11 centers recruiting a large number of patients (e.g. 600 each) was quite different from the usual model in pharmaceutical trials, where there are usually a much larger number of clinical investigators, each recruiting a smaller number of patients. The stated advantages of this model include the following:

1. Using only large clinical centers with experienced investigators and research teams, most of them were full-time on the study so that they could all concentrate on it. Therefore, quality control and training could be more focused, resulting in higher quality clinical data, thus increasing the power of the study.
2. The smaller number of centers results in more efficient use of resources such as densitometers, maintenance and quality control.
3. With fewer investigators, each would be able to have more significant input into the study design and presentation and analysis of results.

Approximately 1.1 million women were contacted by mail, of whom 25 224 were screened at these study sites, 2027 (101% of goal) were randomized (1005 to placebo and 1022 to alendronate 5 mg). The planning for the trial began in May 1991 and screening began in January 1992. Randomization began in May 1992 and was completed in May 1993. Follow-up visits continued through May 1997.

The assumptions used to calculate power are listed in Table 13.8. For the vertebral deformity trial, with a sample size of 2000, the power of the trial would permit the detection of a 40% reduction in the cumulative incidence of vertebral deformities with 90% and 99% power to detect a 32% reduction. Using the assumptions made in the clinical fracture trial (see above), a sample size of 4000 patients has 90% power to detect a 25% reduction in the cumulative incidence of clinical fractures at the end of the study.

TABLE 13.7 Design features of two key trials of the fracture prevention indication for alendronate

Parameter	Vertebral deformity trial	Clinical fracture trial
Primary endpoint	New vertebral deformities	Clinical fractures
Secondary endpoint	Clinical fractures; change in BMD in hip, spine and forearm (20%); change in height bone markers (20%)	New vertebral deformities; change in BMD in hip, spine and forearm (20%); change in height bone markers (20%); bone quality
Design	Double-blind, randomized, placebo-controlled	Double-blind, randomized, placebo-controlled
Inclusion criteria	55–80 years; BMD at femoral neck −2SD or < 0.68 g/cm^2 (Hologic QDR 2000); postmenopausal > 2 years	55–80 years; BMD at femoral neck −2SD or < 0.68 g/cm^2 (Hologic QDR 2000); postmenopausal > 2 years
Exclusion criteria	Erosive gastro-intestinal disease within 5 years, dyspepsia requiring daily drug(s), recent peptic ulcer disease requiring hospitalization, abnormal renal, hepatic function, major medical problems, severe malabsorption, uncontrolled HBP, MI within 6 months, unstable angina, hypo- or hyperthyroidism, metabolic bone disease, bone-active agents within 6 months, unsuitable anatomy on spinal X-ray, BMD at femoral neck > 3SD below age-specific mean, history of bilateral hip replacement	Erosive gastro-intestinal disease within 5 years, dyspepsia requiring daily drug(s), recent peptic ulcer disease requiring hospitalization, abnormal renal, hepatic function, major medical problems, severe malabsorption, uncontrolled HBP, MI within 6 months, unstable angina, hypo- or hyperthyroidism, metabolic bone disease, bone-active agents within 6 months, unsuitable anatomy on spinal X-ray, BMD at femoral neck > 3SD below age-specific mean, history of bilateral hip replacement
Dose	5 mg	5 mg
Safety		Bone biopsy
Diet supplement	500 mg Calcium, 400 IU vitamin D	500 mg Calcium, 400 IU vitamin D
Sample size	2023 Randomized; 36 months	4434 Randomized; 36 months

TABLE 13.8 Parameters used to calculate power of alendronate trial data

Parameter	Vertebral deformity trial	Clinical fracture trial
Annual incidence in placebo	6.5%	4%
Annual mortality	1.1%	1.1%
Significance level	0.025 at 2 years 0.35 at 3 years	0.05 at 4.25 years
Lag in treatment effect	1 year	1 year
Withdrawal rate	10% at 2 years 15% at 3 years	3%/year

In order to protect patients from excessive bone loss during the trial, criteria for excessive reduction in BMD were predetermined. If a patient demonstrated a decrease in BMD at the total hip or lumbar spine of greater than 8% during year 1, and 10% in year 2, etc., the measurement would be repeated and, if confirmed, the patient was informed and considered for alternative treatments and offered the opportunity to discontinue the trial. Biochemical markers were collected on the predetermined 20% random sample of patients. Those who dropped from the trial were encouraged to report all fractures and to return for annual measurements of BMD and biochemical markers.

The overall structure of these fracture prevention intervention trials was similar to NIH collaborative clinical trials. These studies were directed by a Steering Committee consisting of clinical center investigator, coordinating center investigator and sponsor representatives. Unlike most pharmaceutical studies, the FIT trials involved 11 large clinical centers and a coordinating center, each with investigators and teams experienced in the design and execution of collaborative clinical trials. In addition to the Steering Committee, there were other committees: Executive Committee (to provide leadership); Endpoints Committee, Publications Committee, Ancillary Studies Committee (to develop policies and procedures for ancillary studies). There were several groups essential to the planning and execution of these trials: the Coordinating Center (the mechanism for coordinating and assuring the quality of all aspects of the design and implementation of the study, the analysis and dissemination of findings); Merck Research Laboratories; Nichols Institutes (Central Laboratory); Recruitment Committee (to ensure that all clinics had an adequate recruitment plan); Quality Control Working Group (to develop and monitor a quality control system for all clinical and technical procedures required by the protocol, and to plan and carry out quality control site visits); Compliance Working Group (to monitor compliance and dropouts and to recommend measures to improve adherence to the study protocol); Data and Safety Monitoring Board (to review unmasked results of the trial for evidence of beneficial or adverse effects of the study treatments, using the guidelines proposed in the protocol).

PHARMACO-ECONOMIC ANALYSIS

Why Undertake Pharmaco-economic (PE) Analysis?

Rising health care costs around the world have led to an increased awareness by decision makers regarding the scarcity of resources and the difficult, yet unavoidable, choices they must make. PE analyses are performed to measure the economic value of drug products and to assist in the allocation of scarce resources. PE analyses are currently required by Australia (Commonwealth Department of Human Services and Health, 1995) and Canada (CCOHTA, 1994) for reimbursement of new drugs on their respective national formularies. Increasingly, other European nations are requesting PE studies to accompany traditional new drug submissions (Genduso & Kotsanos, 1996). In the USA, PE analyses are not required by the FDA Division of Drug Marketing, Advertising and Communications (1995) but private payers, especially managed care organizations (Langley & Martin, 1996) are demanding that pharmaceutical companies demonstrate the economic value of their products. PE studies are essential for drugs that treat chronic conditions, since many costs and benefits are not captured within the framework of a randomized clinical trial (RCT). Therefore, it is now imperative that pharmaceutical companies conduct PE analyses—either fully integrated into, or in parallel to, their RCTs—to supplement claims of efficacy and safety.

Dimensions of PE Analysis and QoL Scales

PE analyses generally comprise two broad areas—costs of treatment and quality of life (QoL). The first dimension of PE analysis involves measuring resource utilization and costs associated with the underlying disease or condition. These resources may include medical care (direct and indirect), non-medical care (e.g. social services) and productivity losses, depending on the perspective of the analysis. Estimates of the costs of treatment are then compared to the benefits or effectiveness as part of a cost–benefit or cost–effectiveness analysis. The QoL component attempts to measure qualitative aspects of treatment such as pain, overall health, functionality (physical, mental, social, etc.) and ability to perform daily activities. Generic health instruments are designed to capture a broad spectrum of health domains and can be used across a variety of disease states. There are several validated generic instruments, that is, those with internal and external validity, including the SF-36 (Ware et al, 1993), Sickness Impact Profile (SIP) (Bergner et al, 1976, 1981), and the Nottingham Health Profile (NHP) (Hunt, McEwen & McKenna, 1986; Jenkinson, Fitzpatrick & Argyle, 1988). Preference-based health-related quality of life instruments include the Health Utilities Index (HUI) (Torrance et al, 1995; Feeny, Torrance & Furlong, 1996), the Quality of Well-Being Scale (QWB) (Kaplan, Feeny & Revicki, 1993; Kaplan, Anderson & Ganiats, 1993) and the EuroQol (EuroQol Group, 1990) questionnaire. These instruments allow the analyst to calculate a utility score, which can then be used to measure health-related quality of life. A utility score also can be used as a quality adjustment weight for deriving quality-adjusted life years gained or quality-adjusted life years (QALYs) so that both length of life and 'quality' of life are combined into a single metric. In addition, many disease-specific or disease-targeted instruments have been developed over a wide variety of diseases (e.g. renal disease, chronic back pain, osteoarthritis, cancer, etc.).

QoL and Osteoporosis

The inclusion of QoL instruments into clinical trials is becoming commonplace in many therapeutic areas. In osteoporosis, the introduction of health-related QoL instruments is necessary to capture changes in QoL for several reasons (Greendale et al, 1993). First, osteoporosis is a chronic disease where life expectancy does not adequately measure the impact of the disease. Sequelae include both physical (e.g. pain, physical function) and social outcomes, as well as loss of independence or ability to perform daily activities, and decreased quality of life (Cook et al, 1993). Therapies that are effective in eliminating symptoms of osteoporosis may cause other residual limitations. Thus, a better understanding of the entire impact of a therapy on the patient's physical, social and psychological status can be obtained through the use of QoL instruments (Revicki, 1989).

Second, patients may experience QoL improvements independent of changes in bone density or fracture rates. Without QoL instruments in the clinical trial, such improvements or changes cannot be accurately measured or attributed to changes in clinical markers. And third, QoL dimensions of an osteoporosis treatment may be important in differentiating the product from the field of other competing treatments. To date, there are no known validated QoL instruments specifically designed for osteoporosis (i.e. targeted for this disease), although research in the area has identified 'fear of falling' and 'adaptations to the disease' as important new dimensions of QoL in osteoporosis (Lydick et al, 1997; Martin, Holmes & Lydick, 1997). In general, for an osteoporosis study a QoL analysis must identify and measure important effects this disease has on patients' lives, such as loss of function and pain. Ideally, the osteoporosis QoL instrument should possess the following properties: (a) reliability, (b) responsiveness (c) validity, and (d) interpretability. Reliability refers to detection of differences in health-related QoL above the random error or statistical noise associated with any instrument. Thus, a reliable instrument will generally show that repeated observations on a stable population produce very similar results. Another component of reliability is the internal consistency of questions that contribute to a composite score, and is typically measured using Cronbach's alpha. Responsiveness refers to ability to detect change. A responsive instrument should be able to detect changes in patient scores for patients who have improvement or deterioration in their scores. Validity includes construct validity, face validity and content validity. One component of construct validity is the comprehensiveness of the measure; a second component is the extent to which factors hypothesized to influence the overall result are the true influencing factors. Thus, an instrument with construct validity is one that is measuring what it is intended to measure. Face validity exists if the questionnaire is logically related to the disease and it is able to detect obvious changes in a patient's condition. Content validity refers to the extent to which the domain of interest is thoroughly addressed by the items or questions in the instrument. The fourth key property of a QoL instrument, interpretability, is satisfied if minimally important differences in scores can be assessed and are clinically meaningful. Developing a QoL instrument for osteoporosis which satisfies these properties is clearly an arduous and daunting task that could take several years. An alternative approach for measuring QoL in osteoporosis patients, in the absence of an appropriate osteoporosis QoL instrument, is to use a combination of existing instruments (Greendale et al, 1993). For example, in the risedronate international RCT for hip fractures, an activities of daily living (ADL) instrument is being used, while the vertebral fracture RCTs combine the use of a generic instrument (i.e. the SF-36) and a disease-specific instrument (i.e. the Study of Osteoporotic Fractures back pain interview instrument).

Process for Integrating PE Analyses into an RCT for Osteoporosis Treatment

The initial step toward integrating a PE analysis plan into an RCT for osteoporosis is to understand the costs and outcomes of the standard treatment. Ideally, this would occur very early in the product development process in Phases I and II, rather than commencing in Phase III. PE hypotheses must be generated and clearly articulated and should be based on sound medical evidence. A PE model should be developed to form the framework of the PE analysis plan. The type of data needed must then be identified, as well as the reason for and timing of its collection, the setting in which the data will be collected, and how these data will be analyzed. At this point it is critically important that the rationale behind the PE analysis plan be clearly demonstrated to key decision makers within the pharmaceutical company. The next step is to adapt the clinical program to accommodate PE data collection by modifying the clinical protocols. For example, CRFs may need to be revised to gather medical care utilization or QoL data, or modifications could be done to include the addition of an active comparator arm in Phase III. The rationale for the PE plan can be included in the clinical protocol or in a separate, parallel PE protocol. If QoL is to be measured then an appropriate, validated instrument must be selected or developed and incorporated into the protocol.

REGULATORY GUIDELINES

Several national and international guidelines have been developed in order to facilitate standardization of methods and procedures for both preclinical and clinical investigations of drugs for the management of osteoporosis.

1. Consensus Development Conference: diagnosis, prophylaxis and treatment of osteoporosis (1993).
2. WHO assessment of fracture risk and its application to screening for postmenopausal osteoporosis (1994).
3. FDA guidelines for preclinical and clinical evaluation of agents used in the prevention and treatment of postmenopausal osteoporosis (1994).

4. FDA HRT Working Group. Guidance for clinical evaluation of combination estrogen/progestin-containing drug products used for hormone replacement therapy of postmenopausal women (1995).
5. Summary of the draft Japanese guidelines for the evaluation of agents for treating osteoporosis (1995).
6. Recommendations for the registration of new chemical entities used in the prevention and treatment of osteoporosis (1995).
7. National Osteoporosis Foundation assessing vertebral fractures. A report by the NOF Working Group (1995).
8. Note for guidance on involutional osteoporosis in women (draft—European Committee for Proprietary Medicinal Products (1996).

Highlights of Regulatory Issues Relative to Preclinical and Clinical Trials

The FDA draft guidelines document provides details of both preclinical and clinical requirements for the assessment of anti-osteoporotic agents in general. At the time when this document was prepared by the Agency, only antiresorptive drugs were approved for either prevention (estrogens) or treatment of osteoporosis (calcitonin), or investigated in clinical trials (bisphosphonates). Fluoride and parathyroid hormone were the only bone-forming agents which were under investigation. For fluoride, the clinical primary efficacy endpoint was long determined to be antifracture efficacy. Both preclinical and clinical requirements for bone-forming agents and for others with ill-defined mechanisms of action on skeletal tissue are individually addressed and appropriate guidelines are developed with the collaboration from the industry or individual sponsors.

The procedures adopted by the Agency for the approval of alendronate for the prevention and treatment of postmenopausal osteoporosis clearly set up specific preclinical and clinical requirements for other investigational bisphosphonates for similar indications and usage. In general, various regulatory issues relative to investigational evaluation of anti-osteoporotic agents can be summarized as follows:

1. *Preclinical evaluation.* Regulatory guidelines exist for the preclinical studies of new drugs, including pharmacokinetics and toxicology (ICH-S3B, 1995; ICH-M3, 1997). Pharmacodynamic and kinetic studies should be carried out according to the Agency's current draft guidelines. For specific estrogen receptor modulators (SERMs) and bone-forming agents, issues relative to preclinical studies need to be discussed with the Agency. The flow chart for preclinical regulatory aspects essentially depicts the scheduling of all studies (including bone quality) relative to clinical development of a new drug (see FDA Guidelines, 1994).
2. *Clinical evaluation.* Routine Phase I and II studies should be carried out according to the Agency's current guidelines. Biochemical markers of bone turnover should be measured along with vertebral BMD in dose-ranging Phase II studies. Sponsors are encouraged to discuss with the Agency regarding

specific markers of bone resorption and formation that need to be monitored. Assay procedures for these markers should be carefully validated. Bone biopsy with quantitative static and dynamic histomorphometry is an important endpoint of Phase II studies, particularly with bisphosphonates and fluoride.

In Phase III studies, the targeted population (postmenopausal women) for prevention and treatment of osteoporosis should be defined according to the WHO classification of osteoporosis (WHO, 1994).

The recommended primary efficacy endpoints of Phase III prevention and treatment studies for estrogens and non-estrogens are in the Agency's current guidelines. Details of other relevant issues of Phase III studies are according to the Agency's guidelines, and sponsors are encouraged to discuss these issues with the Agency during the drug development process.

In recent years, the usefulness of ultrasound measurement of bone mass has been emphasized in numerous reports. The diagnostic and prognostic uses of both DXA and ultrasound need to be discussed with the Agency prior to the initiation of Phase II and Phase III clinical trials.

Although BMD is considered to be the best predictor of osteoporotic fractures, a variety of qualitative changes have been reported to increase skeletal fragility (Marcus, 1996). Attempts should be made to incorporate, in clinical trials, procedures to provide evidence in support of improvement in bone quality in addition to improved BMD in response to therapy.

For assessment of the antifracture efficacy of an anti-osteoporotic agent, sponsors are encouraged to discuss with the Agency the study design, target population, criteria for defining new and recurrent vertebral fractures, the criteria for evaluation of spinal deformity, and non-vertebral fractures.

Current FDA guidelines for postmenopausal osteoporosis are essentially followed for all investigational drugs for osteoporosis. When a particular situation arises due to a unique pharmacological property of a new chemical entity, the relevant issues need to be discussed with the Agency for a satisfactory resolution.

Histomorphometric Indices of Bone Turnover

In certain situations bone biopsy is indicated in the evaluation of agents for the prevention and treatment of osteoporosis; e.g. (a) to rule out confounding diagnosis; (b) to understand the mechanism of treatment response; and (c) to assess the safety of the drug in terms of quality of bone formed during long-term treatment. The following histomorphometric indices of bone turnover are particularly recommended for evaluation: osteoid volume, osteoid thickness, mineral apposition rate, mineralization surface, and bone formation rate. The nomenclature and symbols of histomorphometric parameters should be those recommended by the Bone Histomorphometry Nomenclature Committee of the American Society for Bone and Mineral Research (Parfitt et al, 1987).

Testing of Combined Drug Regimens

For hormone replacement therapy, see FDA Working Group Guidance (FDA HRT Working Group, 1995). For other combined drug regimens, trials with multiple treatment arms need to be performed. Study design should be discussed with the Agency prior to initiation.

Research Priorities

1. To search for more sensitive bone-specific markers of formation and resorption with improved assay procedures. Biochemical markers of bone turnover provide information relevant to the entire skeleton. Development of specific bone markers sensitive to small changes in remodeling in response to therapy is useful in the investigation of anti-osteoporotic drugs.
2. Role of risk factors other than BMD in identifying high-risk subjects with accelerated bone mass loss.
3. Objective assessment of vertebral deformity.
4. Improving the sensitivity and specificity of assessment of prevalent and incident vertebral fractures. Development of a consensus algorithm.
5. Development of techniques for automated evaluation of vertebral deformity/fracture.
6. Development of a non-invasive technique for assessment of bone quality during clinical trials.
7. Assessment of quality of life in clinical trials.
8. Secondary osteoporosis and osteoporosis in men. Beside endocrinopathies (e.g. Cushing's syndrome, hyperparathyroidism, thyrotoxicosis) and drug-induced osteoporosis (e.g. by glucocorticoids, anticonvulsants, and excess of thyroid hormone) research efforts need to be devoted to improve our insights into the pathophysiology of osteopenia associated with other secondary causes. Many questions remain unanswered regarding the epidemiology, pathophysiology, risk factors and clinical manifestations of osteoporosis in men (Seeman, 1996).

REFERENCES

Aarden EM, Burger EH, Nijweide PJ. Function of osteocytes in bone. *J Cell Biochem* 1994; **55**: 287–99.

Adami S, Passeri M, Ortolani S et al. Effects of oral alendronate and intranasal salmon calcitonin on bone mass and biochemical markers of bone turnover in postmenopausal women with osteoporosis. *Bone* 1995; **17**(4): 383–90.

Addadi L, Moradian J, Shay E et al. A chemical model for the cooperation of sulfates and carboxylates in calcite crystal nucleation: relevance to biomineralization. *Proc Natl Acad Sci USA* 1987; **84**: 2732–6.

Ahmad LA, Eckhoff DG, Kramer AM. Outcome studies of hip fractures. *Orthoped Rev* 1994; 19–24.

Al-Humidan A, Ralston SH, Hughes DE et al. Interleukin-6 does not stimulate bone resorption in neonatal mouse calvariae. *J Bone Mineral Res* 1991; **6**: 3–7.

Ali SY, Sajdera SW, Anderson HC. Isolation and characterization of calcifying matrix vesicles from epiphyseal cartilage. *Proc Natl Acad Sci USA* 1970; **67**: 1513–20.

Aloia JF, Vaswani A, Yeh JK et al. Calcium supplementation with and without hormone replacement therapy to prevent postmenopausal bone loss. *Ann Intern Med* 1994; **120**: 97–103.

Andersson G, Ek-Rylander B, Hammarstrom LE et al. Immunocytochemical localization of a tartrate-resistant and vanadate-sensitive acid nucleotide tri- and diphosphatase. *J Histochem Cytochem* 1986; **34**: 293.

Bagi CM, Brommage R, Deleon L et al. Benefit of systemically administered rhIGF-I/IGFBP-3 on cancellous bone in ovariectomized rats. *J Bone Mineral Res* 1994; **9**: 1301–12.

Baron R, Neff L, Brown W et al. Polarized secretion of lysosomal enzymes: co-distribution of cation-independent mannose-6-phosphate receptors and lysosomal enzymes along with osteoclast exocytic pathway. *J Cell Biol* 1988; **106**: 1863–72.

Baron R, Neff L, Brown W et al. Selective internalization of the apical plasma membrane and rapid redistribution of lysosomal enzymes and mannose 6-phosphate receptors during osteoclast inactivation by calcitonin. *J Cell Sci* 1990; **97**: 439–47.

Baron R, Neff L, Louvard D, Courtoy PJ. Cell-mediated extracellular acidification and bone resorption: evidence for a low pH in resorbing lacunae and localization of a 100 kD lysosomal membrane protein at the osteoclast ruffled border. *J Cell Biol* 1985; **101**: 2210–22.

Baron R, Neff L, Roy C et al. Evidence for a high and specific concentration of $(Na^+, K^+)ATPase$ in the plasma membrane of the osteoclast. *Cell* 1986; **46**: 311–20.

Baron R, Ravesloot J-H, Neff L et al. Cellular and molecular biology of the osteoclast. In M Noda (ed.) *Cellular and Molecular Biology of Bone* 1993, p 483; San Diego, CA: Academic Press.

Bekker PJ, Gay CV. Characterization of a calcium ATPase in osteoclast plasma membrane. *J Bone Mineral Res* 1990a; **5**: 557–67.

Bekker PJ, Gay CV. Biochemical characterization of an electrogenic vacuolar proton pump in purified chicken osteoclast plasma membrane vesicles. *J Bone Mineral Res* 1990b; **5**: 569–79.

Bellows CG, Aubin JE, Heersche JNM. Physiological concentrations of glucocorticoids stimulate formation of bone nodules from isolated rat calvaria cells in vitro. *Endocrinology* 1987; **121**: 1985–92.

Bellows CG, Heersche JNM, Aubin JE. Determination of the capacity for proliferation and differentiation of osteoprogenitor cells in the presence and absence of dexamethasone. *Dev Biol* 1990; **140**: 132–8.

Bergner M, Bobbitt RA, Carter WB, Gilson BS. The Sickness Impact Profile: development and final revision of a health status measure. *Med Care* 1981; **19**: 787–805.

Bergner M, Bobbit RA, Pollard WE et al. The Sickness Impact Profile: validation of a health status measure. *Med Care* 1976; **14**: 57–67.

Bianco P, Fisher LW, Young MF et al. Expression and localization of the two small proteoglycans biglycan and decorin in developing human skeletal and non-skeletal tissues. *J Histochem Cytochem* 1990; **38**: 1549–63.

Bianco P, Riminucci M, Silvestrini G et al. Localization of bone sialoprotein (BSP) to Golgi and post-Golgi secretory structures in osteoblasts and to discrete sites in early bone matrix. *J Histochem Cytochem* 1993; **41**: 193–203.

Bidwell JP, Carter WB, Fryer MJ, Heath H III. Parathyroid hormone (PTH)-induced intracellar Ca^{2+} signaling in naive and PTH-desensitized osteoblast-like cells (ROS 17/

2.8): pharmacological characterization and evidence for synchronous oscillation of intracellular Ca^{2+}. *Endocrinology* 1991; **129**: 2993–3000.

Black K, Garrett IR, Mundy GR. Chinese hamster ovarian cells transfected with the murine interleukin-6 gene cause hypercalcemia as well as cachexia, leukocytosis and thrombocytosis in tumor-bearing nude mice. *Endocrinology* 1991; **128**: 2657–9.

Black LJ, Jones CD, Falcone JF. Antagonism of estrogen action with a new benzothiophene derived antiestrogen. *Life Sci* 1983; **32**: 1031–6.

Black DM, Reiss TF, Nevitt MC et al. Design of the fracture intervention trial. *Osteoporosis Int* 1993; **3** (suppl 3): S29–39.

Black LJ, Sato M, Rowley ER et al. Raloxifene (LY139481 HCI) prevents bone loss and reduces serum cholesterol without causing uterine hypertrophy in ovariectomized rats. *J Clin Invest* 1994; **93**: 63–9.

Blair HC, Teitelbaum SL, Ghiselli R, Gluck S. Osteoclastic bone resorption by a polarized vacuolar proton pump. *Science* 1989; **245**: 855–7.

Boonekamp PM, van der Wee-Pals LJA, van Wijk-van Lennep MLL et al. Two modes of action of bisphosphonates on osteoclastic resorption of mineralized matrix. *Bone Mineral* 1986; **1**: 27–39.

Boskey AL, Wians FJ Jr, Hauschka PV. The effect of osteocalcin on in vitro lipid-induced hydroxyapatite formation and seeded hydroxyapatite growth. *Calcif Tiss Int* 1985; **37**: 57–62.

Boyce BF, Aufdemorte TB, Garrett IR. Effects of interleukin-1 on bone turnover in normal mice. *Endocrinology* 1989; **125**: 1142–50.

Canalis E, Centrella M, Bruch W, McCarthy TL. Insulin like growth factor I mediates selective anabolic effects of parathyroid hormone in bone cultures. *J Clin Invest* 1989; **83**: 60–65.

CCOHTA (Canadian Coordinating Office for Health Technology Assessment). *Guidelines for Economic Evaluation of Pharmaceuticals*, 1st edn, 1994; Ottawa: CCOHTA.

Centrella M, Massague J, Canalis E. Human platelet-derived transforming growth factor-B stimulates parameters of bone growth in fetal rat calvariae. *Endocrinology* 1986; **119**: 2306–12.

Centrella M, McCarty TL, Canalis E. Transforming growth factor is a bifunctional regulator of replication and collagen synthesis in osteoblast-enriched cell cultures from fetal rat bone. *J Biol Chem* 1987; **262**: 2869–74.

Centrella M, McCarty TL, Canalis E. Parathyroid hormone modulates transforming growth factor B activity and binding in osteoblast-enriched cell cultures from fetal rat parietal bone. *Proc Natl Acad Sci USA* 1988; **85**: 5889–93.

Chakraborty M, Su Y, Nathanson M et al. The effects of calcitonin in rat osteoclasts and in a kidney cell line (LLC-PK1) are mediated via an inhibition of the Na^+/H^+ antiporter. *J Bone Mineral Res* 1991; **6**: S134.

Chambers TJ. The cellular basis of bone resorption. *Clin Orthoped Rel Res* 1980; **151**: 283–93.

Chambers TJ, Fuller K, Carby JA et al. Monoclonal antibodies against osteoclasts inhibit bone resorption in vitro. *Bone Mineral* 1986; **1**: 127–35.

Chapuy MC, Arlot ME, Duboeuf F et al. Vitamin D3 and calcium to prevent hip fractures in elderly women. *N Engl J Med* 1992; **327**: 1637–42.

Chen TL, Bates RL, Dudley A et al. Bone morphogenetic protein-2b stimulation of growth and osteogenic phenotypes in rat osteoblast-like cells: comparison with TGF-B1. *J Bone Mineral Res* 1991; **6**: 1387–93.

Chenu C, Pfeilschrifter J, Mundy GR, Roodman GD. Transforming growth factor-B inhibits formation of osteoclast-like cells in long-term human marrow cultures. *Proc Natl Acad Sci USA* 1988; **85**: 5683–7.

Chevalley T et al. Effects of calcium supplementation on femoral bone mass density and vertebral fracture rate in vitamin D replete elderly patients with and without a recent hip fracture: a prospective placebo controlled study. *J Bone Mineral Res* 1992; **7** (suppl 1): 322.

Chevalley T, Rizzoli R, Nydegger V et al. Effects of calcium supplements on femoral bone mineral density and vertebral fracture rate in vitamin-D-replete elderly patients. *Osteoporosis Int* 1994; **4**(5): 245–52.

Chiang CP, Nilsen-Hamilton M. Opposite and selective effects of epidermal growth factor and human platelet transforming growth factor-B on the production of secreted proteins by murine 3T3 cells and human fibroblasts. *J Biol Chem* 1986; **261**: 10478–81.

Christiansen C. Postmenopausal bone loss and the risk of osteoporosis. *Osteoporosis Int* 1994; **4** (suppl 1): S47–51.

Commonwealth Department of Human Services and Health. *Guidelines for the Pharmaceutical Industry on Preparation of Submissions to the Pharmaceutical Benefits Advisory Committee* 1995; Canberra, ACT: Australian Government Publishing Service.

Consensus Development Conference. Diagnosis, prophylaxis and treatment of osteoporosis. *Am J Med* 1993; **94**: 646–50.

Cook DJ, Guyatt GH, Adachi JD et al. Quality of life issues in women with vertebral fractures due to osteoporosis. *Arth Rheum* 1993; **36**(6): 750–56.

Cooper C, Campion G, Melton LJ III. Hip fractures in the elderly: a world-wide projection. *Osteoporosis Int* 1992; **2**: 285–9.

Creek KE, Sly WS. The role of the phosphomannosyl receptor in the transport of acid hydrolases to lysosomes. In Dingle JT, Dean RT, Sly WS (eds) *Lysosomes in Biology and Pathology* 1984, pp 63–82; Amsterdam: Elsevier.

Daughaday WH, Hall K, Raben MS et al. Somatomedin: proposed designation for sulfation factor. *Nature* 1972; **235**: 107.

David P, Nguyen H, Barbier A, Baron R. The bisphosphonate tiludronate is a potent inhibitor of the osteoclast vacuolar H^+-ATPase. *J Bone Mineral Res* 1996; **11**: 1498–1507.

Davies J, Warwick J, Totty N et al. The osteoclast functional antigen, implicated in the regulation of bone resorption, is biochemically related to the vitronectin receptor. *J Cell Biol* 1989; **109**: 1817–26.

Dawson-Hughes B et al. A controlled trial of the effect of calcium supplementation on bone density in postmenopausal women. *N Engl J Med* 1990; **323**: 878–83.

Delaisse JM, Vaes G. Mechanism of mineral solubilization and matrix degradation in osteoclastic bone resoprtion. In Rifkin BR, Gay CV (eds) *The Biology and Physiology of the Osteoclast* 1992; Boca Raton, FL: CRC Press.

Delaisse JM, Ledent P, Vaes G. Biology of the osteoclast. In *Biochem J* (ed.) *Cellular and Molecular Biology of Bone* 1991, p 463; New York: Academic Press.

Dempster DW. Bone remodeling. In Riggs LB, Melton J III (eds) *Osteoporosis: Etiology, Diagnosis and Management*, 2nd edn, 1997, pp 67–91; Philadelphia: Lippincott-Raven.

Dempster DW, Cosman F, Parisien M et al. Anabolic actions of parathyroid hormone on bone. *Endocr Rev* 1993; **14**: 690–709.

Devogelaer JP, Broll H, Correa-Rotter R et al. Oral alendronate induces progressive increases in bone mass of the spine, hip and total body over 3 years in postmenopausal women with osteoporosis. *Bone* 1996; **18**(2): 141–50.

Doty SB, Schoefield BH. Electron microscopic localization of hydrolytic enzymes in osteoclasts. *Histochem J* 1972; **4**: 245–58.

Draper MW, Flowers DE, Huster WJ et al. A controlled trial of raloxifene (LY139481) HCI: impact on bone turnover and serum lipid profile in healthy postmenopausal women. *J Bone Mineral Res* 1996; **11**: 835–42.

Eeckhout Y, Vaes G. Further studies on the activation of procollagenase, the latent precursor of bone collagenase. Effects of lysosomal cathepsin B, plasmin and kallikrein, and spontaneous activation. *Biochemistry* 1977; **166**: 21–31.

Endocrinologic and Metabolic Drugs Advisory Board on Alendronate, Dept. of Health and Human Services, Public Health Service, 1995; Bethesda, MD: FDA.

Endocrinologic and Metabolic Drugs Advisory Board on Estraderm, Dept. of Health and Human Services, Public Health Service, December 1985; Bethesda, MD: FDA.

Eriksen EF. Normal and pathological remodeling of human trabecular bone: three-dimensional reconstruction of the remodeling sequence in normals and in metabolic bone disease. *Endocr Rev* 1986; **7**: 379–408.

Eriksen EF, Colvard DS, Berg NJ et al. Evidence of estrogen receptors in normal human osteoblast-like cells. *Science* 1988; **241**: 84–6.

Eriksen EF, Mosekilde L, Melsen F. Effect of sodium fluoride, calcium, phosphate, and vitamin D2 on trabecular bone balance and remodeling in osteoporotics. *Bone* 1985; **6**: 381–9.

European Committee for Proprietary Medicinal Products. *Note for Guidance on Involutional Osteoporosis in Women* (Draft), 1996; London.

EuroQoL Group. EuroQoL—a new facility for the measurement of health-related quality of life. *Health Policy* 1990; **16**: 199–208.

Everitt EA, Sage EH. Expression of SPARC is correlated with distinct morphologies in F9 murine embryonal carcinoma cells. *Exp Cell Res* 1992; **199**: 134–46.

FDA, Division of Drug Marketing, Advertising, and Communications. *Principles for the Review of Pharmacoeconomic Promotion* (draft guidelines), 1995; Bethesda, MD: FDA.

FDA. *Guidelines for Preclinical and Clinical Evaluation of Agents Used in the Prevention and Treatment of Postmenopausal Osteoporosis* (draft) 1994.

FDA. HRT Working Group. Guidance for clinical evaluation of combination estrogen/progestin-containing drug products used for hormone replacement therapy of postmenopausal women. *Menopause* 1995; **2**: 131–6.

Feeny DH, Torrance GW, Furlong WJ. Health Utilities Index. In Spilker B (ed.) *Quality of Life and Pharmacoeconomics in Clinical Trials*, 2nd edn, 1996; Philadelphia, PA: Lippincott-Raven.

Felix R, Cecchini MG, Fleisch H. Macrophage colony stimulating factor restores in vivo bone resorption in the OP/OP osteopetrotic mouse. *Endocrinology* 1990; **127**: 2592–4.

Feyen JH, Elford P, Dipadova FE, Trechsel U. Interleukin-6 is produced by bone and modulated by parathyroid hormone. *J Bone Mineral Res* 1989; **4**: 633–8.

Flanagan AM, Chambers TJ. Dichloromethylenebisphosphonate (CI2MBP) inhibits bone resorption through injury to osteoclasts that resorb CI2MBP-coated bone. *Bone Mineral* 1989; **6**: 33–43.

Fogelman I, Poser JW, Smith ML et al. Alterations in skeletal metabolism following oophorectomy. In Christiansen C, Arnaud CD, Nordin BEC et al (eds) *Osteoporosis: Proceedings of Copenhagen International Symposium on Osteoporosis* 1984, pp 519–21; Glostrup, Denmark: Aalborg Stiffsbogtrykkeri.

Frost HM. Perspectives: the role of changes in mechanical usage set points in the pathogenesis of osteoporosis. *J Bone Mineral Res* 1992; **7**: 253–72.

Funk SE, Sage EH. The Ca2–binding glycoprotein SPARC modulates cell cycle progression in bovine aortic endothelial cells. *Proc Natl Acad Sci USA* 1991; **88**: 2648–52.

Funk SE, Sage EH. Differential effects of SPARC and cationic SPARC peptides on DNA synthesis by endothelial cells and fibroblasts. *J Cell Physiol* 1993; **154**: 53–63.

Gallagher JC, Riggs BL, Jerpbak CM, Arnaud CD. The effect of age on serum immunoreactive parathyroid hormone in normal and osteoporotic women. *J Lab Clin Med* 1980; **95**: 373–85.

Garrett IR, Black KS, Mundy GR. Interactions between interleukin-6 and interleukin-1 in osteoclastic bone resorption in neonatal mouse calvariae. *Calcif Tissue Int* 1990; **46**.

Garrett IR, Boyce BF, Oreffo ROC et al. Oxygen-derived free radicals stimulate osteoclastic bone resorption in rodent bone in vitro and in vivo. *J Clin Invest* 1990; **85**: 632–9.

Gay CV, Mueller WJ. Carbonic anhydrase and osteoclasts: localization by labelled inhibitor autoradiography. *Science* 1974; **183**: 432–4.

Gehron Robey P, Young MF, Fisher LW, McClain TD. Thrombospondin is an osteoblast-derived component of mineralized extracellular matrix. *J Cell Biol* 1989; **108**: 719–27.

Genduso LA, Kotsanos JG. Review of health economic guidelines in the form of regulations, principles, policies, and positions. *Drug Info J* 1996; **30**(4): 1003–16.

Ghosh-Choudry N, Christy B, Harris MA et al. Structure of the mouse bone morphogenetic protein 2 gene and promoter analysis in primary fetal rat calvarial osteoblasts. *J Bone Mineral Res* 1992; **7**.

Girasole G, Jilka RL, Passeri G et al. 17B-Estradiol inhibits interleukin-6 production by bone marrow-derived stromal cells and osteoblasts in vitro: a potential mechanism for the antiosteoporotic effect of estrogens. *J Clin Invest* 1992; **89**: 883–91.

Glimcher MJ. Mechanisms of calcification in bone: role of collagen fibrils and collagen–phosphoprotein complexes in vitro and in vivo. *Anat Rec* 1989; **224**: 139–53.

Glowacki J, Lian J. Impaired recruitment of osteoclast progenitors in deficient osteocalin-depleted bone implants. *Cell Differ* 1987; **21**: 247–54.

Gonnelli S, Cepollaro C, Pondrelli C et al. The usefulness of bone turnover in predicting the response to transdermal estrogen therapy in postmenopausal osteoporosis. *J Bone Mineral Res* 1997; **12**(4): 624–31.

Gowen M, Meikle MC, Reynolds JJ. Stimulation of bone resorption in vitro by a non-prostanoid factor released by human monocytes in culture. *Biochim Biophys Acta* 1983; **762**: 471–4.

Grampp S, Genant HK, Mathur A et al. Comparisons of noninvasive bone mineral measurements in assessing age-related loss, fracture discrimination, and diagnostic classification. *J Bone Mineral Res* 1997; **12**(5): 697–711.

Greendale GA, Silverman, SL, Hays RD et al. Health-related quality of life in osteoporosis clinical trials. *Calcif Tissue Int* 1993; **53**: 75–7.

Grills BL, Gallagher JA, Allan EH et al. Identification of plasminogen activator in osteoclasts. *J Bone Mineral Res* 1990; **5**: 499–505.

Hall TJ, Chambers TJ. Optimal bone resorption by isolated rat osteoclasts requires chloride/bicarbonate exchange. *Calcif Tissue Int* 1989; **45**: 378–80.

Heaney RP. Design considerations for osteoporosis trials. In Goldberg M, Feldman D, Kelsey J (eds) *Osteoporosis* 1996, p 1125; New York: Academic Press.

Heath JK, Rodan SB, Yoon KG, Rodan GA. Rat calvarial cell lines immortalized with SV-40 large T-antigen. Constitutive and retinoic acid-inducible expression of osteoblastic features. *Endocrinology* 1989; **124**: 3060–68.

Heine U, Munoz EF, Flanders KC et al. Role of transforming growth factor-B in the development of the mouse embryo. *J Cell Biol* 1987; **105**: 2861–76.

Hilliard TJ, Meadows G, Kahn AJ. Lysozyme synthesis in osteoclasts. *J Bone Mineral Res* 1990; **5**: 1217–22.

Holtrop ME, Raisz LG. Comparison of the effects of 1,25–dihydroxycalciferol, prostaglandin E2, and osteoclast activating factor with parathyroid hormone on the ultrastructure of osteoclasts in cultured long bones of fetal rats. *Calcif Tissue Int* 1979; **29**: 201–5.

Holtrop ME, Raisz LG, Simmons HA. The effects of parathyroid hormone, colchicine, and calcitonin on the ultrastructure and the activity of osteoclasts in organ culture. *J Cell Biol* 1974; **60**: 346–55.

Horne W, Moya M, Neff L et al. A band 3-related chloride/bicarbonate exchanger is highly expressed at the basolateral membrane of osteoclasts. *J Bone Mineral Res* 1991; **6**: S95.

Horne W, Neff L, Chatterjee D et al. Osteoclasts express high levels of pp60 c-scr in association with intracellular organelles. *J Cell Biol* 1992; **119**: 1003–13.

Horowitz MC, Coleman DL, Flood PM et al. Parathyroid hormone and lipopolysaccharide induce murine osteoblast-like cells to secrete a cytokine indistinguishable from granulocyte-macrophage colony-stimulating factor. *J Clin Invest* 1989; **83**: 149–57.

Hruska KA, Rolnick F, Duncan RL et al. Signal transduction in osteoblasts and osteoclasts. In Noda M (ed.) *Cellular and Molecular Biology of Bone* 1993, pp 413–44; San Diego, CA: Academic Press.

Hughes DE, MacDonald BR, Russell RGG, Gowen M. Inhibition of osteoclast-like cell formation by bisphosphonates in long-term cultures of human bone marrow. *J Clin Invest* 1989; **83**: 1930–35.

Hughes DE, Wright KR, Uy HL et al. Bisphosphonates promote apoptosis in murine osteoclasts in vitro and in vivo. *J Bone Mineral Res* 1995; **10**: 1478–87.

Hughes FJ. Chemotactic effects of BHPZ on osteoclastic and fibroblastic cell lines. *J Dental Res*; **71**: 730.

Hunt SM, McEwen J, McKenna SP. *Measuring Health Status* 1986; London: Croom Helm.

Hunter SJ, Schraer H, Gay CV. Characterization of the cytoskeleton in isolated chick osteoclasts: effects of calcitonin. *J Histochem Cytochem* 1989; **37**: 1529–37.

ICH-M3 *Non-clinical Safety Studies for the conduct of human clinical trials for pharmaceuticals.* International Conference on Harmonization, July 1997; London, ICH Technical Coordination.

ICH-S3B Guidelines for Industry. *Pharmacokinetics: Guidance for repeated dose tissue distribution studies.* International Conference on Harmonization, March 1995; London, ICH Technical Coordination.

Jee WSS, Ke HZ, Li XJ. Long-term anabolic effects of prostaglandin-E2 on tibial diaphyseal bone in male rats. *Bone Mineral* 1991; **15**: 33–55.

Jenkinson C, Fitzpatrick R, Argyle M. The Nottingham Health Profile. An analysis of its sensitivity in differentiating illness groups. *Soc Sci Med* 1988; **27**: 1411–14.

Johansson AG, Lindh E, Ljunghall S. Insulin-like growth factor I stimulates bone turnover in osteoporosis. *Lancet* 1992; **339**: 1619.

Johnell O et al. The apparent incidence of hip fracture in Europe: a study of national register sources. *Osteoporosis Int* 1992; **2**: 298–302.

Jotereau FV, LeDouarin NM. The developmental relationships between osteocytes and osteoclasts. A study using the quail-chick nuclear markers in endochondral ossification. *Dev Biol* 1978; **63**: 253–65.

Joyce ME, Roberts AB, Sporn MB, Bolander ME. Transforming growth factor-B and the initiation of chondrogenesis and osteogenesis in the rat femur. *J Cell Biol* 1990; **110**: 2195–2207.

Juppner H, Abou-Samra A-B, Freeman M et al. A G protein-linked receptor for parathyroid hormone and parathyroid hormone-related peptide. *Science* 1991; **254**: 1024–6.

Kahn AJ, Simmons JJ. Investigation of cell lineage in bone using a chimera of chick and quail embryonic tissue. *Nature* 1975; **258**: 325–7.

Kanis JA, Passmore R. Calcium supplementation of the diet: not justified by present evidence. *Br Med J* 1989; **298**: 137–40, 205–8.

Kanis JA, Pitt F. Epidemiology of osteoporosis. *Bone* 1992; **31** (suppl 1): S7–15.

Kaplan RM, Anderson JP, Ganiats TG. The Quality of Well-Being Scale: rationale for a single quality of life index. In Walker SR, Rosser RM (eds) *Quality of Life Assessment: Key Issues in the 1990s* 1993, pp 65–94; London: Kluwer Academic.

Kaplan RM, Feeny D, Revicki DA. Methods for assessing relative importance in preference based outcome measures. *Qual Life Res* 1993; **2**: 467–75.

Kassem M, Blum W, Risteli L et al. Growth hormone stimulates proliferation and differentiation of normal human osteoblast-like cells in vitro. *Calcif Tissue Int* 1993; **52**: 222–6.

Kassem M, Mosekilde L & Eriksen EF. Effects of fluoride on human bone cells in vitro:

differences in responsiveness between stromal osteoblast precursors and mature osteoblasts. *Eur J Endocrinol* 1994; **130**: 381–6.

Keeting PE, Rifas L, Harris SA et al. Evidence for interleukin-1B production by cultured normal human osteoblast-like cells. *J Bone Mineral Res* 1991; **6**: 827–33.

Kenzora JE, McCarthy RE, Lowell JD, Sledge CB. Hip fracture mortality: relation to age, treatment, preoperative illness, time of surgery, and complications. *Clin Orthoped* 1984; **186**: 45–56.

Key LL, Ries WL, Taylor RG et al. Oxygen-derived free radicals in osteoclasts: The specificity and location of the nitroblue tetrazolium reaction. *Bone* 1990; **11**: 115–19.

Kimmel DB. An evaluation of existing normal iliac trabecular bone volume (Bv/Tv) data. In Takahashi HE (ed.) *Bone Morphometry: The Fifth International Congress on Bone Morphometry* 1990, pp 208–15; Japan: Nishimura.

Klein B, Wijdenese J, Zhang XG et al. Murine anti-interleukin-6 monoclonal antibody therapy for a patient with plasma cell leukemia. *Blood* 1991; **78**: 1198–204.

Kodama H, Yamasaki A, Nose M et al. Congenital osteoclast deficiency in osteopetrotic (op/op) mice is cured by injections of macrophage colony-stimulating factor. *J Exp Med* 1991; **173**: 269–72.

Komm BS, Terpening CM, Benz DJ et al. Estrogen binding, receptor mRNA, and biologic response in osteoblast-like osteosarcoma cells. *Science* 1988; **241**: 81–4.

Kruska KA, Moskowitz D, Esbrit P et al. Stimulation of inositol trisphosphate and diacylglycerol production in renal tubular cells by parathyroid hormone. *J Clin Invest* 1987; **79**: 230–39.

Laiho M, Saksela O, Andreasen PA, Keski-Oja J. Enhanced production and extracellular deposition of the endothelial-type plasminogen activator inhibitos in cultured human lung fibroblasts by transforming growth factor-B. *J Cell Biol* 1986; **103**: 2403–10.

Lane TF, Sage EH. Functional mapping of SPARC: peptides from two distinct Ca^{++}-binding sites modulate cell shape. *J Cell Biol* 1990; **111**: 3065–76.

Langley P, Martin R. *Guidelines for Formulary Submissions* 1996; Rancho Cordova, CA: Integrated Pharmaceutical Services and Foundation Health Corporation.

Lau KH, Farley JR, Freeman TK, Baylink DJ. A proposed mechanism of the mitogenic action of fluoride on bone cells: inhibition of the activity of an osteoblastic acid phosphatase. *Metabolism* 1989; **38**: 858–68.

LeBaron RG, Zimmermann DR, Ruoslahti E. Hyaluronate binding properties of versican. *J Biol Chem* 1992; **267**: 10003–10.

Liberman UA, Weiss SR, Broll J et al. Effect of oral alendronate on bone mineral density and the incidence of fractures in postmenopausal osteoporosis. The Alendronate Phase III Osteoporosis Treatment Study Group. *N Engl J Med* 1995; **333**(22): 1437–43.

Lin HY, Harris TL, Flannery MS et al. Expression cloning of anadenylate cyclase-coupled calcitonin receptor. *Science* 1991; **254**: 1022–4.

Lopez-Casillas F, Wrana JL, Massague J. Betaglycan presents ligand to the TGF-beta signaling receptor. *Cell* 1993; **73**: 1435–44.

Lorenzo JA, Sousa SL, Brink-Webb SE, Korn JH. Production of both interleukin-1a and B by newborn mouse calvarial cultures. *J Bone Mineral Res* 1990; **5**: 77–83.

Lowik CWGM, van der Pluijm G, van der Wee-Pals LJA et al. Migration and phenotypic transformation of osteoclast precursors into mature osteoclasts: the effect of a bisphosphonate. *J Bone Mineral Res* 1988; **3**: 185–92.

Lucas PA, Price PA, Caplan AI. Chemotactic response of mesenchymal cells, fibroblasts and osteoblast-like cells to bone gla protein. *Bone* 1988; **9**: 319–23.

Lucht U. Acid phosphatase of osteoclasts demonstrated by electron microscopic histochemistry. *Histochemie* 1971; **28**: 103–17.

Lydick E, Zimmerman SI, Yawn B et al. Development and validation of a discriminative quality of life questionnaire for osteoporosis (the OPTQoL). *J Bone Mineral Res* 1997; **12**(3): 456–63.

Magaziner J, Simonsick EM, Kashner M et al. Survival experience of aged hip fracture patients. *Amer J Pub Health* 1989; **79**: 274–8.

Majeska RJ, Rodan GA. The effect of 1,25(OH)2D3 on alkaline phosphatase in osteoblastic osteosarcoma cells. *J Biol Chem* 1982; **257**: 3362–5.

Maliakal JC, Hauschka PV, Sampath TK. Recombinant human osteogenic protein (hOp-1) promotes the growth of osteoblasts and stimulates expression of the osteoblast phenotype in culture. *J Bone Mineral Res* 1991; **6**.

Malone JD, Teitelbaum SL, Griffin GL et al. Recruitment of osteoblast precursors by purified bone matrix constituents. *J Cell Biol* 1982; **92**: 227–30.

Marchisio PC, Cirillo D, Teti A et al. Rous sarcoma virus-transformed fibroblasts and cells of monocytic origin display a peculiar dot-like organization of cytoskeletal proteins involved in microfilament-membrane interactions. *Exp Cell Res* 1987; **169**: 202–14.

Marchisio PC, Naldini L, Cirillo D et al. Cell-substratum interaction of cultured avian osteoclasts is mediated by specific adhesion structures. *J Cell Biol* 1984; **99**: 1696–1705.

Marcus R. The nature of osteoporosis. *J Clin Endocrinol Metab* 1996; **81**: 1–5.

Mark MP, Prince CW, Osawa T et al. Immunohistochemical demonstration of a 44-KD phosphoprotein in developing rat bones. *J Histochem Cytochem* 1987; **35**: 707–15.

Martin A, Holmes R, Lydick E. Fears, knowledge, and perceptions of osteoporosis among women. *Drug Info J* 1997; **31**: 301–6.

McKee MD, Farach-Carson MC, Butler WT et al. Ultrastructural immunolocalization of noncollagenous (osteopontin and osteocalcin) and plasma (albumin and alpha2 HS-glycoprotein) proteins in rat bone. *J Bone Mineral Res* 1993; **8**: 485–96.

Melsen F, Mosekilde L, Christensen MS. Interrelationship between bone histomorphometry, S-iPTH and calcium phosphorous metabolism in primary hyperparathyroidism. *Calcif Tissue Res* 1977; **24** (suppl): 16.

Melton LJ III. Epidemiology of fractures. In Riggs BL, Melton LJ III (eds) *Osteoporosis: Etiology, Diagnosis, and Management* 1988, pp 133–54; New York: Raven Press.

Melton LJ III. Differing patterns of osteoporosis across the world. In Chestnut CH III (ed.) *New Dimensions in Osteoporosis in the 1990s* 1991, pp 13–18; Hong Kong: Excerpta Medica Asia.

Melton LJ. How many women have osteoporosis now? *J Bone Mineral Res* 1995; **10**(2): 175–7.

Melton LJ III, Khosla S, Atkinson EJ et al. Relationship of bone turnover to bone density and fractures. *J Bone Mineral Res* 1997; **12**(7): 1083–91.

Merry K, Dodds R, Littlewood A, Gowen M. Expression of osteopontin mRNA by osteoclasts and osteoblasts in modelling adult human bone. *J Cell Sci* 1993; **104**: 1013–20.

Meunier PJ, Sellami S, Briancon D, Edouard C. Histological heterogeneity of apparently idiopathic osteoporosis. In DeLuca HF, Frost HM, Jee WSS et al (eds) *Osteoporosis: Recent Advances in Pathogenesis and Treatment* 1981, pp 293–301; Baltimore: University Park Press.

Miller SC. Rapid activation of the medullary bone osteoclast cell surface by parathyroid hormone. *J Cell Biol* 1978; **76**: 615–18.

Miller SC, Bowman BM, Smith JM. Characterization of endosteal bone-lining cells from fatty marrow bone sites in adult beagles. *Anat Rec* 1980; **198**: 163–73.

Miyauchi A, Alvarez J, Greenfield E et al. Matrix protein binding to the osteoclast adhesion integrin mediates a reduction in Ca. *J Bone Mineral Res* 1991; **6**: S96.

Mundy GR, Poser JW. Chemotactic activity of the gamma-carboxyglutamic acid containing protein in bone. *Calcif Tissue Int* 1983; **35**: 164–8.

Nagata T, Todescan R, Goldberg HA et al. Sulfation of secreted phosphoprotein I (SPP1, osteopontin) is associated with mineralized tissue formation. *Biochem Biophys Res Commun* 1989; **165**: 234–40.

National Osteoporosis Foundation. Assessing vertebral fractures. A Report by the NOF Working Group. *J Bone Mineral Res* 1995; 10–58.

Neff L, Horne W, Male P et al. A cyclic RGD peptide induces a wave of tyrosine phosphorylation and the translocation of a c-src substrate (p85) in isolated rat osteoclasts. *J Bone Mineral Res* 1992; **7**: S106 (abstract).

Nelson RD, Guo X-L, Masood K et al. Selectively amplified expression of an isoform of the vacuolar H$^+$ATPase 56-kDa subunit in renal intercalated cells. *Proc Natl Acad Sci USA* 1992; **89**: 3541–5.

Ng KW, Gummer PR, Michelangeli VP et al. Regulation of alkaline phosphatase expression in a neonatal and rat calvarial cell strain by retinoic acid. *J Bone Mineral Res* 1988; **3**: 53–61.

Nijweide PJ, Burger EH, Feyen JH. Proliferation, differentiation and hormonal regulation. *Physiol Rev* 1986; **66**: 855–86.

Oldberg A, Franzen A, Heinegard D. Cloning and sequence analysis of rat bone sialoprotein (osteopontin) cDNA reveals an Arg-Gly-Asp cell binding sequence. *Proc Natl Acad Sci USA* 1986; **83**: 8819–23.

Oreffo RO, Mundy GR, Seyedin SM, Bonewald LF. Activation of the bone-derived latent TGF-B complex by isolated osteoblasts. *Biochem Biophys Res Commun* 1989; **158**: 817–23.

Oursler MJ, Osdoby P, Pyfferoen J et al. Avian osteoclasts as estrogen target cells. *Proc Natl Acad Sci USA* 1991; **88**: 6613–17.

Oursler MJ, Pederson L, Fitzpatrick L et al. Human giant cell tumors of the bone (osteoclastomas) are estrogen target cells. *Proc Natl Acad Sci USA* 1994; **91**: 5227–31.

Overall CM, Wrana JL, Sodek J. Independent regulation of collagenase, 72 kDa-progelatinase, and metalloendoproteinase inhibitor (TIMP) expression in human fibroblasts by transforming growth factor-B. *J Biol Chem* 1989; **264**: 1860–69.

Overgaard K, Hansen MA, Jensen SB et al. Effect of salcatonin given intranasally on bone mass and fracture rates in established osteoporosis: a dose–response study. *Br Med J* 1992; **305**: 556–61.

Pacifici R, Rifas L, McCracken R et al. Ovarian steroid treatment blocks a postmenopausal increase in blood monocyte interleukin-1 release. *Proc Natl Acad Sci USA* 1989; **86**: 2398–2402.

Pacifici R, Rifas L, Teitelbaum S et al. Spontaneous release of interleukin-1 from human blood monocytes reflects bone formation in idiopathic osteoporosis. *Proc Natl Acad Sci USA* 1987; **84**: 4616–20.

Parfitt AM. Use of bisphosphonates in the prevention of bone loss and fractures. *Am J Med* 1991; **91**: 42S.

Parfitt AM. The physiologic and pathogenetic significance of bone histomorphometric data. In Coe FL, Favus MJ (eds) *Disorders of Bone and Mineral Metabolism* 1992, pp 475–89; New York: Raven.

Parfitt AM, Drezner MK, Glorieux FH et al. Bone histomorphometry: standardization of nomenclature, symbols, and units. *J Bone Mineral Res* 1987; **2**: 595–610.

Parfitt AM, Mundy GR, Roodman GD et al. A new model for the regulation of bone resorption, with particular reference to the effects of bisphosphonates. *J Bone Mineral Res* 1996; **11**: 150–59.

Pfeilschifter J, Seyedin SM, Mundy GR. In vivo effects of human recombinant transforming growth factor-B on bone resorption in fetal rat long bone cultures. *J Clin Invest* 1988; **82**: 680–85.

Poli V, Balena R, Fattori E et al. Interleukin-6 deficient mice are protected from bone loss caused by estrogen depletion. *EMBO J* 1994; **13**: 1189–96.

Praemer A, Furner S, Rice DP. *Musculoskeletal Conditions in the United States* 1992; Park Ridge, IL: American Academy of Orthopedic Surgeons.

Puopolo K, Kumamoto C, Adachi I et al. Differential expression of the 'B' subunit of the vacuolar H$^+$-ATPase in bovine tissues. *J Biol Chem* 1992; **267**: 3696–3706.

Ray NF, Chan JK, Thamer M, Melton LJ III. Medical expenditures for the treatment of osteoporotic fractures in the United States in 1995: report from the National Osteoporosis Foundation. *J Bone and Min Res* 1997; **12**(1).

Recommendations for the registration of new chemical entities used in the prevention and treatment of osteoporosis. *Calcif Tissue Int* 1995; **57**: 247–50.

Reid IR, Ams RW, Evans MC et al. Effect of calcium supplementation on bone loss in postmenopausal women. *N Engl J Med* 1993; **328**: 460–64.

Reinholt FP, Hultenby K, Oldberg A, Heinegard D. Osteopontin—a possible anchor of osteoclasts to bone. *Proc Natl Acad Sci USA* 1990; **87**: 4473–5.

Revicki DA. Health-related quality of life in the evaluation of medical therapy for chronic illness. *J Fam Pract* 1989; **29**(4): 377–80.

Reinholt FP, Mengarelli-Wildhom S, Ek-Rylander B, Andersson G. Ultrastructural localization of a tartrate-resistant acid ATPase in bone. *J Bone Mineral Res* 1990; **5**: 1055.

Roberts AB, Anzano MA, Lamb LC et al. New class of transforming growth factors potentiated by epidermal growth factor. *Proc Natl Acad Sci USA* 1981; **78**: 5339–43.

Rogers MJ, Chilton KM, Coxon FP et al. Bisphosphonates induce apoptosis in mouse macrophage-like cells in vitro by a nitric oxide-independent mechanism. *J Bone Mineral Res* 1996; **11**: 1482–91.

Ross, Davis JW, Epstein R, Wasnich RD. Pre-existing fractures and bone mass predict vertebral fracture incidence in women. *Ann Intern Med* 1991; **114**: 919–23.

Ross PD, Davis JW, Vogel JM, Wasnich RD. A critical review of bone mass and the risk of fractures in osteoporosis. *Calcif Tissue Int* 1990; **46**: 149–61.

Rowe DJ, Hausmann E. The alteration in osteoclast morphology by diphosphonates in bone organ culture. *Calcif Tissue Res* 1976; **20**: 53–60.

Rowe DJ, Hausmann E. The effects of calcitonin and colchicine on the cellular response to diphosphonate. *Br J Exp Path* 1980; **61**: 303–9.

Rowe DJ, Hays SJ. Inhibition of bone resorption by difluoromethylene diphosphonate in organ culture. *Metab Bone Dis Rel Res* 1983; **5**: 13–16.

Sage EH, Bornstein P. Extracellular proteins that modulate cell–matrix interactions: SPARC, tenascin, and thrombospondin. *J Biol Chem* 1991; **266**: 14831–4.

Sauer P, Leidig G, Minne HW et al. Spine deformity index (SDI) versus other objective procedures of vertebral fracture identification in patients with osteoporosis: a comparative study. *J Bone Med* 1991; **6**(3): 227–38.

Schenk R, Spiro D, Wiener J. Cartilage resorption in tabial epiphyseal plate of growing rats. *J Cell Biol* 1967; **34**: 275–91.

Scheven BAA, Visser JWM, Nijweide PJ. In vitro osteoclast generation from different bone marrow fractions, including a highly enriched haematopoietic stem cell population. *Nature* 1986; **321**: 79–81.

Schneider EL, Guralnik JM. The aging of America. Impact on health care costs. *J Am Med Assn* 1990; **263**: 2335–40.

Seeley DG, Browner WS, Nevitt MC et al. Which fractures are associated with low appendicular bone mass in elderly women? *Ann Intern Med* 1991; **115**: 837–42.

Seeman E. Advances in the study of osteoporosis in men. In Papapoulos SE et al (eds) *Osteoporosis* 1996, pp 341–58; Amsterdam: Elsevier Science.

Shiraga H, Min W, VanDuen WJ et al. Inhibition of calcium oxalate crystal growth in vitro by uropontin: another member of the aspartic acid-rich protein superfamily. *Proc Natl Acad Sci USA* 1992; **89**: 426–30.

Simonet WS, Lacey DL, Dunstan CR et al. Osteoprotegerin: A novel secreted protein involved in the regulation of bone density. *Cell* 1997; **89**: 309–19.

Skjodt H, Russell G. Bone cell biology and the regulation of bone turnover. In Gowen M (ed.) *Cytokines and Bone Metabolism* 1992, pp 1–70; Boca Raton, FL: CRC Press.

Sly WS, Hewett-Emmett D, Whyte MP et al. Carbonic anhydrase II deficiency identified as the primary defect in the autosomal recessive syndrome of osteopetrosis with renal tubular acidosis and cerebral calcification. *Proc Natl Acad Sci USA* 1983; **80**: 2752–6.

Soriano P, Montgomery C, Geske R, Bradley A. Targeted disruption of the c-src proto-oncogene leads to osteopetrosis in mice. *Cell* 1991; **64**: 693–702.

Sporn MB, Roberts AB, Shull AB et al. Polypeptide transforming growth factor isolated from bovine sources and used for wound healing in vivo. *Science* 1983; **219**: 1329–31.

Steiniche T, Hasling C, Charles P et al. A randomized study on the effects of ostrogen/gestagen or high dose oral calcium on trabecular bone remodeling in postmenopausal osteoporosis. *Bone* 1989; **10**: 313–20.

Storm T, Thamsborg G, Steiniche T et al. Effect of intermittent cyclical etidronate therapy on bone mass and fracture rate in women with postmenopausal osteoporosis. *N Engl J Med* 1990; **322**: 1265–71.

Summary of draft Japanese guidelines for the evaluation of agents for treating osteoporosis. *Ed Semin Rec* 1995; **11**(11–12): 14–18.

Termine JD, Belcourt AB, Conn KM, Kleinman HK. Mineral and collagen-binding proteins of fetal calf bone. *J Biol Chem* 1981; **256**: 10403–8.

Termine JD, Kleinman HK, Whitson SW et al. Osteonectin, a bone-specific protein linking mineral to collagen. *Cell* 1981b; **26**: 99–105.

Teti A, Blair HC, Teitelbaum SL et al. Cytoplasmic pH regulation and chloride bicarbonate exchange in avian osteoclasts. *J Clin Invest* 1989; **84**: 227–33.

Teti A, Marchisio PC, Zambonin-Zallone A. Clear zone in osteoclast function: role of podosomes in regulation of bone-resorbing activity. *Am J Physiol* 1991; **261**: C1–7.

Torrance GW, Furlong W, Feeny D, Boyle M. Multi-attribute preference functions: Health Utilities Index. *PharmacoEconomics* 1995; **7**(6): 503–20.

Udagawa N, Takahashi N, Akatsu T et al. Origin of osteoclasts: mature monocytes and macrophages are capable of differentiating into osteoclasts under a suitable micro-environment prepared by bone marrow-derived stromal cells. *Proc Natl Acad Sci USA* 1990; **87**: 7260–64.

US Congress, Office of Technology Assessment. *Hip Fracture Outcomes in People Age 50 and Over—Background Paper* 1994; OTA-BP-H-120, Washington, DC: US Government Printing Office.

Vaananen HK, Karhukorpi EK, Sundquist K et al. Evidence for the presence of a proton pump of the vacuolar H^+-ATPase type in the ruffled border of osteoclasts. *J Cell Biol* 1990; **111**: 1305–11.

Vogel KG, Trotter JA. The effect of proteoglycans on the morphology of collagen fibrils formed in vitro. *Collagen Rel Res* 1987; **7**: 105–14.

Wang EA, Rosen V, D'Alessandro JS et al. Recombinant human bone morphogenetic protein induces bone formation. *Proc Natl Acad Sci USA* 1990; **87**: 2220–4.

Ware JE, Snow KK, Kosinski M, Gandek B. *SF-36 Health Survey Manual and Interpretation Guide* 1993; Boston: New England Medical Center, The Health Institute.

Watts NB, Harris St, Genant HK et al. Intermitten cyclical etidronate treatment of postmenopausal osteoporosis. *N Engl J. Med* 1990; **323**(2): 73–9.

Weinreb M, Shinar D, Rodan GA. Different pattern of alkaline phosphatase, osteopontin and osteocalcin in developing rat bone visualized by in situ hybridization. *J Bone Mineral Res* 1990; **5**: 831–42.

Wergedal JE, Mohan S, Lundy M, Baylink DJ. Skeletal growth factors and other growth factors known to be present in matrix stimulate proliferation and protein synthesis in human bone cells. *J Bone Mineral Res* 1990; **5**: 179–86.

WHO (World Health Organization). *Assessment of Fracture Risk and Its Application to Screening for*

Postmenopausal Osteoporosis, 1994, pp 3–63; WHO Technical Report Series #843. Geneva: WHO.

Whyte MP. Alkaline phosphatase: physiological role explored in hypophosphatasia. In Peck WA (ed.) *Bone and Mineral Research* 1989, pp 175–218; New York: Elsevier.

Wuthier RE, Register TC. Role of alkaline phosphatase, a polyfunctional enzyme, in mineralizing tissues. In Butler WT (ed.) *The Chemistry and Biology of Mineralized Tissues* 1985, pp 113–24; Birmingham, AL: Ebsco Media.

Yamaguchi A, Kahn AJ. Clonal osteogenic cell lines express myogenic and adipocytic developmental potential. *Calcif Tissue Int* 1991; **49**: 221–5.

Yeh CK, Rodan GA. Tensile forces enhance prostaglandin E synthesis in osteoblastic cells grown on collagen ribbons. *Calcif Tissue Int* 1984; **36**: S67–71.

Yoshida H, Hayashi SI, Kunisada T et al. The murine mutation osteopetrosis is in the coding region of the macrophage colony stimulating factor gene. *Nature* (London) 1990; **345**: 442–4.

Zambonin-Zallone A, Teti A, Grano M et al. Immunocytochemical distribution of extra-cellular matrix receptors in human osteoclasts: a B3 integrin is colocalized with vinculin and talin in the podosomes of osteoclastoma giant cells. *Exp Cell Res* 1989; **182**: 645–52.

14

Breast Cancer

Eleni Diamandidou[1], Aman U. Buzdar[1] and Paul Pluorde[2]

[1]University of Texas, Houston, TX, and [2]Zeneca Pharmaceuticals Group, Wilmington, DE, USA

INTRODUCTION

The development of breast cancer involves a complex interaction of susceptibility factors, both inherited and acquired, as well as endogenous and exogenous factors. The best way to control breast cancer is to find ways to prevent it, which involves understanding its etiology, various risk factors and natural history, and establishing effective screening programs.

EPIDEMIOLOGY

Women in North America and northern European countries have the highest risk of breast cancer, women in southern European and Latin American countries are at intermediate risk, and women in African and Asian countries have the lowest risk. However, rapid increases in incidence rates—mostly among women younger than 50 years—have been noted in recent years in many Asian, central European and South American countries. If the increases in incidence rates in these previously low-risk countries continue, the annual worldwide incidence of breast cancer will be more than 1 000 000 cases per year by 2000 (Miller & Bulbrook, 1986). This year, for the first time, the estimates of new cancer cases in the USA are based on computations using a quadratic function with an autoregressive model, which was found to be better for cancer statistics (Miller et al, 1994). The estimated number of new breast cancer cases for 1995 in the USA was 182 000 with 46 000 deaths expected from breast cancer.

The probability of developing breast cancer is 1 in 217 from birth to 39 years of age, 1 in 26 from 40 to 59 years and 1 in 15 from 60 to 79 years. The cumulative probability of developing breast cancer from birth to death is 1 in 8. Reported deaths from breast cancer in 1991 were 660 for ages 15–34, increasing to 9188 for ages 35–54 and 19 900 for ages 55–74; deaths dropped to 13 834 for ages 75

Drug Development for Women. Edited by V.V. Ragavan. © 1998 John Wiley & Sons Ltd.

years and older. The lifetime risk of dying of breast cancer is 1 in 30. Fifty-five percent of all breast cancer cases are localized at diagnosis; 35% present with regional metastasis and 6% with distant metastasis (National Center for Health Statistics, 1994). The 5 year survival rate for the years 1983–1990 was 82% for all stages, 95% for localized disease, 75% for regional metastasis, and 19% for distant metastasis. In comparison, the 5 year survival rate for all stages for 1960–1963 was 63%, for 1970–1973 68%, for 1974–1976 75%, for 1980–1982 77%, and for 1983–1990 82% (National Center for Health Statistics, 1994).

From 1973 to 1990, incidence rates rose approximately 21%, with rates leveling off in recent years. The majority of this increase (60%) has been attributed to increased screening with early detection of prevalent cases, but an underlying true increase of about 1% per year is estimated based on Connecticut incidence rates (Feuer et al, 1993). The breast cancer increase has been confined mainly to early stage disease (Miller, Feuer & Hankey, 1993). The incidence of larger tumors and those with regional or distant metastases at diagnosis has not changed (Hankey et al, 1993). This trend might ultimately lead to declining breast cancer mortality, although mortality trends can be expected to lag behind incidence variations (Tarone & Chu, 1992). The rise in breast cancer incidence without an increase in mortality could be the result of improved survival due to detection of more cases of early stage disease detected by screening and/or effect of systemic adjuvant therapies (Tarone & Chu, 1992).

Changes in other factors, including certain reproductive variables, diet, alcohol consumption and long-term use of estrogen in menopausal patients, also may have contributed to the rise in breast cancer incidence (Kelsey, 1993). The majority of newly diagnosed cases of breast cancer are estrogen receptor-positive (ER+) tumors, particularly those among older women, suggesting that some of the changes are related to hormonal factors (Glass & Hoover, 1990). Although the increase in the incidence of breast cancer cases is largely the result of early diagnosis by mammography, there has been a true small increase in ER+ tumors, especially among postmenopausal women. Also there has been no change in the incidence of advanced disease, which indicates that no major decline in mortality rates should be expected in the near future.

RISK FACTORS

Various risk factors for developing BC have been recognized over the years. Rates of breast cancer vary more than fivefold among countries (Armstrong & Doll, 1975) and over time within countries (Prentice & Sheppard, 1990), and the rates of breast cancer increase among populations migrating from countries with low incidence to those with high incidence increase (Buell, 1973). These findings suggest that there are potentially modifiable, non-genetic, environmental risk factors for breast cancer.

Diet

Diet has been prominent among hypothesized environmental factors, but after several decades of study, few if any dietary constituents can be confidently associated with an increase or decrease in the risk of breast cancer.

Fat

The dominant diet–breast cancer hypothesis has been that high fat intake increases breast risk. Increased risk of breast cancer with increased fat consumption was first demonstrated in animals by Tannenbaum (1942). Subsequent animal studies showed that this effect occurs with both saturated and unsaturated fats (Carroll, 1986). Albanes (1987), in a meta-analysis of diet and mammary cancer experiments in mice, observed a strong positive association with total energy intake, while fat composition was weakly inversely associated with mammary tumor incidence. However, the relevance of rodent models to human experience has been questioned.

A number of case-control studies of diet and breast cancer in humans have been reported, with varying results. The largest study so far is that of Graham et al (1982), who reported no increased risk of breast cancer in association with fat intake. Goodwin & Boyd (1987) reviewed the published results from 14 case-control studies and concluded that the results are inconsistent with respect to an association between fat intake and breast cancer risk. Two cohort studies conducted in Japan (Hirayama, 1978, 1979) showed positive associations between markers of fat intake, such as meat in the diet, and risk of breast cancer, whereas three cohort studies in the USA failed to find an association of breast cancer either with markers of fat intake or with fat intake itself (Willet et al, 1987). Howe et al (1990), in a meta-analysis of 12 small case-control studies, reported a significant positive association of breast cancer incidence with both total fat intake and saturated fat intake. The relative risk was stronger for postmenopausal women. However, a prospective American Nurse Health Study (Willet et al, 1992) reported no evidence of any association of breast cancer with total fat, saturated fat, linoleic acid or cholesterol.

Almost all case-control and cohort studies have focused on the influence of current diet on fairly short-term (up to 10 years) breast cancer risk in adults. It remains possible that dietary fat intake during childhood and adolescence affects breast cancer risk decades later, and the hypothesis that diet and energy intake during early life are associated with breast cancer risk is interesting but unproven.

Randomized trials of fat reduction have been proposed to resolve the uncertainty about the association between dietary fat and breast cancer. The Women's Health Initiative sponsored by the US National Institutes of Health has commenced with the goal of enrolling and randomizing thousands of women, half of whom will be trained to reduce their total fat intake to 20% of calories.

Fiber

It has been hypothesized that diets high in fiber may be protective against breast cancer, most likely because fiber may reduce the intestinal reabsorption of estrogen excreted via the biliary system. Howe et al (1990) reported a statistically significant relative risk (RR) of 0.85 for a 20 g/day increase in dietary fiber, and Rohan et al (1993) observed a marginally significant inverse association between dietary fiber and breast cancer risk. Two other studies (Graham et al, 1992; Willet et al, 1992) observed no protective effect for fibers. Although there are few data on fruit or vegetable intake and risk of breast cancer, there is some support for an inverse association of breast cancer risk with these dietary components (La Vecchia et al, 1987).

Vitamins and Minerals

Most of the human studies of vitamin A intake and breast cancer have been case-control studies. Of the four studies that reported data for total vitamin A intake (retinol and carotenoids with vitamin A activity), all reported a protective association. Graham et al (1982) reported a significantly reduced risk of breast cancer with increased vitamin A consumption. In a meta-analysis of nine other case-control studies, Howe et al (1990) reported a significant increased association between total vitamin A intake and breast cancer. In a recent large prospective study (Hunter et al, 1993), a small inverse association between vitamin A consumption and the incidence of breast cancer during 8 years of follow-up was reported; however, consumption of vitamin A supplements was not associated with a reduced risk except among women in the lowest quintile group for vitamin A intake from food.

Relatively few studies have reported on the association between dietary vitamin E intake and breast cancer (Hunter & Willet, 1993). None of the three published prospective studies reported a significant inverse association. The Nurses' Health Study (Hunter et al, 1993), the largest study done, showed no evidence of a protective effect from consumption of vitamin E supplements. Vitamin E is sometimes recommended for the treatment of benign breast disease (Abrams, 1965).

Vitamin C has been postulated to decrease the risk of cancer in general (Cameron, Pauling & Liebovitz, 1979) and breast cancer in particular (Howe et al, 1990). Of three prospective studies reporting on the relationship between vitamin C and breast cancer risk (Hunter et al, 1993), only the study by Graham et al (1992) observed a non-significant inverse association. The available prospective data do not support the hypothesis of an inverse association.

Selenium has been claimed to have chemoprotective properties (Thompson, Herbst & Meeker, 1986). Results of the first case-control studies pointed to decreased selenium levels in the serum of women with breast cancer (Stamberger et al, 1973). Meyer & Verreault (1987) observed a positive association between erythrocyte selenium level and breast cancer risk. However, Hunter et al (1990), in their 4-year follow-up study, did not find any association between selenium and breast cancer risk. A study from Finland (Knekt et al, 1989) showed evidence of an increased risk of breast cancer with low levels of selenium, but in a recent study by van Noord et al (1993), selenium was not found to have any role in preventing breast cancer.

Alcohol

The results of epidemiologic studies of the association between alcohol consumption and risk of breast cancer have been inconsistent. The association between alcohol intake and risk of breast cancer was examined among participants in the Canadian National Breast Screening Study (Friedenreich et al, 1993). Among women who were premenopausal, the risk of breast cancer increased with increasing alcohol intake; there was a RR of 1.88 for women consuming more than 30 g/day compared with non-drinkers. No increased risk with alcohol consumption was observed among women who were postmenopausal. A meta-analysis based on four cohort studies and 12 case-control studies demonstrated a dose-dependent increase in breast cancer risk with increased alcohol consumption (Longhecker et al, 1988). However, a combined analysis of six previously published case-control studies of diet and breast cancer found no increase in risk at moderate levels of alcohol intake, but daily consumption of 40 g or more of alcohol was associated with a significantly elevated risk of breast cancer (Howe et al, 1991). In a population-based, case-control study conducted in Spain (Martin-Moreno et al, 1993), a modest but significantly increased risk of breast cancer with alcohol consumption was observed. Recently, Rosenberg et al, in a review article, concluded that the observed associations between alcohol and breast cancer have been weak and inconsistent (Rosenberg, Metzger & Palmer, 1993).

Caffeine

Caffeine consumption does not appear to be related to breast cancer risk (Jacobsen et al, 1986). A cohort study of 34 388 Iowa women did not find any association between breast cancer and caffeine intake (Folsom et al, 1993). In a case-control study, no association was found between regular vs. decaffeinated coffee and risk of breast cancer (Martin-Moreno et al, 1993). A possibly adverse effect of caffeine intake on fibrocystic breast disease (Marshall, Graham & Swanson, 1982) has not been entirely ruled out.

Cigarette Smoking

Evidence for a protective effect of cigarette smoking—possibly mediated through smoking-related changes in estrogen metabolism and age at menopause—has been contradictory and inconclusive (Baron et al, 1987; O'Connell et al, 1987). Palmer and Rosenberg (1993), in a review of all published epidemiologic studies of cigarette smoking and risk of breast cancer found either no association or a very small positive association (decreased breast cancer risk), for ever smoking, current smoking, or heavy smoking. Most of the studies did not provide any data on the age of smoking initiation or identify any relationship between age and smoking-related risk of breast cancer (Palmer & Rosenberg, 1993).

Body Size: Height and Obesity

The relationship between height and breast cancer has been extensively studied. In a follow-up study of 7259 postmenopausal women in The Netherlands (de Waard & Baanders van Halewijn, 1974), the observed risk of breast cancer was increased more than twofold for a 15 cm difference in height; similar results have been reported in the NHANES I study (Swanson et al, 1988). The Nurses' Health Study (London et al, 1989) showed a significant positive association between height and breast cancer risk for postmenopausal women but not for premenopausal women. In several large cohort studies conducted in Scandinavia, a significant association was found between height and breast cancer risk (Hunter & Willet, 1993).

The association between obesity and breast cancer has been examined in numerous studies. Available data suggest an interaction between obesity and menopausal status (Hunter & Willet, 1993). The prospective data, so far, support the possibility of an inverse association between obesity and breast cancer risk for premenopausal women. The Nurses' Health Study (London et al, 1989) reported an inverse association between weight at age 18 and risk of breast cancer in premenopausal women, but no association was found for postmenopausal women. On the other hand, Willet et al (1985) reported that in postmenopausal women, obesity has a weak but clinically unimportant positive association with the incidence of breast cancer but has a stronger association with mortality from breast cancer, due in part to delayed diagnosis among obese women.

Exercise and Breast Cancer

Women who are physically active at an early age may have a reduced risk of breast cancer: this needs to be evaluated. Evidence indicates that even moderate physical activity at an early age decreases the frequency of ovulatory menstrual cycles (Bernstein, Ross & Lobo, 1987) and that moderate physical activity in young adults depresses luteal progesterone levels (Ellison & Lager, 1986). The changes could theoretically lead to a reduction in breast cancer risk.

Chemicals

Chemicals have long been suspected to play a prominent role in the risk of breast cancer. The possibility that organochlorine residues may be related to breast cancer arises from several studies. Both DDT and polychlorinated biphenyls (PCBs) have been shown to be tumor promoters and to have estrogenic activity (IARC, 1991; Silberhorn, Glanert & Robertson, 1990). However, environmental exposure to PCBs has not been associated with an increased breast cancer risk (Kamrin & Fischer, 1991). Kreiger et al (1994) found organochlorine levels to be significantly higher among Black and Asian women compared with White women; however, no association has been found between serum levels of DDT and PCBs and the risk of developing breast cancer. It has been suggested that the high breast cancer mortality among premenopausal Israeli women prior to 1976, which was followed by a significant reduction in mortality after 1976, may have been related to high pesticide levels in milk prior to 1978 (Westin & Richter, 1990). The concentration of aromatic hydrocarbons in mammary adipose tissue has been hypothesized to play a role in breast carcinogenesis (Morris & Seifter, 1992). Wolff et al (1993) found elevated levels of serum DDE, the primary metabolite of DDT, and PCBs in newly diagnosed patients with breast cancer, compared with control subjects. DDE exhibited a dose–response relationship with the risk of breast cancer; the relationship between PCBs and breast cancer suggested a possible threshold effect.

Radiation

It is known that relatively high doses of ionizing radiation can cause breast cancer. Extensive follow-up of radiation-exposed populations has shown that breast tissue is very sensitive to the effects of radiation (National Research Council, 1990). The effects of radiation are greatly dependent on the age at exposure. It was traditionally believed that the susceptibility of the breast to the carcinogenic effects of radiation was maximal between ages 10 and 20 years, when breast tissue is rapidly developing, and decreased after age 30, with little or no risk before age 10 or after 40 (Land et al, 1980; Boice et al, 1979). However, two groups of investigators have reported excess breast cancer risks among women who were younger than 10 years at the time of exposure. In one study, women treated with radiation in infancy for enlarged thymus glands had a threefold increased risk of breast cancer (Hildreth, Shore & Dvortskey, 1989). It is still not known whether in utero radiation exposure increases breast cancer risk (Yoshimoto, Kato & Schull, 1988).

Most (Storm et al, 1992) but not all (Hankey et al, 1983) studies of women with primary breast cancer found no increased risk of cancer of the contralateral breast among those treated with radiation.

Few data are available on the risk of breast cancer from very low radiation doses from occupational (Stebbings, Lucas & Stehney, 1984) and medical diagnostic exposure; however, most suggest that diagnostic radiography has a small effect on the occurrence of breast cancer (Evans, Wennberg & McNeil, 1986). No studies are available for evaluation of the potential risk of breast cancer associated with radiation exposure from mammography.

Endogenous Hormonal Factors

Nulliparity, early age at menarche, late age at menopause, and late age at first full-term pregnancy have been known for many years to be associated with an increased risk of breast cancer. Recently, it has been suggested that other hormonal variables, including multiparity, age at births other than first, and breast feeding, may also affect breast cancer risk.

Menarche

Early menarche is a well-established but weak risk factor for breast cancer (Kampert, Whittemore & Paffenbarger, 1988). The relative risk of developing breast cancer is 1.2 for women in whom menarche occurred before the age of 12 years, compared with those in whom it occurred at the age of at least 14 (Howard, 1987). This may account for the differences seen between countries for breast cancer risk; in China, the average age at menarche is 17 years (Chen et al, 1990) as compared with 12.8 years in the USA (Wyshak & Frisch, 1982).

Pregnancy

Nulliparity and late age at first birth both increase the lifetime incidence of breast cancer (White, 1987; MacMahon et al, 1970). The risk of breast cancer among women who have their first child after the age of 30 years is about twice as high as that among those who have their first child before the age of 20, and those who have their first child after the age of 35 have a slightly higher risk than nulliparous women (MacMahon et al, 1970).

The hormonal changes associated with pregnancy have little, if any, influence on the prognosis of breast cancer in patients diagnosed with early stage, operable breast cancer. A recent study (Schoultz et al, 1995) showed that the relative hazard for women who became pregnant after diagnosis of breast cancer compared with women without a subsequent pregnancy was 0.48, which suggests a possible decreased risk of distant dissemination. In a review of 109 patients, Clark & Reid (1978) reported an improved survival rate in women with breast cancer and a subsequent pregnancy. Other studies on pregnancy following primary breast cancer therapy have shown similar results (Peters, 1968; Rissanen, 1968; Ariel & Kempner, 1989; Harvey et al, 1981; Sutton, Buzdar & Hortobagyi, 1990).

Breast-feeding

A recent study (UK National Case Control Study Group, 1993) examined the association between duration of breast-feeding and risk of breast cancer. The investigators reported a decreased risk of breast cancer with increasing duration of breast-feeding, but hormonal suppression of lactation was not related to the risk of breast cancer. Review of several studies (Byers et al, 1985) also suggested that breast-feeding may reduce breast cancer risk among women younger than 50 years. However, some other case-control and cohort studies have reported little or no association, between breast-feeding and breast cancer risk (Brignone et al, 1987; Kvale & Heuch, 1987).

Menopause

The older a woman's age at menopause, the higher her risk of breast cancer; for every 5 years of difference in age at menopause, the risk of breast cancer increases by about 17% (Hsieh et al, 1990). This elevation in risk may be due to existing tumors having an increased growth rate at the time of menopause. Bilateral oophorectomy before age 40 is associated with a lifetime decrease in risk of breast cancer of about 50% compared with natural menopause (Brinton et al, 1988; Irwin et al, 1988). The increased risks associated with early age at menarche and late age at menopause suggest that the longer the exposure to sex hormones during the reproductive years, the higher the risk of breast cancer (Henderson et al, 1985).

Abortion

Parazzini, La Vecchia & Negri (1991) and Remennick (1990) reviewed most of the studies addressing whether spontaneous or induced abortion increase the risk of breast cancer. Most of the studies were inconclusive and controversial; it is difficult to reach definitive conclusions from these studies because of the inconsistency of the results and data.

Menstrual Cycle Characteristics

Several studies have addressed the issue of whether certain characteristics of the menstrual cycle, tenderness and distention of the breasts before menstruation, duration of bleeding, and consistency of cycle length, play a role in the risk of breast cancer (Kelsey, Gammon & John, 1993). The results have been controversial. A preliminary report (Dupont & Page, 1985) suggested that a large number of menstrual cycles prior to the first full-term pregnancy may play a unfavorable role. However, the results of other studies did not support that observation (Kelsey,

Gammon & John, 1993). It has been suggested (Henderson et al, 1985) that women with shorter cycles spend more of their reproductive years in the luteal phase, when estrogen and progesterone are high and when mitotic activity reaches its peak, than women with longer cycles, and this may increase the risk of breast cancer.

BENIGN BREAST DISEASE

A history of benign breast disease has long been known to increase the risk of breast cancer. However, the term 'benign breast disease' encompasses a hetero-geneous group of histopathologic entities and needs to be defined specifically (Dupont & Page, 1985; London et al, 1992). Benign breast conditions are identified primarily among premenopausal women. Estimates of the prevalence of the various benign proliferative lesions differ; some of these cases might represent precursor lesions in cancer-free patients, but identification of such lesions is complicated by the fact that patients are usually asymptomatic, and do not seek medical attention. The definitive diagnosis requires microscopic review of the breast tissue.

Proliferative Disease and Atypical Hyperplasia

An increasing relative risk of developing breast cancer has been associated with the degree of proliferation and atypical hyperplasia in the lobules or ducts of the breast tissue (Dupont & Page, 1985; Krieger & Hiatt, 1992).

Adenosis and Intraductal Papilloma

There is a positive association between the presence of adenosis or intraductal papilloma and the risk of subsequent breast cancer (Krieger & Hiatt, 1992). Occasionally, an association between adenosis and the presence of hyperplasia and atypical hyperplasia has been found (McDivett et al, 1992; Bodian et al, in press).

Fibroadenoma

Fibroadenoma forming a clinically detectable lump has not been associated with an increased incidence of breast cancer (Dupont & Page, 1985). However, fibro-adenoma associated with hyperplasia doubles the risk of breast cancer (McDivett et al, 1992; Bodian et al, in press).

Gross Cystic Disease

Gross cystic disease is defined as the formation of cysts larger than 3 mm in diameter. Davis, Simons & Davis (1964) reported a modest association between cystic disease and breast cancer risk; however, there is some controversy regarding their findings (Page & Dupont, 1985).

Two studies (Bodian, Lattes & Perzin, 1992; Bundred et al, 1991) reported an increase in relative risk for patients with multiple aspirated cysts. Another study, however, found no increase in risk of breast cancer (Harrington & Lesnick, 1981).

EXOGENOUS HORMONES

The association between exogenous hormone use and breast cancer continues to be investigated.

Oral Contraceptive Use

Although a significant amount of epidemiologic data has been published on the oral contraceptive (OC)/breast cancer issue, controversy continues. Most of the studies published before 1984 found little indication of increased incidence of breast cancer with OC use (Malone, Daling & Weiss, 1993); this may be explained in part by the relatively small number of subjects who had used these hormones for a long period. Studies conducted after 1984 suggested an increased risk of breast cancer among specific subgroups of OC users (Malone, Daling & Weiss, 1993). A positive association between OC use and breast cancer risk has been reported in several subgroups of women, but not consistently. Nevertheless, there is convincing evidence that long-term OC use increases the risk of developing breast cancer before age 35 or 45 (Delgado-Rodriguez et al, 1991; Lubin et al, 1982; Merrik et al, 1986; Miller et al, 1989; Olsson, Moller & Ranstam, 1989; Peto, 1989; Rushton & Jones, 1992; Ursin et al, 1992).

A study carried out in New Zealand reported an increased risk of breast cancer with 10 or more years of OC use among women younger than 35, but little suggestion of risk for women aged 35–44 (Paul, Skegg & Spears, 1990). The largest case-control study of breast cancer, the CASH study, originally reported RR estimates of 1.2, 1.4 and 1.2, respectively, for durations of OC use of 4–7 years, 8–11 years, and more than 11 years among women younger than 45 (Stadel & Schlesselman, 1986). In contrast, a final report from a case-control study conducted in northern Italy, where the prevalence of OC use is low (15%), found no association between duration of OC use and breast cancer in women younger than 60 years (Tavani et al, 1993). Investigators (Paffenbarger, Kampert & Chang, 1980; Pike et al, 1981, 1983) have proposed that OC use beginning at a young age, when breast development is ongoing, might be associated with breast cancer.

Four studies observed an increased risk of breast cancer with early age at first OC use (Olsson, Moller & Ranstam, 1989; UK National Case-Control Study Group, 1989; Clare et al, 1991; Weinstein et al, 1991); yet other studies reported no evidence of such an association (Merrick et al, 1986; Paul, Skegg & Spears, 1990; Cancer and Steroid Hormone Study, 1986; Ronan & McMichael, 1988). Studies have reported the relationship between breast cancer risk and duration of OC use before age 25. Three of these studies have shown no indication of a relationship between use before age 25 and increased breast cancer risk (Miller et al, 1989; Stadel et al, 1985; McPherson et al, 1987), but six have suggested a positive association (Merrick et al, 1986; Olsson, Moller & Ramstam, 1989; Pike et al, 1983; Weinstein et al, 1991; WHO Collaborative Study, 1990; Wingo et al, 1991). Thomas (1991) estimated a 1.5-fold excess risk for the longest duration of OC use before age 25. Three studies have reported RR estimates between 1.6 and 4.0 for ever use of OC after age 40 (Romieu et al, 1989; Yuan et al, 1988; Thomas & Noonan, 1991), and one study found no indication of increased or decreased risk (Rosenberg et al, 1984).

The most consistent positive associations between OC use and breast cancer risk have been observed in studies of women younger than 45. The association with duration of OC use before first full-term pregnancy, or age 25, or overall long duration of use is suggestive of a relationship between OC use and breast cancer in younger women.

The association between hormone treatment and breast cancer was similar for women with and without a family history of breast cancer (RRs 1.07 and 1.11, respectively) based on combined data from 10 studies.

Women with a history of benign breast disease had an estimated RR of breast cancer of 1.11 from exogenous hormone use based on data from 12 studies (Helzlsouer, 1994). Thomas (1991) reported that exogenous estrogen taken prior to diagnosis of the initial benign lesion did not alter the risk of cancer. Subsequent use, however, appeared to increase the risk of breast cancer.

More studies are needed to determine the risk, if any, between benign breast lesions, OC use and risk of breast cancer.

ESTROGEN REPLACEMENT THERAPY (ERT)

Epidemiologic studies of the risk of breast cancer after treatment with estrogen for the symptoms of menopause have given conflicting results (Kelsey et al, 1981; Kaufman et al, 1984; Wingo et al, 1987; Brinton, Hoover & Fraumeni, 1986; La Vecchia et al, 1986). Most of the studies have failed to show an overall excess risk of breast cancer (Kelsey et al, 1981; Laufman et al, 1984; Wingo et al, 1987), whereas few have indicated an increased risk after long-term use (Brinton, Hoover & Fraumeni, 1986; La Vecchia et al, 1986). In a recent meta-analysis, Colditz et al (1993) found no statistically significant association between ever using ERT and risk of breast cancer. Data from five studies reported that compared with never-users, women using less than 1.25 mg/day of conjugated estrogens had a RR of 1.05 and those using 1.25 mg/day or more had a RR of 0.94. Results from nine other studies reported a RR of 1.05 with ERT. The RR for ever using ERT in three European studies was 1.31, but outside Europe, the combined RR was 1.01. Most studies support the absence of relationship (Wingo et al, 1987); however, three studies reported slightly elevated RRs of borderline statistical significance: 1.4, 1.2 and 1.1, respectively (Hoover et al, 1976, 1981; Brinton et al, 1981).

In an update of the Nurses' Health Study, Colditz et al (1995) reported an increased risk of breast cancer in postmenopausal women who had used ERT for 5–9 years (RR 1.46; 95% CI 1.22–1.74), and a similarly increased risk in current users for a total of 10 or more years (RR 1.46; 95% CI 1.20–0.76). The risk was higher for women older than 60 years. The addition of progestins did not affect the risk of breast cancer.

Another issue addressed in several studies is the use of ERT and breast cancer risk in naturally and surgically menopausal women. Wingo et al (1987) reported that surgically menopausal women had a slightly higher but not significantly different risk of breast cancer, compared with women with intact ovaries. Colditz et al (1993) analyzed different studies addressing the role of oophorectomy in the breast cancer risk in ERT users. Analysis of seven studies of hormone use in women with menopause from bilateral salpingo-oophorectomy showed a RR of 1.18; however, analysis of another five studies of women who had bilateral oophorectomy found a RR of 0.86. Brinton et al (1981) reported increasing breast cancer risk with increasing duration of ERT use among oophorectomized women; the hypothesis from most studies is that the protective effect of bilateral oophorectomy against breast cancer is reversed among women who have used ERT (Wingo et al, 1987).

Another issue is the use of synthetic vs. conjugated estrogens. Most of the studies conducted in the USA that failed to demonstrate significantly increased risk of breast cancer were of users of conjugated estrogens. However, the two large studies, one conducted in Denmark and the other in Sweden (Ewertz, 1988; Bergkvist et al, 1989) showed a significant trend of increasing risk of breast cancer with increasing duration of ERT, with synthetic estrogens. The Denmark study (Ewertz, 1988) reported an estimated RR of 2.3 for use of synthetic estrogens for at least 12 years, and the Sweden study (Bergkvist et al, 1989) showed a 70% increase in risk among women who had used primarily estradiol compounds for at least 109 months. These reports address the possibility that estradiols have a different effect on breast tissue than do conjugated estrogens.

The effects on the breast of the addition of cyclic progestins to estrogen have been difficult to assess (Hunt et al, 1987). Gambrell (1984) suggested that the addition of progestin to estrogen reduced the RR of breast cancer to 0.3. However, a recent review of research on endogenous and exogenous hormonal factors in the causation of breast cancer, reported that the combination treatment may in fact increase the risk of breast cancer (Key & Pike, 1988). Combined data from four studies reported a RR of 1.13 in those treated with a combination of progestins and estrogens (Colditz et al, 1993, 1995).

Most studies (Colditz et al, 1993, 1995) have failed to demonstrate an increased risk of breast cancer with ERT in subgroups with a family history of the disease. Among women with a family history of breast cancer, the RR for ERT users was 1.07 and for women without a family history it was 1.11. Thomas et al (1982) and Brinton et al (1986) reported a higher risk among women whose benign breast disease preceded first estrogen use; these authors suggested a promotional effect of estrogen on benign breast pathology. However, Dupont & Page (1991), in their review of five studies, and Colditz et al (1993, 1995), in a review of 12 studies, reported no significant increase in risk of breast cancer with ERT use (RR 1.11).

There is limited information about women who develop breast cancer while receiving ERT. A small number of studies have suggested that the subgroup of women who develop breast cancer while receiving ERT may have a better outcome than non-users of ERT (Byrd, Burch & Vaughn, 1977; Hunt, Vessey & McPherson, 1990; Bergkvist et al, 1989). This may be because women receiving ERT have earlier stage disease at the time of diagnosis (Brinton et al, 1986).

The issue of whether physiologic doses of ERT are harmful to the patient who has been treated for breast cancer is under investigation. As more young women treated for breast cancer are reaching menopause, and given the known metabolic consequences of prolonged estrogen deficiency, it is essential to define whether ERT has any real impact on disease outcome. In the small number of women who have elected to receive ERT after the diagnosis of breast cancer, no adverse effects have been reported (Wile, Opfell & Marigileth, 1993).

Currently, clinical studies are under way to establish the safety of ERT in breast cancer patients.

HORMONAL REGULATORY MECHANISMS/ROLE IN CARCINOGENESIS

The concept that estrogens are the major adverse factor in breast cancer has been a principal hypothesis in carcinogenesis studies (Henderson, Ross & Bernstein, 1988; Vessey, 1989). This hypothesis is based on several observations: (a) the mitogenic effect of estrogens on established breast cancer cell lines (Dickson & Lippman, 1988); (b) the reduction of breast cancer risk with early menopause, whether it occurs naturally or with bilateral oophorectomy; (c) the increased risk of breast cancer with postmenopausal obesity but decreased risk with premenopausal obesity; (d) the ability of estrogen to generate mammary tumors in rodents (Welsch, 1982). Progesterone also has been shown to increase breast cancer risk in both premenopausal (Thomas, 1991) and postmenopausal women (Bergkvist et al, 1989).

In a recent prospective study, Toniolo et al (1995) showed a positive association between serum levels of estrone and estradiol and increased risk of breast cancer in postmenopausal women. The authors calculated risk for both estradiol and albumin-bound estradiol. Their findings also showed that estradiol bound to

SHBG was inversely related to breast cancer risk. Similar studies (Bulbrook et al, 1986; Wysowski et al, 1987; Garland et al, 1992; Moore et al, 1986) reported no such association; the number of cases, however, was small and might have influenced the results.

Different agents are known to influence different stages of carcinogenesis, and the same agent can have different effects, depending on the stage of progression at the time of exposure. Although neoplastic development is a multifactorial process, one feature, proliferation, is common. The effects of estrogen and progesterone on promotion of proliferation in normal breast epithelium and breast cancer cells are believed to be mediated through transcriptional activation of specific sets of genes recognized by their particular receptor proteins (Press, in press). The estrogen receptor (ER) gene has been localized to the long arm of chromosome 6 (Kumar et al, 1987) and the progesterone receptor (PR) gene to the long arm of chromosome 11 (Law et al, 1987). Some studies have shown that hormone sensitivity changes as the cells progress from the normal to the neoplastic state (King, 1991). In normal breast epithelium, however, there are some data supporting an additional estrogen effect on proliferation via induction of PRs. There are not sufficient data to indicate whether the proliferative effects of progestins change during progression to breast cancer. Even though ERs are very difficult to detect in normal human breast tissue—correlating with the poor mitogenic action of estrogens in the normal breast—there is a strong estrogen mitogenic effect on established cancer tissue, which could be associated with up-regulation of ERs (King, 1991).

There are also data indicating that estrogens indirectly influence tumor growth through the secretion of growth factors produced at distant sites (Ikeda, Danielpour & Sirbasku, 1984). Evidence has also shown that, in addition to steroid hormones, polypeptide hormones and growth factors may play a role in the regulation of breast cancer growth. Certain cultured human breast cancer cell lines have been shown to respond to physiologic concentrations of insulin, and it has also been shown that breast cancer cells express specific high-affinity membrane insulin receptors (Osborne et al, 1978). Receptors for the insulin-like growth factors (IGFs) have been found in human breast cancer specimens (Pekonen et al, 1988). IGF-I and IGF-II were found to be potent mitogens for breast cancer cells (Karey & Sirbasku, 1988). Another group of factors, epidermal growth factor (EGF) and transforming growth factor-α (TGF-α) may modulate breast cancer proliferation (Osborne, Hamilton & Nover, 1982; Arteaga, Coronado & Osborne, 1988). TGF-α has been shown to be mitogenic for cultured human breast cancer cells. Recent studies have reported that breast cancer cells have the capacity to make growth factors that potentially could stimulate their own growth in an autocrine fashion (TGF-α or IGFs) or that could affect stromal tissues or tumor invasiveness by paracrine mechanisms (Huff et al, 1988; Peres et al, 1987; Salomon et al, 1984). TGF-β polypeptides have been shown to have growth-inhibitory effects on epithelial cells in breast cancer lines (Sporn et al, 1986). TGF-α and IGFs are stimulated by estrogen and inhibited by anti-estrogens, whereas the reverse is true for TGF-β, a potential tumor inhibitor. A hypothesis has been formed that the growth effects of estrogen and anti-estrogens may be mediated by these poly-peptides. Moreover, the growth advantage in ER-tumors may be due to the production of autocrine growth factors (Lippman et al, 1987).

There is some evidence that breast cancer growth is controlled not only by growth factors produced by the tumor but also by the mesenchymal stromal elements (fibroblasts, mononuclear cells and endothelial cells) that comprise normal breast tissue. Malignant breast cells secrete peptides such as TGF-β and platelet-derived growth factor (PDGF) that stimulate the growth of stromal cells. Similarly, stromal elements secrete proteins that may stimulate the growth of breast cancer cells (Picard, Rolland & Poupon, 1986; Clemmons et al, 1986).

TUMOR SUPPRESSOR GENES/ONCOGENES/IMMUNOBIOLOGY

Tumor-suppressor genes appear to be important in cell cycle regulation and cell growth. Mutated tumor-suppressor genes lose their regulatory function, potentially contributing to malignant transformation. Genetic factors contribute to about 5% of all breast cancer cases but to approximately 25% of cases diagnosed before age 30 (Claus, Thompson & Risch, 1991).

Mutation of one gene, BRCA1, is believed to be present in about 45% of families with significantly high breast cancer incidence and at least 80% of families with an increased incidence of early-onset breast cancer and ovarian cancer (Easton et al, 1993). BCRA1 was first mapped to chromosome arm 17q in 1990 (Hall et al, 1990). A second locus, BRCA2, recently mapped to chromosome arm 13q (Wooster et al, 1994), appears to contribute to early onset breast cancer. Several studies of sporadic breast tumors have suggested that BRCA1 mutations also play an important role in the development of non-inherited breast cancer (Cannon-Albright et al, 1994). BRCA1 appears to encode a tumor-suppressor protein that acts as a negative regulator of tumor growth; however, mutated BRCA1 encodes proteins that are absent, non-functional, or reduced in function (Smith et al, 1993; Kelsell et al, 1993). The functional BRCA1 protein is absent in some breast tumors.

Of particular relevance to breast cancer is the p53 gene. This gene was the first tumor-suppressor gene identified, and it appears to be one of the most frequently mutated genes in human breast tumors (Hollstein et al, 1991). It is involved in the development of both sporadic and some hereditary breast tumors. In its unmutated form, p53 acts as a tumor suppressor gene, but it can lose its negative growth control or acquire oncogenic activity when mutated (Lane & Benchimol, 1990).

Although germline mutations in the p53 gene carry a high risk of early-onset breast cancer, it is not usually the initiating genetic event in most breast tumors. Mutations in the p53 gene and protein are associated with increased protein stability, which prolongs the protein's half-life. The incidence of p53 immuno-histochemical positivity in sporadic human breast cancers ranges from 20% to 62%

(Bartek et al, 1990, 1991). However, the presence of mutations does not always result in positive immunohistochemical staining (Eeles, 1993); and immunohistochemical positivity does not always equate with mutation (Vojtesek & Lane, 1993).

The oncogenes most frequently implicated in the development and progression of breast cancer are the membrane-bound growth factor receptors c-erbB-2 (HER 2/neu), which is over-expressed in 20–30% of breast tumors (Mool & Peterse, 1992), and the epidermal growth factor receptor (EGFR, erbB-1), which is overexpressed in about 30–60% of breast tumors (Nicholson et al, 1993). Coexpression of EGFR and c-erbB-2 occurs in about 10% of human breast cancers and correlates with poorer survival and increased number of early recurrences, suggesting a functional interaction between these proteins (Barker & Vincent, 1990). Nicholson et al (1993), in a recent study, reported that expression of the EGFR and the c-erbB-2 proteins correlates with loss of hormone sensitivity in breast cancer. EGFR has been shown to be more strongly associated with hormonal insensitivity than c-erbB-2 proteins.

FAMILY HISTORY AND BREAST CANCER RISK

A family history of breast cancer consistently has been shown to increase a woman's risk of developing breast cancer. An inherited component to breast cancer has long been suspected based on anecdotal reports of families with many affected individuals, consistent with dominant inheritance, and systemic epidemiologic studies of familial risk, which have shown that the risk of breast cancer is higher in the relatives of breast cancer patients than in the general population (Claus, Risch & Thompson, 1990). Even though the majority of breast cancers are sporadic, 5–10% may be due to inheritance of a highly penetrate gene (Claus, Risch & Thompson, 1991).

Hereditary breast cancer is defined as a pattern of distribution within a family that is consistent with the autosomal dominant disease susceptibility gene (Lynch, 1990). Inheritance in these families follows the classic mendelian pattern of autosomal dominant transmission, with 50% of children of carriers inheriting BRCA1 mutations. Female mutation carriers are estimated to have an 85% lifetime risk of developing breast and/or ovarian cancer, with an increased incidence of bilateral breast cancer and more than a 50% risk of developing breast cancer before the age of 50 years (Easton et al, in press).

Familial breast cancer is defined as two or more relatives having breast cancer in the absence of hereditary breast cancer. The association between the development of breast cancer and a family history of breast cancer was examined using the Utah Population Database and the Utah Cancer Registry (Slattery & Kerber, 1993). First-degree relatives are mothers and sisters; second-degree relatives are grandmothers and aunts; third-degree relatives are cousins; and fourth- and fifth-degree relatives include more distant relatives. The calculation of the family risk was based on the percentage of family members with breast cancer. Researchers observed a threefold increased risk of breast cancer in those with the highest family history score (6% of cases). About 12% of the breast cancer cases had a first-degree relative as their closest relative with breast cancer; a slightly lower risk estimate was observed for this variable—2.45. Additionally, a slightly greater risk of breast cancer was noted if a woman's mother was the first-degree relative with breast cancer, as compared with her sister. Based on the results from Utah study, about 17–19% of cases of breast cancer in the population could be attributed to family history.

The association between the development of breast cancer and the family history and age of breast cancer onset among first-degree relatives was examined in a retrospective study using data from the Nurses' Health Study (Colditz et al, 1993). The risk of developing breast cancer ranged from 1.5 (95% CI 1.1–2.2) for a maternal diagnosis of breast cancer after the age of 70 to 2.5 (95% CI 1.5–4.2) for women with a family history of breast cancer in mother and sister. For a 40 year-old woman with a sister who had breast cancer, the probability of being diagnosed with breast cancer before the age of 70 was about 12%; similar cumulative risk was observed when the mother was diagnosed with breast cancer before the age of 50 years. The risk decreased to 9% for those whose mother was older than 60 years at the time of diagnosis. The rate of women with a positive family history of breast cancer, undergoing mammography, was 8% higher than among those without a family history. Additionally, among all breast cancer cases, a higher proportion of diagnosed breast cancers (9.2%) were in situ lesions among those with a family history of breast cancer than among those without family history (6.1%). According to this study, the elevated risk of breast cancer in those with a family history of breast cancer may, in fact, be due to greater surveillance and consequently earlier detection of tumors. A report from the prospective Iowa Women's Health Study showed a lower RR of 1.5 (95% CI 1.2–1.9) (Sellers et al, 1992). Houlston et al (1992) analyzed 254 consecutive pedigrees and found a RR of breast cancer of 1.85 in patients with first-degree relatives with breast cancer.

Family history is one of the most consistent factors identified as increasing the risk of breast cancer. Based on current knowledge, it is likely that family history represents a combination of genetic and environmental factors. Although having a family history of breast cancer is not a modifiable risk factor, a better understanding of family history within the population might improve our knowledge of breast cancer etiology.

SCREENING

Early diagnosis of breast cancer by screening may reduce mortality by identifying tumors before they metastasize. The difference in mortality between screened and control groups is the only indicator of the effectiveness of screening (Miller et al, 1991) and takes several years (usually more than 10) of follow-up to detect.

Screening will detect some occult lesions of questionable malignant potential, which usually would not have become clinically apparent during a patient's lifetime (overdiagnosis bias) (Pollei et al, 1987), lesions that grow more slowly than those that are diagnosed between screenings (length bias), and also lethal cancers at earlier stages (lead time bias).

The main modalities for earlier detection of breast cancer are mammography, clinical breast examination and breast self-examination. Studies of breast cancer screening that include mammography, clinical breast examination and breast self-examination have been conducted for at least 30 years. Studies (Tabar, Duffy & Kruseino, 1987) comparing screening mammography with clinical breast examination have shown that screening mammography detects the majority of breast cancers at a smaller size and earlier stage than does clinical breast examination. The International Workshop on Screening for breast cancer recently summarized the results of eight major randomized controlled clinical trials of breast cancer screening (Fletcher et al, 1993). These trials included the Health Insurance Plan (HIP), Swedish Two-County, Malmo and Stockholm, the First Canadian National Breast Screening Study, Edinburgh and Gotenburg studies. These trials varied in frequency of screening, duration of follow-up, compliance, and the screening test used (mammography alone vs. combination of mammography and breast self-examination with or without clinical examination). The most important issue addressed in the workshop was the effectiveness of screening in different age groups of women.

The most controversial issue is the effectiveness of mammography in women aged 40–49. For this age group, based on the results of the above studies, there is no evidence of a reduction in mortality, attributable to screening in the first 5–7 years. However, there is some evidence of a marginal reduction in mortality seen after 10–12 years of screening in five of the eight trials (King, 1994). The mortality reduction ranges from 22% in the Edinburgh trial, 23% in the HIP trial, and 25% in the Kopparberg trial, to 40% in the Gothenburg trial and 49% in the Malmo trial (Kopans & Feig, 1993). The meta-analysis of these trials showed a 'statistically significant' benefit from screening in women aged 40–49 (Smart et al, 1995). The remaining three trials, including the Canadian trial, failed to demonstrate a statistically significant benefit in mortality reduction from screening women aged 40–49 (Kopans, 1995).

Even though the current recommendation from the National Cancer Institute for breast cancer screening with mammography does not include women aged 40–49, stating that there are not enough data to support a benefit from screening in this group, the above studies support that screening mammography is as effective in reducing mortality for women younger than 50 as for women 50 and older (Kopans, 1995).

In a recent study (Kerlikowske et al, 1993) done to evaluate the positive predictive value (PPV) of screening mammography by age, the authors reported that the overall PPV of first-screening mammography was 8.5% and that this increased significantly with age from 0.03 for those aged 30–39 years to 0.19 for those aged

70 years or older; for those aged 50–59 years the PPV was 0.09, and for those 40–49 it was 0.04. The women aged 60 years or older had the highest PPV, 0.17–0.19. The higher PPV of women aged 50 and older, compared with those younger than 50, is most likely due to the high prevalence of breast cancer in the older age group. In another study addressing the PPV for screening mammography, the reported results were lower than those reported by Kerlikowske et al (1993). The observed increase in PPV of screening mammography with increasing age could in part also be due to lower sensitivity of mammography in younger women. The sensitivity of screening mammography in younger women has been reported to be 60–84% compared with 86–95% in older women (Tabar et al, 1992; Elwood et al, 1993). This is most likely because of different breast tissue quality (denser, less fat) in younger women compared to older ones (less dense, higher proportion of fat).

For women aged 50–69, the evidence presented at the workshop indicates a benefit of screening mammography in mortality reduction. The observed reduction in mortality ranged between 30–40%.

A family history of breast cancer has a significant impact on breast cancer prevalence. Kerlikowske et al (1993) reported the PPV of screening mammography to be three times higher in women aged 40–49 years and 50–59 years who had a family history of breast cancer than in comparably aged women without a family history of breast cancer (0.13 vs. 0.04 and 0.22 vs. 0.09, respectively). The PPV of screening mammography for women aged 30–39, 60–69, and 70 years or older with family history of breast cancer was similar to that of the same age groups without a family history of breast cancer. Screening only high-risk women aged 40–49, however, will not benefit the majority of women (60–95%) who develop breast cancer but do not belong to the high-risk groups (Kopans, 1995).

The current American Cancer Society guidelines for breast cancer detection include breast self-examination every month, starting at age 20, clinical breast examination every 3 years from the age of 20 and every year from the age of 40, and screening mammography every 1–2 years from age 40–49 and every year from 50 (Mettlin et al, 1993). However, if mammography is to be done in women aged 40–49, the data available to date suggest that it should be performed every year, because of the shorter preclinical phase of breast cancer in this subgroup (Bassett et al, 1991; Tabar et al, 1987).

To achieve maximal results from mammography, quality control of the images and the reading must be maintained. Currently, there are no standard recommendations regarding whether single-view mammography is as good as double-view (adding craniocaudal to the mediolateral oblique projection); when results from the eight major trials (Fletcher et al, 1993) were compared, it was not clear whether the number of views had an impact on sensitivity or effectiveness. More studies are needed to resolve this issue.

It is too early to determine whether screening mammography has had any impact on the mortality rate from breast cancer, since the lead time is limited, and it is unlikely that the statistical benefit will appear in the near future. However, the National Cancer Institute, having analyzed mortality data for the past 50 years, reported that there is a decline in the mortality rate from breast cancer for women younger than 50 (Moskowitz, 1986).

PROGNOSTIC FACTORS

Adjuvant systemic therapy for early breast cancer significantly reduces the annual rates of disease recurrence and death (Early Breast Cancer Trialist Collaborative Group, 1992). However, despite adjuvant therapy, 25–30% of patients with node-negative disease will have relapses and eventually die of metastatic disease; this subgroup requires additional definitions of prognostic factors to optimize adjuvant chemotherapy (Cooper, 1991).

Nodal Status

The axillary lymph node status generally is accepted as the most powerful prognostic indicator of risk of breast cancer recurrence. The risk of recurrence increases as the number of lymph nodes involved increases (Nemoto et al, 1980). After surgery and radiation therapy, patients with node-negative disease after surgery and radiation therapy have a 10-year survival probability of about 70%, significantly higher than that of patients with node-positive disease (McGuire et al, 1990).

Approximately one-half of patients with node-positive disease belong to high-risk groups with more than a 50% probability of developing metastases within 5 years (Nemoto et al, 1980). Patients with 10 or more positive lymph nodes are considered to be at very high risk for relapse and death and are eligible for high-dose therapy with bone marrow or peripheral stem cell support, or colony-stimulating factors.

Tumor Size

The relationship between the size of the primary tumor and tumor recurrence and patient survival has been well proven in many studies. Fisher et al (1969) found that increasing tumor size was associated with an increasing likelihood of recurrence. The largest series of cases examining the role of tumor size in axillary node-negative (ANN) breast cancer patients is from the SEER program of the National Cancer Institute. Between 1977 and 1982, a total of 13 464 ANN breast cancer patients were studied to address the issue of the prognostic value of tumor size; patients with tumors smaller than 2 cm had a 5-year survival rate of 92% (Carter, Allen & Henson, 1989). Recently Rosen et al (1993) reported their experience with prognostic factors in ANN patients. The recurrence-free survival rate for patients with tumors 1.00 cm or smaller was 88%; for those with tumors 1.1–2.0 cm, 74%; and for those with tumors 2.1–3.0 cm, 72%. The worst recurrence-free survival rate was in women with tumors measuring 3.1–5.0 cm (61%).

The most favorable subgroup (< 1 cm) in most studies represents about 25% of all patients with ANN. For this particular subgroup of patients, the current recommendation, supported both by National Cancer Institute consensus (NIH, 1991) and world-wide overview (Early Breast Cancer Trialist Collaborative Group, 1992), and based on these patients' proven excellent prognosis, is that they do not require adjuvant chemotherapy (in contrast to the patients with tumors > 1 cm).

The selection of the tumor mass of 1 cm or smaller as prognostic indicator for survival is not arbitrary. Based on the Delbruck–Luria model demonstrated by Law to be applicable to cancer cells, and popularized by Goldie & Goldman, this is the tumor size at which the probability of finding a biologically important mutation changes rapidly from very low to very high (Norton & Day, 1991). Size is related to the number of malignant cells contained within the mass. Therefore, tumors measuring more than 1 cm have an increased probability of having already metastasized at the time of diagnosis.

Histologic Grade

To date, histologic grading in breast cancer has not been widely and routinely utilized by pathologists and oncologists in therapeutic decision making. The two most frequently used histologic grading systems are those of Scarff–Bloom–Richardson and Fisher et al; both take into account the architectural arrangement of cells, the degree of nuclear differentiation, and the mitotic grade (Bloom & Richardson, 1957; Scarff & Toroni, 1968; Fisher, Redmond & Fisher, 1980). The histologic grading system of Fisher et al (1980) involves the combined assessment of nuclear grade and the presence of tubule or gland formation. The nuclear grade component is determined by a modification of the method of Black et al (1955).

The role of these grading systems has been recently evaluated in ANN patients (Fisher et al, 1988). The data show a statistically significant difference in both recurrence and survival between patients with high nuclear grade and those with low nuclear grade.

Ploidy and Cellular Proliferation

Ploidy is a measure of the genetic stability of the tumor; a tumor's ploidy status can be determined by flow cytometry. Data in the literature have shown that operable breast cancers with a DNA index of 1 ('diploid') have a more favorable prognosis but that the advantage over tumors showing aneuploidy is small (Hedley et al, 1993). To date, in different studies, DNA index has failed to achieve independent prognostic significance. In contrast, cellular proliferation is an important indicator of prognosis in ANN patients. A low thymidine labeling index in ANN patients has been shown to predict prolonged disease-free survival (DFS) and low rates of recurrence, independently of tumor size, ER status and histologic grade (McGuire et al, 1990). However, measurements of thymidine-labeling index are not practical because they can be performed only on fresh tissue. For this reason, the DNA synthesis phase (S-phase) determined by flow cytometry is performed on frozen or formalin-fixed material. Several studies have shown statistically superior DFS and overall survival for patients with diploid vs. aneuploid tumors and low S-phase vs. high S-phase tumors (McGuire, 1990). In a recent study done by Clark et al (1989), the actuarial 5 years DFS rates were 90% for patients with diploid and low S-phase tumors, 74% for patients with aneuploid tumors regardless of S-phase fraction, and 70% for patients with diploid and high S-phase tumors.

Estrogen and Progesterone Receptors

Steroid hormones have been shown to be involved in the growth regulation of breast cancer. The mechanism of action of estrogen on breast cancer and the development of hormone independence or resistance is not fully understood. Estrogens have many effects on the expression of various genes, on growth factor secretion, on growth factor receptor expression, and on the production of a number of estrogen-regulated proteins such as PR, PS2, cathepsin D, and plasminogen activators (Klijn, Berns & Foekens, 1993). Patients with high tumor levels of ER and PR receive more benefits from adjuvant endocrine therapy than do patients with ER/PR− tumors (Carter, Allen & Henson, 1989).

Some studies have shown (Klijn, Berns & Foekens, 1993) that steroid receptor status is also indicative of response to chemotherapy. Most of the data in the literature do not support this.

In patients with metastatic disease, the response to endocrine therapy has been about 10% for ER− tumors, 50% in ER+ tumors, and 75% in ER+ and PR+ tumors. The PR status might be especially predictive of response to therapy with antiprogestins (Horwitz, 1992; Klijn et al, 1989). Metastases to the liver and brain are more frequent with ER− tumors (Alexieva-Figusch et al, 1988). In combined series of 2853 ANN patients, the 5-year DFS of patients with ER+ tumors and those with ER− tumors was highly significantly different, although the magnitude of the difference was only 8–9% (Fisher et al, 1988; Benner, Clark & McGuire, 1988). This might indicate that ER by itself is not a strong prognostic factor for response to therapy (McGuire, 1988).

Resistance to endocrine therapy can be present from the beginning, regardless of receptor status, or can develop later during disease progression (Klijn, 1991).

Oncogenes, Tumor Suppressor Genes

The HER-2/neu proto-oncogene encodes a putative growth factor receptor that has been shown to be amplified in 25–30% of primary human breast cancers (Slamon et al, 1990). A recent study showed that breast cancer patients whose tumors had Her-2/neu over-expression had a significantly worse overall survival compared with women whose tumor did not over-express HER-2/neu (Merkel & Osborne, 1989). In a multivariate analysis, HER-2/neu over-expression was the second most important independent predictor of survival after nodal status (Paik et al, 1990). There are increasing data on the value of HER-2/neu in predicting response to endocrine therapy. These data show that HER-2/neu-positive tumors have a poor response to endocrine therapy (Nicholson et al, 1990). The data on the relationship between HER-2/neu and response to chemotherapy are conflicting (Benz et al, 1992).

C-myc

C-myc has been found to be amplified in 20% of breast cancer patients in several studies (Berns et al, 1992a). C-myc amplification has been shown to be highly predictive for short-term relapse and overall survival, especially among node-negative or steroid receptor-positive patients (Berns et al, 1992b). C-myc amplified tumors have been reported to have a response to therapy opposite to that of HER-2/neu-amplified tumors (Berns et al, 1992a, b).

p53

The p53 gene functions as a negative regulator of cell growth. p53 mutation and over-expression can reflect a more advanced stage of disease with a higher proliferation rate. Tumors that over-express p53 might have a higher likelihood of micrometastases, so over-expression of p53 might be useful as a prognostic factor for recurrence after primary therapy. In a large study (Allred et al, 1993) including ANN patients, p53 over-expression was detected in tumors of patients who had a worse overall survival and DFS rates at 5 years. A negative association with ER and prognosis has been found. A recent study showed that abnormalities of the p53 gene were more prevalent in the ER-group and in about half of the cases were associated with amplification of c-myc and HER-2/neu oncogenes (Klijn, Berns & Foekens, 1993).

Growth Factors

TGF-α, EGF

Transforming-growth factor-α (TGR-α) and epidermal growth factor (EGF) are growth-regulatory proteins that interact with a membrane-bound protein kinase known as EGFR. TGF-α has been shown to induce a transient malignant phenotype in vitro (Todato, Fryling & Delarco, 1980). This observation led to the autocrine theory, in which it was hypothesized that a cell could exhibit autonomous growth by responding to endogenously produced growth factors (Sporn & Torado, 1980); the cell that expresses both the growth factor and its receptor would escape normal growth-regulatory control. Recent studies have shown that increased expression of EGFR in breast tumors predicts for significantly worse DFS and overall survival rates (Merkel & Osborne, 1989). Multivariate analysis of survival using axillary node status, tumor grade, size, EGFR and ER showed that nodes were the most significant factor and EGFR the only other independent factor (Sainsbury et al, 1987). In node-negative patients, only EGFR was significant for overall survival. A recent study (Klijn et al, in press) showed that EGFR positivity is twice as high in ER– or PR– tumors than in ER+ or PR+ tumors. Some investigators hypothesized that EGFR expression may allow escape from endocrine control by enhancing responsiveness to residual TGF-α after anti-estrogen treatment (Nicholson et al, 1989). In recent studies (Nicholson et al, 1989, 1990) it was reported that expression of EGFR is associated with a lack of response to endocrine therapy in recurrent breast cancer.

IGF-I, IGF-II

Insulin-like growth factors (IGF-I and IGF-II) are potent mitogens for breast cancer cells (Clarke, Dickson & Lippman, 1992). At present, there is no clear indication of the prognostic value of IGF-IR. Some studies have suggested that both very low (Bonneterre et al, 1990) or very high levels (Berns et al, 1992c) of these receptors may predict poor survival.

FGF

Although there are few data on the prognostic significance of fibroblast-growth factor (FGF) and breast cancer, these data suggest a possible role of FGFs in the progression of breast cancer to an estrogen-independent state (McLeskey et al, 1993). High FGF receptor levels in primary breast cancer may predict a poor response to endocrine therapy (Peyrat et al, 1992).

Cathepsin D

Cathepsin D, a lysosomal protease, is one of the newer prognostic factors for ANN breast cancer. It has been suggested that cathepsin D may play a part in the metastatic process (Liotta, 1988). In a recent study (Mandelonde et al, 1988), it was shown that levels of cathepsin D were correlated with ER status in breast cancer.

Tandon et al (1990) reported that in patients with ANN breast cancer, those with higher levels of cathepsin D had statistically shorter DFS and overall survival than those with lower levels of the protein, independent of other prognostic factors.

The development of prognostic factors that can reliably predict both the subset of patients who will benefit from adjuvant chemotherapy and the development of drug resistance is a challenging and expanding field. The development of such predictive parameters would have important clinical utility.

HORMONAL APPROACH TO BREAST CANCER THERAPY

Tamoxifen

Tamoxifen, a non-steroidal anti-estrogen, has been established to be effective as an adjuvant therapy in node-positive and node-negative patients (Early Breast Cancer Trialist Collaborative Group, 1992). The US Food and Drug Administration (FDA) has approved the use of tamoxifen for the advanced disease (1978) and as an adjuvant therapy with chemotherapy (1986) and alone (1988) in node-positive postmenopausal and pre- and postmenopausal node-negative patients with ER+ disease (1990).

Walpole (Harper & Walpole, 1966) was the ICI scientist who first suggested that tamoxifen might be useful to treat breast cancer. Cole was the first clinician who tested tamoxifen clinically.

The mechanism of action of tamoxifen is not fully known, but most studies have shown that tamoxifen competes with estrogen for cytoplasmic ERs in breast tissue; the tamoxifen–ER complex prevents estrogen/ER-mediated DNA synthesis, proliferation, cancer cell growth (30%) and induction of autocrine polypeptides such as TGF-α, EFF and IGF (Osborne, 1988; Imai et al, 1989).

Tamoxifen may act in part by inducing secretion of TGF-β in hormone-dependent breast cancer cells (Kuabbe et al, 1987). It has been shown that anti-estrogens increase TGF-β secretion in fibroblasts by a mechanism that does not involve the ER (Colletta et al, 1990). Other mechanisms of tamoxifen action also have been suggested. Tamoxifen binds with high affinity to a microsomal protein called anti-estrogen-binding site (Sutherland et al, 1980). However, the functional importance of this protein is not known. Tamoxifen also increases antibody formation (Nagy & Berez, 1986), which enhances natural killer cell activity (Benry, Green & Matheson, 1987), and inhibits suppressor T-cell lymphocytes (Mandeville, Ghali & Chasseau, 1984). These non-ER-mediated actions of tamoxifen may in part explain the inhibition of tumor growth by tamoxifen in 10–15% of ER– tumors. Tamoxifen also has been shown to inhibit angiogenesis (Gagliardi & Collins, 1993).

Tamoxifen is considered to act in part as a tumoristatic rather than tumoricidal agent, and eventually a subset of tumor cells might overcome this growth inhibition and begin to grow during tamoxifen treatment.

Tumors treated with tamoxifen could become hormone-independent. These tumors may or may not continue to maintain expression of ER. Estrogen receptor-positive but non-responsive tumors may account for the patients with ER+ breast cancers that fail to respond to tamoxifen therapy. This observation led to the proposal that not all ER+ tumors contain functional ERs (Horwitz & McGuire, 1975). Tamoxifen-resistant tumors may contain aberrant receptor forms that could interfere with normal receptor function (McGuire, Chamness & Fuqua, 1991). Several reports of naturally occurring mutant or variant ER forms (Murphy, 1990) and polymorphic forms of the ER gene (Hill et al, 1989) have been described. Several of the variant ERs described contain deletions of some or all of the hormone-binding domain (Murphy & Dotzlow, 1989; Graham et al, 1990). An alternative mechanism that could lead to failure of anti-estrogen therapy is the stimulation of tumor growth by tamoxifen. One hypothesis suggests that tamoxifen-stimulated tumors acquire the ability to modify tamoxifen or its metabolites to act as potent estrogens. Tamoxifen-stimulated tumors are capable of actively lowering the intracellular concentration of tamoxifen and its anti-estrogenic metabolites. Another hypothesis suggests that changes within the tumors cause a subset of cells to respond to tamoxifen as stimulators (Osborne et al, 1992; Wiebe et al, 1992).

Tamoxifen for Treatment of Early and Metastatic Breast Cancer

Over the past decade, many randomized trials of adjuvant systemic therapy with tamoxifen in early breast cancer have shown an improvement in disease-free survival, and some have shown an improvement in overall survival in women with ER+ and/or PR+ tumors.

The Nolvadex Adjuvant Trial Organization (NATO) initiated a study in 1977 to investigate the role of tamoxifen in women with early breast cancer (Nolvadex, 1988). Over a period of 3.5 years, 1131 patients were enrolled. Included were premenopausal node-positive cases and postmenopausal node-positive and node-negative cases.

The Cancer Research Campaign Adjuvant Trial for Early Breast Cancer began recruitment in 1980. This trial was designed to repeat both the NATO trial of adjuvant tamoxifen and the Scandinavian Adjuvant Chemotherapy Study Group's trial of peri-operative cyclophosphamide (CRC Adjuvant Breast Trial Working Party, 1988).

The Stockholm Adjuvant Tamoxifen trial (Rutqvist et al, 1987) was initiated more than 15 years ago. It was designed to evaluate the effect of adjuvant tamoxifen in early breast cancer only on recurrence-free survival and overall survival.

An ECOG trial (Cummings et al, 1985, 1993) investigated maintenance tamoxifen after postoperative induction chemotherapy in node-positive breast cancer patients.

The Italian Cooperative Group (GROCTA-I) (Boccardo et al, 1992) studied prolonged tamoxifen treatment in early breast cancer.

Other European and American trials also investigated the role of tamoxifen given at different doses and different durations as adjuvant treatment for early breast cancer (Breast Cancer Trials Committee, 1987; Ribeiro & Swindell, 1988; Rose et al, 1985; Fisher et al, 1989; Ludwig Breast Cancer Study Group, 1984). Most of the data are for postmenopausal women (limited data for premenopausal women) treated for 1–2 years. Most of these trials failed to present sufficient data on hormone receptor status. Some of these studies combined tamoxifen with chemotherapy (Ludwig Breast Cancer Study Group, 1984) and ovarian irradiation (Ribeiro & Swindell, 1988).

The National Surgical Adjuvant Breast and Bowel Project (NSABP B14, Fisher et al, 1989; NATO (Nolvadex, 1988), Scottish (Breast Cancer Trials Committee, 1987) and Christie (Ribeiro & Swindell, 1988) studies have shown a significant improvement in overall survival with adjuvant tamoxifen. The Nolvadex Adjuvant Trial Organization (1988), Scottish (CRC Adjuvant Breast Trial Working Party, 1987), Stockholm (Rutqvist et al, 1987) and NSABP B14 (Fisher et al, 1989) trials have shown reduction in distant metastasis and in local recurrence. These benefits were for both node-negative and node-positive tumors. The addition of chemotherapy to tamoxifen in node-positive postmenopausal women offered a statistically significant survival advantage only in the NSABP B14 study (Fisher et al, 1989).

The Early Breast Cancer Trialist Cooperative Group (EBCTCG: 1992) trial combined results from 133 trials evaluating 30 000 women treated with adjuvant tamoxifen vs. no adjuvant treatment and tamoxifen plus chemotherapy vs. chemotherapy alone. The beneficial effects of tamoxifen were higher for women 50 years and older. The reductions in the risk of recurrence and death for women 50 years and older were $29 \pm 2\%$ and $20 \pm 2\%$, respectively, whereas the reductions were only $12 \pm 4\%$ and $6 \pm 5\%$ in women younger than 50 years. No significant differences in recurrence-free and overall survival were found at various tamoxifen doses. The standard 20 mg/day dose was recommended. The optimal duration of adjuvant tamoxifen has not been defined.

The role of tamoxifen in treating metastatic breast cancer was initially evaluated in postmenopausal women (Cole, Jones & Todd, 1971). Most of the studies have shown that more than 50% of the patients with metastatic disease and ER+ tumors achieved a complete or partial response with a median duration of response ranging from 9 to 13 months (Rose & Mouridsen, 1984; Ingle et al, 1991). The data on the use of tamoxifen in premenopausal women with advanced breast cancer are limited. The reported response rates range between 20% and 45% with a median duration of response of 2.5–36 months (Manni & Pearson, 1980; Hoogstraten et al, 1982).

There are some controversial data addressing the issue of oophorectomy vs. tamoxifen in premenopausal women. Some studies have (Ingle et al, 1986) suggested no difference in overall response rate or survival, whereas other studies favored oophorectomy over tamoxifen. A Southwest Oncology Group (SWOG) trial (Hoogstraten et al, 1982) reported that some women who failed to respond to tamoxifen responded to oophorectomy; however, it was hypothesized that the observed response to oophorectomy was actually due to tamoxifen withdrawal effect (Canney et al, 1987).

Acute and Late Side Effects of Tamoxifen

Tamoxifen is a non-steroidal anti-estrogen that possesses both partial agonist and partial antagonist properties. The side effects are related to its differential anti-estrogenic and estrogenic properties in various target tissues. Most data on tamoxifen toxicity are from the adjuvant therapy trials (Nolvadex, 1988; Ludwig Breast Cancer Study Group, 1984); fewer than 5% of patients in such trials withdrew from therapy because of toxic effects (Breast Cancer Trials Committee, 1987; Ribeiro & Swindell, 1988).

The adverse effect most consistently reported by patients receiving tamoxifen was vasomotor instability (hot flashes). Hot flashes probably represent an anti-estrogenic effect of tamoxifen; within the target cell exposed to tamoxifen, there is an apparent decrease in estrogen activity at the receptor level, and this can lead to symptoms similar to those observed in perimenopausal women (Manni & Pearson, 1980). The incidence of hot flashes in premenopausal women is higher than in postmenopausal women (Fisher et al, 1989). If hot flashes are severe enough, coadministration of a progestin such as oral medroxyprogesterone acetate (MPA) at 20 mg/day is recommended to decrease them (Schiff et al, 1988). Alternatively, injection of Depo-provera at 150 mg every 3 months may also decrease hot flashes. It has been reported that MPA may decrease the effectiveness of tamoxifen in some cases (Mouridsen et al, 1979). Clonidine also has shown some ability to reduce the incidence of hot flashes (Nagamani, Kelver & Smith, 1987).

In the NSABP B14 trial, nausea was reported in 25.7% of patients with tamoxifen and 23.9% with placebo.

The effect of tamoxifen on bone mineral density is not clear; some studies have shown no reduction in bone density (Powles et al, 1990), and two clinical trials in postmenopausal women have shown a beneficial effect (Love et al, 1992; Turken et al, 1989).

Patients treated with tamoxifen have shown significant reduction in total serum cholesterol, LDL cholesterol, and apoliprotein B levels (Love et al, 1991). All these effects are associated with significant reduction in cardiovascular risk.

Other potential adverse reactions to tamoxifen therapy include ocular effects. Cases of retinopathy (Griffiths, 1991), optic neuritis (Pubesgaard & Van Eyben, 1986) and keratopathy (Kaiser-Kupfer & Lippman, 1978) have been reported in patients receiving tamoxifen.

Other side effects include vaginal bleeding or discharge, fluid retention and irregular menses. Depression, nausea, irritability, headache, dizziness, nervousness, inability to concentrate, sleep disturbance and fatigue have been rarely reported in women taking tamoxifen (Margreiter & Wiegle, 1984).

Thrombosis is an uncommon but serious complication of tamoxifen therapy. The available data from the adjuvant studies (Nolvadex, 1988; Breast Cancer Trials Committee, 1987) indicate a 1–3% incidence of thrombo-embolic events (Cummings et al, 1985, 1993; Fisher et al, 1989). Thrombosis occurs more frequently in patients receiving chemotherapy (Saphner, Tormey & Gray, 1991) and tamoxifen than in patients receiving chemotherapy only. Patients with evidence of a thrombo-embolic event should consider discontinuing tamoxifen therapy. However, previous clotting disorders are not a contraindication to tamoxifen therapy. Tamoxifen has been shown to decrease antithrombin III levels in some studies (Rieche, 1986) but not in others (Auger & Mackie, 1988).

A rare complication of tamoxifen therapy, hypercalcemia, has been observed in patients with metastatic bone disease (Gibson, 1990).

Tamoxifen has been shown to promote the growth of liver tumors in rats (Dragon, Xu & Pitot, 1991). However, there are few clinical data on hepatic complications in women receiving tamoxifen. In one adjuvant tamoxifen trial (Rutqvist et al, 1995), three cases of hepatocellular carcinoma were reported in patients taking tamoxifen and one in the observation group.

Cholestasis has been rarely reported in women treated with tamoxifen.

The association between tamoxifen and endometrial cancer is based upon clinical observations during the past decade. In 1985 Killackey et al (1985) first described endometrial cancer in three patients treated with tamoxifen. Over the last 8–9 years, a series of about 25 reports (Seoud, Johnson & Weed, 1993; Segna et al, 1992) presented about 100 cases of endometrial cancer in patients treated with tamoxifen. Since all the breast cancer studies were not designed to determine the risk of endometrial cancer with tamoxifen, precise quantitation of RR is not possible. However, it would appear that the incidence is low and the risk is two- to three-fold higher than the general population (Fisher et al, 1994). Patients should have routine gynecological care and report any abnormal vaginal bleeding or pelvic symptoms to their physicians.

OTHER HORMONAL AGENTS

The hormonal approach so far applied to the treatment of breast cancer, including tamoxifen, GnRH analog and aromatase inhibitors, has not achieved complete inhibition of all stimulatory actions of estrogens in breast cancer patients. The search is ongoing for new agents or combinations of these agents to completely block the stimulatory effect of estrogens with an improved toxicity profile.

In postmenopausal women with metastatic breast cancer, second-line treatment with another hormonal drug is feasible when first-line therapy fails. Research efforts are also ongoing to find drugs which show improved efficacy and tolerability over existing agents.

Anti-estrogens

Toremifene, a chlorinated triphemylethylene derivative chemically related to tamoxifen, has been evaluated in a number of trials in women with advanced breast cancer (Pyrhonen, 1990). These trials have not demonstrated any added benefit in either efficacy or safety over the comparator, tamoxifen, when given as first-line treatment for advanced breast cancer. Some clinical studies (Ebbs, Roberts & Baum, 1987) have shown that high-dose toremifene may be active against tumors for which tamoxifen is ineffective. Preclinical studies (Kangas et al, 1986) have shown that high-dose toremifene may act against tumors without estrogen receptors. A trial from the UK (Ebbs, Roberts & Baum, 1987) reported a significant response rate (25%), whereas other studies, including the USA study (Vogel et al, 1993) and the Helsinki study (Pyrhonen et al, 1994), showed response rates at the level of 4.5%. The Swedish study (Jonsson, 1991) showed no responses in patients who did not respond to tamoxifen.

Droloxifene is another derivative of tamoxifen with anti-estrogenic activity which is currently being tested in clinical trials. Relative to tamoxifene, droloxifene has a 10–60-fold higher binding affinity to the estrogen receptor (Roos et al, 1983) and with lower estrogenic effects on the rat uterus (Loser et al, 1985). In a large multicenter trial, the drug produced an overall response rate of 39% (Bruning, 1992), which is similar to response rates that have been reported with tamoxifen.

A new anti-estrogen, ICI 182780, offers potential advantages over tamoxifen in the treatment of breast cancer. ICI 182780 is a steroidal analog which has high affinity for the estrogen receptor comparable with estradiol and 100-fold greater than tamoxifen (Wakeling, Dukes & Bowler, 1991). In vitro studies with human breast cancer cell lines and in vivo studies in animals have demonstrated potent anti-estrogenic and antitumor activity while having no measurable estrogenic activity (Wakeling, Dukes & Bowler, 1991). Of significance is the antitumor activity in breast cancer cell lines resistant to tamoxifen. These preclinical studies suggest potential advantages over tamoxifen, such as more rapid and complete tumor inhibition; longer duration before relapse; significant antitumor activity after tamoxifen resistance develops; decreased potential for tumor flare with the initiation of treatment; and decrease potential for estrogenic activity on reproductive organs. Early clinical trials with ICI 182780 have been encouraging. In a study reported by Howell et al (1995), 19 postmenopausal women with advanced breast cancer who had clinical progression while on tamoxifen were treated with ICI 182780. Thirteen (69%) received treatment for a median duration of 18 months, and nine were still continuing treatment at the time of this report. Further studies are necessary, but the early results offer promise of greater efficacy of ICI 182780 in both first- and second-line treatment.

Aromatase Inhibitors

Aromatase inhibitors represent another approach to the treatment of advanced breast cancer in postmenopausal women. They decrease circulating estrogens by inhibiting their biosynthesis via the aromatase enzyme, which catalyzes the final step in estrogen production in humans (Thompson & Siiteri, 1974). There are two main types of aromatase inhibitors; the competitive type and the mechanism-based or suicide inhibitors. The competitive inhibitors bind reversibly to the enzyme complex and prevent production of estrone from androstenedione; suicide inhibitors compete with androstenedione and testosterone and irreversibly bind to the action sites of aromatase (Santen, 1990, 1991).

Aminoglutethimide, an aromatase inhibitor, is a widely used second-line agent for the treatment of advanced breast cancer in postmenopausal patients. Tamoxifen and aminoglutethimide have been shown to produce comparable response rates in postmenopausal women with advanced breast cancer. However, tamoxifen lacks the significant side effects associated with aminoglutethimide (Petru & Schmahl, 1987). In particular, aminoglutethimide requires the concomitant use of glucocorticoids and in some patients mineralocorticoids due to the inhibition of cytochrome P-450 enzymes other than aromatase. A number of newer aromatase inhibitors are currently being clinically evaluated (Goss et al, 1994; Jonat et al, 1995). Not only are these agents showing an improved safety profile, but greater decreases in estrogen levels have been reported. Both ICI-D1033 (Arimidex) and CGS-20267 (Letrozole) have shown estradiol levels suppressed to the quantitation limits of sensitive assays without inhibition of adrenal steroidal synthesis. Jonat et al (1995) have recently reported, in a large phase III trial with Arimidex in post-menopausal women with advanced breast cancer who progressed on tamoxifen, that efficacy was similar to the comparator, megestrol acetate, but Arimidex was better tolerated.

GnRH Analogs

Gonadrotropin releasing hormone (GnRH) analogs offer another approach to the hormonal treatment of premenopausal women with breast cancer (Schally, Redding & Cumaru-Schally, 1984). Continuous administration of these agents leads to the desensitization of the pituitary and a subsequent decrease in luteinizing (LH) and follicle-stimulating hormone (FSH) secretion. This in turn reduces the circulating estrogen level to the postmenopausal range, similar to that seen with oophorectomy.

Goserelin acetate (Zoladex), a long-acting GnRH analog, has recently received approval by the FDA for use in premenopausal women with hormonal-sensitive breast cancer. The drug leads to significant suppression of estradiol by the ovaries (Furr, 1987). Clinical results haved shown goserelin to be as effective as oophor-ectomy and thereby eliminates the need for this surgery (Blamey et al, 1992; Boccardo et al, 1994).

Progestational Agents

The use of progestational agents, including high-dose oral or intramuscular medroxyprogesterone acetate (MPA), and megestrol acetate, has been shown to produce response rates ranging from 21% to 54%. These response rates are not significantly different from those produced by tamoxifen (Petru & Schmahl, 1987; Kiang et al, 1980; Nemoto et al, 1984; Ingle et al, 1981; Matelski et al, 1985; Van Veelen et al, 1986). A recent Swiss study (Gastiglione-Gertsch et al, 1993) reported higher response rates with high-dose parenteral MPA, but overall survival was not significantly different than in patients treated with tamoxifen.

The toxicity associated with the use of currently available progestins have limited their use. Undesired weight gain, fluid retention and thrombo-embolic events are the commonly reported adverse events.

Newer progestins are being evaluated to determine whether efficacy can be improved with a better side effect profile. The antiprogestin, mifepristone (RU486), has been shown to inhibit mammary cancer cell growth in cell lines and in DMBA-induced breast cancers in rats (Michna et al, 1992). Early clinical trials have also demonstrated some beneficial activity in postmenopausal women (Michna et al, 1992). Other anti-progesterone agents, such as Onapristone and ZK112993, have less anti-glucocorticoid activity and may be less toxic than current agents (Michna et al, 1992).

Estrogen and Androgen Analogs

Diethylstilbestrol (DES) and ethinylestradiol were used in the past as initial treatment for postmenopausal women with advanced disease (Ingle et al, 1981; Matelski et al, 1985); they have been shown to produce response rates of about 30%; similar response rate, response duration and overall survival have been shown in women treated with tamoxifen as first-line therapy. However, adverse effects, including nausea, vomiting, and water retention, were reported to be two to four times higher in patients treated with DES instead of tamoxifen.

PREVENTION

The term 'chemoprevention' was introduced about 20 years ago by Sporn to define the inhibition or reversal of carcinogenesis by the use of natural nutrients or non-toxic pharmacologic compounds that protect against the development and progression of malignancy (Sporn, 1976). Development of cancer involves a multistep process 'defined' as carcinogenesis (Sporn, 1991). Carcinogenesis may arise as a result of chemical, physical, biologic and/or genetic insults to cells (Weinstein, 1991). Inhibitors of carcinogenesis can be classified by the point in the carcinogenic process at which they act: (a) they may prevent the formation or absorption of carcinogens; (b) they may prevent carcinogens from reaching or reacting with cellular targets; or (c) they may suppress the expression of neoplasia (Wattenberg, 1985). Primary prevention and secondary prevention, e.g. screening or early detection, are currently employed to reduce breast cancer mortality. As few alterable risk factors for breast cancer have been identified, efforts have focused on using a drug or combination of drugs to prevent breast cancer (chemoprevention).

To initiate any chemoprevention trial, an agent or combination that can block the carcinogenic process and has very low toxicity needs to be identified. Furthermore, the ability to identify accurately women at high risk for breast cancer is essential. Any selected agent must have proven efficacy and be non-toxic to the healthy women, who may be required to take the agent for many years. Currently, two pharmacologic agents are being tested, the anti-estrogen tamoxifen (Lerner & Jordan, 1990) and retinoids (Moon & Mehta, 1990).

The biologic rationale for using tamoxifen as a chemopreventive agent is provided by data showing a reduced incidence of second primary breast cancers in women with stage I and II breast cancer treated with adjuvant tamoxifen. In the largest tamoxifen studies, including the Stockholm trial (Rutqvist et al, 1995), NSABP B14 trial (Fisher et al, 1994), Cancer Research Campaign trial (CRC Adjuvant Breast Trial Working Party, 1988), and Scottish trial (Breast Cancer Trials Committee, 1987), the reported reduction in contralateral breast cancers ranged between 40% and 50%.

Retinoids are potent regulators of cell differentiation and proliferation, essentially in all epithelia that are sites for development of invasive cancer. Retinoids have been shown to induce premalignant lesions to differentiate (Sporn, 1991; Sporn & Roberts, 1983). The retinoids may potentially control the replication of both estrogen-dependent and estrogen-independent disease, based on preclinical data; very little clinical experience with retinoids is available (Moon & Mehta, 1990).

Currently there are four ongoing breast cancer prevention studies, three involving tamoxifen and one using the retinoid N-4-hydroxyphenyl retinamide (4-HPR).

In a pilot study and the subsequent trial at the Royal Marsden Hospital (Powles et al, 1989, 1990), 2000 high-risk women were randomized to receive either tamoxifen 20 mg/day or placebo for 3 years. High-risk women were defined as those with at least one first-degree relative diagnosed with premenopausal breast cancer or bilateral breast cancer at any age, or with at least two first-degree relatives with breast cancer at any age, a personal history of unilateral breast cancer or atypical hyperplasia, or age over 40.

A trial conducted by NSABP (Fisher, 1992) is studying about 16 000 high-risk women, older than 35 years, randomized to receive either tamoxifen 20 mg/day or placebo for an initial period of 5 years. High-risk women are those older than 60 years, with or without risk factors, or 35–59 years old with risk factors, including breast biopsy-proven lobular carcinoma in situ or atypical hyperplasia, first-degree relative with breast cancer, age more than 25 years before birth of first child, no children, or menarche before age 12.

The other two chemoprevention trials are being conducted in Italy. The first trial is using 4-HPR; 3000 women have been enrolled in the study. High-risk women are defined as those with unilateral T1 or T2, and node-negative breast carcinomas who did not receive adjuvant chemotherapy or hormonal therapy.

The second trial has enrolled 1000 patients; criteria for participation include age older than 45 years with a history of hysterectomy. The trial has been designed to enroll a total of 20 000 women. Randomization is between 20 mg/day of tamoxifen and placebo for 5 years.

REFERENCES

Abrams AA. Use of vitamin E in chronic cystic mastitis. *N Engl J Med* 1965; **272**: 1080–81.

Albanes D. Total calories, body weight, and tumor incidence in mice. *Cancer Res* 1987; **47**: 1987–92.

Alexieva-Figusch J, Van Putten WL, Blankenstein MA et al. The prognostic value and relationships of patient characteristics, estrogen and progestin receptors, and site of relapse in primary breast cancer. *Cancer* 1988; **61**: 758–68.

Allred DC, Clark GM, Elledge RM et al. Accumulation of mutant p53 is associated with increased proliferation and poor clinical outcome in node (–) breast cancer. *J Natl Cancer Inst* 1993; **85**: 200–6.

Ariel IM, Kempner R. The prognosis of patients who become pregnant after mastectomy for breast cancer. *Int Surg* 1989; **74**: 185–7.

Armstrong B, Doll R. Environmental factors and cancer incidence and mortality in different countries, with special reference to dietary practices. *Int J Cancer* 1975; **15**: 617–31.

Arteaga CL, Coronado E, Osborne CK. Blockade of the EGF receptor inhibits TGF-alpha induced but not estrogen-induced growth of hormone-dependent human breast cancer. *Mol Endocrinol* 1988; **2**: 1064–9.

Auger MJ, Mackie MJ. Effect of tamoxifen in blood coagulation. *Cancer* 1988; **61**: 1316–19.

Barker S, Vincent GP. EGF in breast cancer. *Int J Biochem* 1990; **22**: 939–45.

Baron JA, Byers T, Greenberg ER et al. Cigarette smoking in women with cancer of the breast and reproductive organs. *J Natl Cancer Inst* 1987; **77**: 677–80.

Bartek J, Bartkova J, Vojtesek B et al. Aberrant expression of the p53 oncoprotein is a common feature of wide spectrum of human malignancies. *Oncogene* 1991; **6**: 1699–1703.

Bartek J, Bartkova J, Vojtesek B et al. Patterns of expression of the p53 tumour suppressor in human breast tissues and tumours in situ and in vitro. *Int J Cancer* 1990; **46**: 839–44.

Bassett LW, Liu TH, Giuliano AC et al. The prevalence of carcinoma in palpable vs impalpable mammographically detected lesions. *Am J Radiol* 1991; **157**: 21–4.

Benner SE, Clark GM, McGuire WL. Review: steroid receptors, cellular kinetics and LN status as prognostic factors in breast cancer. *Am J Med Sci* 1988; **296**: 59–66.

Benry J, Green EJ, Matheson DS. Modulation of natural killer cell activity by tamoxifen in stage 1 postmenopausal breast cancer. *Eur J Cancer Clin Oncol* 1987; **23**: 517–20.

Benz CC, Scott GK, Sarup JC et al. Estrogen-dependent tamoxifen resistant tumorigenic growth of MCF-7 cells transfected with HER 2/neu. *Breast Cancer Res Treat* 1992; **24**: 85–95.

Bergkvist L, Adami H, Persson I et al. Prognosis after breast cancer diagnosis in women exposed to estrogen and estrogen replacement therapy. *Am J Epidemiol* 1989; **130**: 221–8.

Bergkvist L, Adami HO, Persson I et al. The risk of breast cancer after estrogen and estrogen progestin replacement. *N Engl J Med* 1989; **321**: 293–7.

Berns PMJJ, Foekens JA, Van Putten WLJ et al. Prognostic factors in human primary breast cancer. Comparison of c-myc and HER 2/neu amplification. *J Steroid Biochem Mol Biol* 1992a; **43**: 13–19.

Berns PMJJ, Klijn JGM, Van Putten WLJ et al. C-myc amplification is a better prognostic factor than HER 2/neu amplification in primary breast cancer. *Cancer Res* 1992b; **52**: 1107–14.

Berns PMJJ, Klijn JGM, van Staveren IL et al. Sporadic amplification of the insulin-like growth factor I. Receptor gene in human breast tumors. *Cancer Res* 1992c; **52**: 1036–9.

Bernstein L, Ross RK, Lobo RA. The effects of moderate physical activity on menstrual cycle patterns in adolescence: implications for breast cancer prevention. *Br J Cancer* 1987; **55**: 681–5.

Black MM, Opler SR, Speer FD. Survival in breast cancer cases in relation to the structure of the primary tumor and regional LNs. *Surg Gynecol Obstet* 1955; **100**: 543–51.

Blamey R, Jonat W, Kaufmann M et al. Goserelin depot in the treatment of premenopausal advanced breast cancer. *Eur J Cancer* 1992; **28A**: 810–14.

Bloom HJG, Richardson WW. Histological grading and prognosis in breast cancer. *Br J Cancer* 1957; **11**: 359–77.

Boccardo F, Rubagotti A, Amoroso D et al. Chemotherapy vs tamoxifen vs chemotherapy + tamoxifen in node positive estrogen receptor positive breast cancer patients. An update at 7 years of the first GROCTA trial. *Eur J Cancer* 1992; **28**: 673–89.

Boccardo F, Rubagotti A, Perotta A et al. Ovarian ablation versus goserelin with or without tamoxifen in pre-perimenopausal patients with advanced breast cancer: results of a multicentric Italian study. *Ann Oncol* 1994; **5**(4): 337–42.

Bodian CA, Lattes R, Perzin KH. The epidemiology of gross cystic disease of the breast confirmed by biopsy or by aspiration of cyst fluid. *Cancer Detect Prev* 1992; **16**: 7–15.

Bodian CA, Perzin KH, Lattes R et al. Risk of breast cancer after proliferative benign disease. *Cancer* (in press).

Boice JD, Land CE, Shore RE et al. Risk of breast cancer following low-dose radiation exposure. *Radiology* 1979; **131**: 589–97.

Bonneterre J, Peyrat JP, Benscart R et al. Prognostic significance of IGF-1 receptors in human breast cancer. *Cancer Res* 1990; **50**: 6931–5.

Breast Cancer Trials Committee, Scottish Cancer Trials Office: adjuvant tamoxifen in the management of operable breast cancer. The Scottish trial. *Lancet* 1987; **2**: 171–5.

Brignone G, Cusimano R, Dardanomi G et al. A case control study on breast cancer risk factors in a Southern European population. *Int J Epidemiol* 1987; **16**: 356–61.

Brinton LA, Hoover R, Fraumeni JF Jr. Menopausal estrogens and breast cancer risk: an expanded case-control study. *Br J Cancer* 1986; **54**: 825–32.

Brinton LA, Hoover RN, Szklo M et al. Menopausal estrogen use and risk of breast cancer. *Cancer* 1981; **47**: 2517–23.

Brinton LA, Schairer C, Hoover RN et al. Menstrual factors and risk of breast cancer. *Cancer Invest* 1988; **6**: 245–54.

Bruning PF. Droloxifene, a new anti-estrogen in postmenopausal advanced breast cancer: preliminary results of a double-blind dose-finding phase II trial. *Eur J Cancer* 1992; **28A**: 1404–7.

Buell P. Changing incidence of breast cancer in Japanese-American women. *J Natl Cancer Inst* 1973; **51**: 1479–83.

Bulbrook RD, Moore JW, Clarke GM et al. Relation between risk of breast cancer and biological availability of estradiol in the blood: prospective study in Guernsey. *Ann NY Acad Sci* 1986; **464**: 378–88.

Bundred NJ, West RR, O'Dowd J et al. Is there an increased risk of breast cancer in women who have had a breast cyst aspirated? *Br J Cancer* 1991; **64**: 953–5.

Byers T, Graham S, Rzepka T et al. Lactation and breast cancer: evidence for a negative association in premenopausal women. *Am J Epidemiol* 1985; **121**: 664–74.

Byrd BF, Burch JC, Vaughn WK. The impact of long-term estrogen support after hysterectomy: a report of 1016 cases. *Ann Surg* 1977; **185**: 574–80.

Cameron E, Pauling L, Leibovitz B. Ascorbic acid and cancer: a review. *Cancer Res* 1979; **39**: 663–81.

Cancer and Steroid Hormone Study of the Centers for Disease Control and the National Institute of Child Health and Human Development. Oral contraceptive use and the risk of breast cancer. *N Engl J Med* 1986; **315**: 405–11.

Canney PA, Griffiths T, Latiaf TN et al. Clinical significance of tamoxifen withdrawal response. *Lancet* 1987; **1**: 36.

Cannon-Albright L, Thomas A, Goldgar DE et al. Familiality of cancer in Utah. *Cancer Res* 1994; **54**: 2378.

Carroll KK. Experimental studies on dietary fat and cancer in relation to epidemiological data. *Prog Clin Biol Res* 1986; **222**: 231–48.

Carter CL, Allen C, Henson DE. Relation of tumor size, LN status, and survival in 24 740 breast cancer cases. *Cancer* 1989; **63**: 181–7.

Chen J, Campbell TC, Li J, Peto R. *Diet, Life-style and Mortality in China: A Study of the Characteristics of 65 Chinese Counties* 1990, p 750; Oxford: Oxford University Press.

Ciatto S, Cecchini S, Del Turco MR et al. Referral policy and positive predictive value of call for surgical biopsy in the Florence Breast Cancer Screening Program. *J Clin Epidemiol* 1990; **43**: 419–23.

Clark GM, Dressler LG, Owens MA et al. Prediction of relapse or survival in patients with node negative breast cancer by flow cytometry. *N Engl J Med* 1989; **320**: 627–33.

Clark RM, Reid J. Carcinoma of the breast in pregnancy and lactation. *Int J Radiat Oncol Biol Phys* 1978; **4**: 693–8.

Clarke R, Dickson RB, Lippman ME. Hormonal aspects of breast cancer. GF, drugs and stromal interactions. *Crit Rev Oncol/Hematol* 1992; **12**: 1–23.

Claus EB, Risch N, Thompson WD. Age of onset as an indicator of familial risk of breast cancer. *Am J Epidemiol* 1990; **131**: 961–72.

Claus EB, Thompson WD, Risch N. Genetic analysis of breast cancer in the cancer and steroid hormone study. *Am J Hum Genet* 1991; **48**: 232–42.

Clave F, Andrieu N, Gairard B et al. Oral contraceptives and breast cancer: a French case-control study. *Int J Epidemiol* 1991; **20**: 32–8.

Clemmons DR, Elgin RG, Han VKM et al. Cultured fibroblast monolayers secrete a protein that alters the cellular binding of somatomedin-c/IGFI. *J Clin Invest* 1986; **77**: 1548–56.

Colditz GA, Egan KM, Stampfer MJ. Hormone replacement therapy and risk of breast cancer. Results from epidemiologic studies. *Am J Obstet Gynecol* 1993; **168**: 1473–80.

Colditz GA, Hankinson SE, Hunter DJ et al. The use of estrogens and progestins and the risk of breast cancer in postmenopausal women. *N Engl J Med* 1995; **332**: 1589–93.

Colditz GA, Willett WC, Hunter DJ et al. Family history, age, and risk of breast cancer. A prospective data from the Nurses Health Study. *JAMA* 1993; **270**: 338–43.

Cole MP, Jones CTA, Todd IDH. A new antiestrogenic agent in late breast cancer. An early clinical appraisal of ICI 46,474. *Br J Cancer* 1971; **25**: 270–5.

Colletta AA, Wakefield LM, Howell FU et al. Antiestrogens induce the secretion of active TGF-B from human fetal fibroblasts. *Br J Cancer* 1990; **62**: 405–9.

Cooper MR. The role of chemotherapy for node negative breast cancer. *Cancer* 1991; **67**(suppl): 1744–7.

CRC Adjuvant Breast Trial Working Party. Cyclophosphamide and tamoxifen as adjuvant therapies in the management of breast cancer. *Br J Cancer* 1988; **57**: 604–7.

Cummings FJ, Gray R, Davis TE et al. Adjuvant tamoxifen treatment of elderly women with stage II breast cancer. A double blind comparison with placebo. *Ann Intern Med* 1985; **103**: 324–9.

Cummings FJ, Gray R, Tormey DC et al. Adjuvant tamoxifen vs placebo in elderly women with node positive breast cancer. Long term F/U and causes of death. *J Clin Oncol* 1993; **11**: 29–35.

Davis HH, Simons N, Davis JC. Cystic disease of the breast: relationship to carcinoma. *Cancer* 1964; **17**: 957–75.

de Waard F, Baanders van Halewijn EA. A prospective study in general practice of breast cancer risk in postmenopausal women. *Int J Cancer* 1974; **14**: 153–60.

Delgado-Rodriguez M, Sillero-Arenas M, Rodriguez M et al. Oral contraceptives and breast cancer. A meta-analysis. *Rev Epidemiol Sante Publique* 1991; **39**: 165–81.

Dickson RB, Lippman ME. Control of human breast cancer by estrogen, GF, and oncogenes. In Lippman ME, Dickson RB (eds) *Breast Cancer: Cellular and Molecular Biology* 1988, pp 119–65; Boston, MA: Kluwer Academic.

Dragon YP, Xu YD, Pitot HC. Tumor promotion as a target for estrogen/antiestrogen effects in rat hepatocarcinogenesis. *Prev Med* 1991; **20**: 15–26.

Dupont WD, Page DL. Menopausal estrogen replacement therapy and breast cancer. *Arch Intern Med* 1991; **151**: 67–72.

Dupont WD, Page DL. Risk factors for breast cancer in women with proliferative breast disease. *N Engl J Med* 1985; **312**: 146–51.

Early Breast Cancer Trialist Collaborative Group. Systemic treatment of early breast cancer by hormonal, cytotoxic or immune therapy. *Lancet* 1992; **339**: 1–15, 71–85.

Easton DF, Bishop DT, Ford D et al. Genetic linkage analysis in familial breast and ovarian cancer: results from 214 families. The breast cancer linkage consortium. *Am J Hum Genet* 1993; **52**(4): 678–701.

Ebbs SR, Roberts JV, Baum M. Alternative mechanisms of action of antiestrogens in breast cancer. *Lancet* 1987; **ii**: 621.

Eeles RA. Predictive testing for germline mutation in the p53 gene: are all the questions answered? *Eur J Cancer* 1993; **29A**: 1361–5.

Ellison PT, Lager C. Moderate recreational running is associated with lower salivary progesterone profiles in women. *Am J Obstet Gynecol* 1986; **154**: 1000–1003.

Elwood JM, Cox B, Richardson AK et al. The effectiveness of breast cancer screening by mammography in younger women. *Online J Curr Clin Trials* (serial outline) 1993; **2**, Doc NR 32.

Evans JS, Wennberg JE, McNeil BJ. The influence of diagnostic radiography on the incidence of breast cancer and leukemia. *N Engl J Med* 1986; **315**: 810–15.

Ewertz M. Influence of non-contraceptive exogenous and endogenous sex hormones on breast cancer risk in Denmark. *Int J Cancer* 1988; **42**: 832–8.

Feuer EJ, Wun LM, Boring CC et al. The lifetime risk of developing breast cancer. *J Natl Cancer Inst* 1993; **85**: 892–7.

Fisher B, Constantino JP, Redwood CK et al. Endometrial cancer in tamoxifen-treated breast cancer patients: findings from the NSABP B14 Trial. *J Natl Cancer Inst* 1994; **86**: 527–73.

Fisher B, Constantino J, Redwood C et al. A randomized clinical trial evaluating tamoxifen in the treatment of patients with node-negative breast cancer who have estrogen receptor-positive tumors. *N Engl J Med* 1989; **320**: 479–84.

Fisher B, Redmond C, Fisher ER et al. Relative worth of estrogen or progesterone receptor, and pathologic characteristics of differentiation as indicators of prognosis in node (−) breast cancer patients. Findings from National Surgical Adjuvant Breast and Bowel Project, Protocol B-06. *J Clin Oncol* 1988; **6**: 1076–87.

Fisher B, Slack NH, Bross IDJ et al. Cancer of the breast. Size of neoplasm and prognosis. *Cancer* 1969; **24**: 1071–80.

Fisher B. Experimental and clinical justification for the use of tamoxifen in a breast cancer prevention trial. A description of the NSABP effort. *Proc Am Assn Cancer Res* 1992; **33**: A567–8 (abstr).

Fisher ER, Redmond C, Fisher B. Histologic grading of breast cancer. In Sommers SC, Rosen PP (eds) *Pathology Annual* 1980, pp 239–51; Norwalk, CT: Appleton Century Crofts.

Fletcher SW, Balck W, Harris R et al. Report of the International Workshop on Screening for Breast Cancer. *J Natl Cancer Inst* 1993; **85**: 1644–56.

Folsom AR, McKenzie DR, Bisgard KM et al. No association between caffeine intake and postmenopausal breast cancer incidence in the Iowa Women's Health Study. *Am J Epidemiol* 1993; **138**: 380–83.

Friedenreich CM, Howe GR, Miller AB et al. A cohort study of alcohol consumption and risk of breast cancer. *Am J Epidemiol* 1993; **137**: 512–20.

Furr BJA. Pharmacological trials with Zoladex, a novel luteinizing hormone releasing hormone analog. *Roy Soc Med Int Congr Sympos Ser* 1987; **125**: 1–15.

Gagliardi A, Collins DC. Inhibition of angiogenesis by antiestrogens. *Cancer Res* 1993; **53**: 533–5.

Gambrell RD Jr. Hormones in the etiology and prevention of breast cancer and endometrial cancer. *South Med J* 1984; **77**: 1509–15.

Garland CF, Friedlauder NJ, Barrett-Connor E et al. Sex hormones and postmenopausal breast cancer: a prospective study in an adult community. *Am J Epidemiol* 1992; **135**: 1220–30.

Gastiglione-Gertsch M, Pampallona S, Varim M et al. Primary endocrine therapy for advanced breast cancer: to start with tamoxifen or with medroxyprogesterone acetate. *Ann Oncol* 1993; **4**: 735–40.

Gibson TC. Severe hypercalcemia and tamoxifen flares. *Br J Clin Practice* 1990; **44**: 716–17.

Glass AG, Hoover RN. Rising incidence of BC: relationship to stage and receptor status. *J Natl Cancer Inst* 1990; **82**: 693–6.

Goodwin PJ, Boyd NF. Critical appraisal of the evidence that dietary fat intake is related to breast cancer risk in humans. *J Natl Cancer Inst* 1987; **179**: 473–85.

Goss EP, Gwyn MEH et al. Current perspectives in aromatase inhibitors in breast cancer. *J Clin Oncol* 1994; **12**: 2460–70.

Graham ML II, Krett NL, Miller LA et al. T4 Dco cells genetically unstable and containing estrogen receptor mutations are a model for the progression of breast cancers to hormone resistance. *Cancer Res* 1990; **50**: 6208–17.

Graham S, Marshall J, Mettlin C et al. Diet in the epidemiology of breast cancer. *Am J Epidemiol* 1982; **116**: 68–75.

Graham S, Zielezny M, Marshall J et al. Diet in the epidemiology of postmenopausal breast cancer in the NY State Cohort. *Am J Epidemiol* 1992; **136**: 1327–37.

Griffiths MF. Tamoxifen retinopathy at low dosages. *Am J Ophthalmol* 1991; **104**: 185–6.

Hall JM, Lee MK, Newman B et al. Linkage of early-onset familial breast cancer to chromosome 17q21. *Science* 1990; **250**: 1684–9.

Hankey BF, Brinton LA, Kessler LG et al. Breast. In Miller BA, Ries LA, Hankey BF et al (eds) *SEER Cancer Statistics Review 1973–1990* 1993, pp IV.1–IV.24 (NIH Publication 93-2789); Bethesda, MD: National Cancer Institute.

Hankey BF, Curtis RE, Naughton MD et al. A retrospective cohort analysis of second breast cancer risk for primary breast cancer patients with an assessment of the effect of radiation therapy. *J Natl Cancer Inst* 1983; **70**: 797–804.

Harper MJK, Walpole AL. Contrasting endocrine activities of *cis* and *trans* isomers in a series of substituted triphenylethylenes. *Nature* 1966; **212**: 87.

Harrington E, Lesnick G. The association between gross cysts of the breast and breast cancer. *Breast* 1981; **7**: 13–17.

Harvey JC, Rosen PP, Ashikari R et al. The effect of pregnancy in the prognosis of carcinoma of the breast following radical mastectomy. *Surg Gynecol Obstet* 1981; **153**: 723–5.

Hedley DW, Clark G, Cornelisse CJ et al. Consensus review of the clinical utility of DNA cytometry in cancer of the breast. *Breast Cancer Res Treat* 1993; **28**: 55–9.

Helzlsouer KJ. Epidemiology, prevention and early detection of breast cancer. *Curr Opin Oncol* 1994; **6**: 541–8.

Henderson BE, Ross R, Bernstein L. Estrogens as a cause of human cancer. *Cancer Res* 1988; **48**: 246–53.

Henderson BE, Ross RK, Judd HL et al. Do regular ovulatory cycles increase breast cancer risk? *Cancer* 1985; **56**: 1206–8.

Hildreth NG, Shore RE, Dvortsky PM. The risk of breast cancer after irradiation of the thymus in infancy. *N Engl J Med* 1989; **321**: 1281–4.

Hildreth NG, Shore RE, Hempelmann LH. Risk of breast cancer among women receiving radiation therapy in infancy for thymic enlargement. *Lancet* 1983; **2**: 273.

Hill SM, Fuqua SAW, Chamness GC et al. Estrogen receptor expression in human breast cancer associated with an estrogen receptor gene restriction fragment length polymorphism. *Cancer Res* 1989; **49**: 145–8.

Hirayama T. Diet and cancer. *Nutr Cancer* 1979; **1**: 67–81.

Hirayama T. Epidemiology of breast cancer with special reference to the role of diet. *Prev Med* 1978; **7**: 173–95.

Hollstein MC, Sidransky D, Vogelstein B et al. p53 Mutation in human cancers. *Science* 1991; **253**: 49–53.

Hoogstraten B, Fletcher WS, Gad-el-Mawla N et al. Tamoxifen and oophorectomy in the treatment of recurrent breast cancer. A Southwest Oncology Group study. *Cancer Res* 1982; **42**: 4788–91.

Hoover R, Glass A, Finkle W et al. Conjugated estrogens and breast cancer risk in women. *J Natl Cancer Inst* 1981; **67**: 815–20.

Hoover R, Gray L, Cole P et al. Menopausal estrogens and breast cancer. *N Engl J Med* 1976; **295**: 401–5.

Horwitz KB, McGuire WL. Predicting response to endocrine therapy in human breast cancer: a hypothesis. *Science* 1975; **189**: 726–7.

Horwitz KB. The molecular biology of RV 486: is there a role of antiprogestins in the treatment of breast cancer? *Endocr Rev* 1992; **13**: 146–69.

Houlston RS, McCaiter E, Parbhoo S et al. Family history and risk of breast cancer. *J Med Genet* 1992; **29**: 154–7.

Howard J. Using mammography for cancer control: an unrealized potential. *CA Cancer J Clin* 1987; **37**: 34–48.

Howe G, Rohan T, Decarli A et al. The association between alcohol and breast cancer risk: evidence from the combined analysis of six dietary case-control studies. *Int J Cancer* 1991; **47**: 707–10.

Howe GR, Hirohata T, Hislop TG et al. Dietary factors and risk of breast cancer: combined analysis of 12 case-control studies. *J Natl Cancer Inst* 1990; **82**: 561–9.

Howell A, DeFriend D, Robertson J et al. Responses to a specific antiestrogen (ICI 182780) in a tamoxifen-resistant breast cancer. *Lancet* 1995; **345**: 29–30.

Hsieh CC, Trichopoulos D, Kastouyanni K et al. Age at menarche, age at menopause, height and obesity as risk factors for breast cancer: associations and interactions in an international case-control study. *Int J Cancer* 1990; **46**: 796–800.

Huff KK, Knabbe C, Lindsey R et al. Multihormonal regulation of IGF-I related protein in MGF-7 human breast cancer cells. *Mol Endocrinol* 1988; **2**: 200–208.

Hunt K, Vessey M, McPherson K et al. Long-term surveillance of mortality and breast cancer incidence in women receiving hormone replacement therapy. *Br J Obstet Gynaecol* 1987; **94**: 620–35.

Hunt K, Vessey M, McPherson K. Mortality in a cohort of long-term users of ERT: our updated analysis. *Br J Obstet Gynaecol* 1990; **97**: 1080–86.

Hunter DJ, Manson JE, Colditz G et al. A prospective study of the intake of vitamins C, E and A and the risk of breast cancer. *N Engl J Med* 1993; **329**: 234–40.

Hunter DJ, Morris JS, Stampfer MJ et al. A prospective study of selenium status and breast cancer risk. *JAMA* 1990; **264**: 1128–31.

Hunter DJ, Willett WC. Diet, body size, and breast cancer. *Epidemiol Rev* 1993; **15**: 110–32.

IARC (International Agency for Research on Cancer). Occupational exposures in insecticide application and some pepticides. *IARC Monogr Eval Carcinog Risk Chem Man* 1991; **53**: 179–249.

Ikeda T, Danielpour D, Sirbasku DA. Characterization of a sheep pituitary-derived GF for rat and human mammary tumor cells. *J Cell Biochem* 1984; **25**: 213–29.

Imai Y, Leung CKH, Friesen HG et al. Epidermal growth factor receptors and effect of epidermal growth factor on growth of human breast cancer cells in long term tissue cultures. *Cancer Res* 1989; **42**: 4394–8.

Ingle JN, Ahmann DL, Green SJ et al. Randomized clinical trial of DES vs tamoxifen in postmenopausal women with advanced breast cancer. *N Engl J Med* 1981; **304**: 16–21.

Ingle JN, Krook JE, Gren SJ et al. Randomized trial of bilateral oophorectomy vs tamoxifen in premenopausal women with metastatic breast cancer. *J Clin Oncol* 1986; **4**: 178–85.

Ingle JN, Mailliard JA, Schaid DJ et al. A double blind trial of tamoxifen plus placebo in postmenopausal women with metastatic breast cancer. A collaborative trial of the North Central Cancer Treatment Group and Mayo Clinic. *Cancer* 1991; **68**: 34–9.

Irwin KL, Lee NC, Peterson HB et al. Hysterectomy, tubal sterilization, and the risk of breast cancer. *Am J Epidemiol* 1988; **127**: 1192–1201.

Jacobsen BK, Bjelke E, Kvale G et al. Coffee drinking, mortality and cancer incidence: results from a Norwegian prospective study. *J Natl Cancer Inst* 1986; **76**: 823–31.

Jonat W, Howell A, Blomqvist CP et al. A randomized trial of the new specific aromatase inhibitor ARIMIDEX vs megestrol acetate in the treatment of postmenopausal women with advanced breast cancer. *Proc Am Soc Clin Oncol* 1995; abstr 130.

Jonsson PE, Malmberg M, Bergljung L et al. Phase II study of high-dose toremifene in advanced breast cancer progressing during tamoxifen therapy. *Anticancer Res* 1991; **11**: 873–6.

Kaiser-Kupfer MI, Lippman ME. Tamoxifen retinopathy. *Cancer Treat Rep* 1978; **62**: 315–20.

Kampert JB, Whittemore AS, Paffenbarger RS Jr. Combined effects of childbearing, menstrual events and body size on age-specific breast cancer risk. *Am J Epidemiol* 1988; **128**: 962–79.

Kamrin MA, Fischer LJ. Workshop on human health impacts of halogenated biphenyl and related compounds. *Environ Health Perspect* 1991; **91**: 157–64.

Kangas L, Nieminen A-L, Blanco G et al. A new triphenylethylene compound Fc-1157-a II. Antitumor effects. *Cancer Chemother Pharmacol* 1986; **17**: 109–13.

Karey KP, Sirbasku DA. Differential responsiveness of human breast cancer cell lines MCF-7 and T47D to growth factors and 17B-estradiol. *Cancer Res* 1988; **48**: 4083–92.

Kaufman DW, Miller DR, Rosenberg L et al. Noncontraceptive estrogen use and the risk of breast cancer. *JAMA* 1984; **252**: 63–7.

Kelsell DP, Black DM, Bishop DT et al. Genetic analysis of the BRCA1 region in a large breast/ovarian family: refinement of the minimal region containing BRCA1. *Hum Mol Genet* 1993; **2**: 1823–8.

Kelsey J, Gammon M, John E. Reproductive and hormonal risk factors. *Epidemiol Rev* 1993; **15**.

Kelsey JL (ed.). Breast cancer. *Epidemiol Rev* 1993; **15**: 1–263.

Kelsey JL, Fisher DB, Holford TR et al. Exogenous estrogens and other factors in the epidemiology of BC. *J Natl Cancer Inst* 1981; **67**: 327–33.

Kerlikowske K, Grady D, Barclay J et al. Positive predictive value of screening mammography by age and family history of breast cancer. *JAMA* 1993; **270**: 2444–50.

Key TJ, Pike MC. The role of estrogens and progestagens in the epidemiology and prevention of breast cancer. *Eur J Cancer Clin Oncol* 1988; **24**: 29–43.

Kiang DT, Frenning DH, Vosika GJ et al. Comparison of tamoxifen and hypophysectomy in breast cancer treatment. *Cancer* 1980; **45**: 1322–5.

Killackey MA, Hakes TB, Pierce VK. Endometrial adenocarcinoma in breast cancer patients receiving antiestrogens. *Cancer Treat Rep* 1985; **69**: 237–8.

King J. Mammography screening for breast cancer. Letter to the Editor. *Cancer* 1994; **73**: 2003–4.

King RJB. A discussion of the roles of estrogen and progestin in human mammary carcinogenesis. *J Steroid Biochem Mol Biol* 1991; **39**: 811–18.

Klijn JGM, Berns EMJ, Foekens JA. Prognostic factors and response to therapy in breast cancer. *Cancer Surv* 1993; **18**: 165–97.

Klijn JGM, Berns PMJJ, Schmitz PI et al. Epidermal GF receptor in clinical breast cancer: update 1993. *Monographs of Endocrine Reviews* (in press).

Klijn JGM, DeJong FH, Bakker GH et al. Antiprogestins, a new form of endocrine therapy for human breast cancer. *Cancer Res* 1989; **49**: 2851–6.

Klijn JGM. Clinical parameters and symptoms for the progression to endocrine independence of breast cancer. In Berus PMJJ, Romiju JC, Schroder FH (eds) *Mechanisms of Progression to Hormone Independent Growth of Breast and Prostate Cancer* 1991, pp 11–19; Caru Forth: Parthenon.

Knabbe C, Lippman ME, Wakefield LM et al. Evidence that transforming growth factor-B is a hormonally regulated negative growth factor in human breast cancer cells. *Cell* 1987; **48**: 417–28.

Knekt P, Aromaa A, Maatela J et al. Serum selenium and subsequent risk of breast cancer among Finnish men and women. *J Natl Cancer Inst* 1989; **81**: 31–5.

Kopans DB, Feig SA. The Canadian National Breast Screening Study. A critical review. *Am J Radiol* 1993; **161**: 755–60.

Kopans DB. *Mammography Screening for Women Ages 40–49* 1995, pp 260–67; Los Angeles, CA: ASCO Educational Books.

Krieger N, Hiatt RA. Risk of breast cancer after benign breast disease: variation by histologic type, degree of atypia, age of biopsy, and length of follow-up. *Am J Epidemiol* 1992; **135**: 619–31.

Krieger N, Wolff MS, Hiatt RA et al. Breast cancer and serum organochlorines: a prospective study among white, black and Asian women. *J Natl Cancer Inst* 1994; **86**: 589–99.

Kumar V, Green S, Stack G et al. Functional domains of the human estrogen receptor. *Cell* 1987; **51**: 941–51.

Kvale G, Heuch I. Lactation and cancer risk: is there any relation specific to breast cancer. *J Epidemiol Commun Health* 1987; **42**: 30–37.

Land CE, Boice JD Jr, Shore RE et al. Breast cancer risk from low-dose exposures to ionizing radiation. Results of parallel analysis of three exposed populations of women. *J Natl Cancer Inst* 1980; **65**: 353–76.

Lane DP, Benchimol S. p53 Oncogene or anti-oncogene? *Genes Dev* 1990; **4**: 1–8.

La Vecchia C, Decardi A, Franceschi S et al. Dietary factors and the risk for breast cancer. *Nutr Cancer* 1987; **10**: 205–14.

La Vecchia C, Decardi A, Parazzini F et al. Non-contraceptive estrogens and the risk of breast cancer in women. *Int J Cancer* 1986; **38**: 853–8.

Law ML, Kao FT, Wei Q et al. The progesterone receptor maps to human chromosome 11q13, the site of mammary oncogene int-2. *Proc Natl Acad Sci USA* 1987; **84**: 2877–81.

Lerner LJ, Jordan VC. Development of antiestrogens and their use in breast cancer: eighth Cain Memorial Award Lecture. *Cancer Res* 1990; **50**: 4177–89.

Liotta LA. Gene products which play a role in cancer invasion and metastasis. *Breast Cancer Res Treat* 1988; **11**: 113–24.

Lippman ME, Dickson RB, Gelmann EP et al. Growth regulation of human breast cancer occurs through regulated GF secretion. *J Cell Biochem* 1987; **35**: 1–16.

London SJ, Colditz GA, Stampfer MJ et al. Prospective study of relative weight, height and risk for breast cancer. *JAMA* 1989; **262**: 2853–8.

London SJ, Connolly JL, Schmitt SJ et al. A prospective study of benign breast disease and the risk of breast cancer. *JAMA* 1992; **267**: 941–4.

Longhecker MP, Berlin JA, Orza MJ et al. A metaanalysis of alcohol consumption in relation to risk of breast cancer. *JAMA* 1988; **260**: 652–6.

Loser R, Seibel K, Roos W et al. In vivo and in vitro antiestrogenic action of 3-hydroxytamoxifen, tamoxifen and 4-hydroxytamoxifen. *Eur J Cancer Clin Oncol* 1985; **21**: 985–90.

Love RR, Mazess RB, Barden HS et al. Effects of tamoxifen on bone mineral density in postmenopausal women with breast cancer. *N Engl J Med* 1992; **326**: 852–6.

Love RR, Weibe PA, Newcomb PA et al. Effects of tamoxifen on cardiovascular risk factors in postmenopausal women. *Ann Intern Med* 1991; **115**: 860–4.

Lubin JH, Burus PE, Blot WJ et al. Risk factors for breast cancer in women in N. Alberta, Canada, as related to age at diagnosis. *J Natl Cancer Inst* 1982; **68**: 211–17.

Ludwig Breast Cancer Study Group. Randomized trial of chemoendocrine therapy and mastectomy alone in postmenopausal patients with operable breast cancer and axillary node metastases. *Lancet* 1984; **1**: 1256–60.

Lynch HT. The family history and cancer control. Hereditary breast cancer. *Arch Surg* 1990; **125**: 151–2.

MacMahon B, Cole P, Lin TM et al. Age at first birth and breast cancer risk. *Bull WHO* 1970; **43**: 209–21.

Malone KE, Daling J, Weiss N. Oral contraceptives in relation to breast cancer. *Epidemiol Rev* 1993; **15**: 80–97.

Mandelonde T, Khalaf S, Garci M et al. Immunoenzymatic assay of Mr52,000 cathepsin D in 182 breast cancer cytosols: low correlation with other prognostic parameters. *Cancer Res* 1988; **48**: 462–6.

Mandeville R, Ghali SS, Chasseau JP. In vitro stimulation of human NK activity by an estrogen antagonist (tamoxifen). *Eur J Cancer Clin Oncol* 1984; **20**: 983–5.

Manni A, Pearson OH. Antiestrogen-induced remissions in premenopausal women with stage IV breast cancer: effects on ovarian function. *Cancer Treat Rep* 1980; **64**: 779–85.

Margreiter R, Wiegle J. Tamoxifen for premenopausal patients with advanced breast cancer. *Breast Cancer Res Treat* 1984; **4**: 45–84.

Marshall J, Graham S, Swanson M. Caffeine consumption and benign breast disease: a case control comparison. *Am J Public Health* 1982; **72**: 610–12.

Martin-Moreno JM, Boyle P, Gorgojo L et al. Alcoholic beverage consumption and risk of breast cancer in Spain. *Cancer Causes Control* 1993; **4**: 345–53.

Matelski H, Greene R, Huberman M et al. Randomized trial of estrogen vs tamoxifen therapy for advanced breast cancer. *Am J Clin Oncol* 1985; **8**: 128–33.

McDivitt RW, Stevens JA, Lee NC et al. Histologic types of benign breast disease and risk of breast cancer. *Cancer* 1992; **69**: 1408–14.

McGuire WL, Chamness GC, Fuqua SA. Estrogen receptor variants in clinical breast cancer. *Mol Endocrinol* 1991; **5**: 1571–7.

McGuire WL, Tandon AT, Allred DC et al. How to use prognostic factors in axillary node-negative breast cancer patients. *J Natl Cancer Inst* 1990; **82**: 1006–15.

McGuire WL. Estrogen receptor vs nuclear grade as prognostic factors in axillary node negative breast cancer. *J Clin Oncol* 1988; **6**: 1071–2.

McGuire WL. Prognostic factors in axillary node negative breast cancer patients. *Proc Am Assn Cancer Res* 1990; **31**: 469–70.

McLeskey SW, Kurebayashi J, Honig SF et al. Fibroblast growth factor 4 transfection on MCF-7 cells produces cell lines that are tumorigenic and metastatic in ovariectomized or tamoxifen-treated athymic nude mice. *Cancer Res* 1993; **53**: 2168–77.

McPherson K, Vessey MP, Neil A et al. Early oral contraceptive use and breast cancer: results of another case control study. *Br J Cancer* 1987; **56**: 653–70.

Merkel DE, Osborne CK. Prognostic factors in breast cancer. *Hematol/Oncol Clin North Am* 1989; **3**: 641–52.

Merrik O, Lund E, Adami HO et al. Oral contraceptive use and breast cancer in young women. A joint national case-control study in Sweden and Norway. *Lancet* 1986; **2**: 650–59.

Mettlin C, Jones G, Averette H et al. Defining and updating the American Cancer Society guidelines for the cancer-related check-up: prostate and endometrial cancers. *Cancer J Clin* 1993; **43**: 42–6.

Meyer F, Verreault R. Erythrocyte selenium and breast cancer risk. *Am J Epidemiol* 1987; **125**: 917–19.

Michna H, Nishimo Y, Neef G et al. Progesterone antagonist: tumor inhibition potential and mechanism of action. *J Steroid Biochem Mol Biol* 1992; **41**(3–8): 339–48.

Miller AB, Bulbrook RD. VICC multidisciplinary project on breast cancer: the epidemiology, etiology and prevention of breast cancer (BC). *Int J Cancer* 1986; **37**: 173–7.

Miller AB, Chamberlain J, Day NE et al. *Cancer Screening* 1991, pp 1–438; Cambridge: Cambridge University Press.

Miller BA, Feuer EJ, Hankey BF. Recent incidence trends for breast cancer in women and the relevance of early detection. An update. *CA Cancer J Clin* 1993; **43**: 27–41.

Miller BA, Ries LAG, Hankey BF et al. *SEER Cancer Statistics Review: 1973–1991* (NIH Pub. 94-2789) 1994; Bethesda, MD: National Cancer Institute.

Miller DR, Rosenberg L, Kaufman DW et al. Breast cancer before age 45 and oral contraceptive use. New finding. *Am J Epidemiol* 1989; **129**: 269–80.

Mool WJ, Peterse JL. Progress in molecular biology of breast cancer. *Eur J Cancer* 1992; **28**: 623–5.

Moon RC, Mehta RG. Cancer chemoprevention by retinoids: animal models. *Methods Enzymol* 1990; **190**: 395–406.

Moore JW, Clark GM, Hoare SA et al. Binding of estradiol to blood proteins and etiology of breast cancer. *Int J Cancer* 1986; **38**: 625–30.

Morris JJ, Seifter E. The role of aromatic hydrocarbons in the genesis of breast cancer. *Med Hypotheses* 1992; **38**: 177–84.

Moskowitz M. Breast cancer: age-specific growth rates and screening strategies. *Radiology* 1986; **161**: 37–41.

Mouridsen HT, Ellemann K, Mattson W et al. Therapeutic effect of tamoxifen vs tamoxifen combined with medroxyprogesterone acetate in advanced breast cancer in postmenopausal women. *Cancer Treat Rep* 1979; **63**: 171–5.

Murphy LC, Dotzlow H. Variant estrogen receptor mRNA species detected in human breast cancer biopsy samples. *Mol Endocrinol* 1989; **3**: 687–93.

Murphy LC. Estrogen receptor variants in human breast cancer. *Mol Cell Endocrinol* 1990; **74**: C83–6.

Nagamani M, Kelver ME, Smith R. Treatment of menopausal hot flashes with transdermal administration of clonidine. *Am J Obstet Gynecol* 1987; **156**: 561–3.

Nagy E, Berez I. Immunomodulation by tamoxifen and pergolide. *Immunopharmacology* 1986; **12**: 145–53.

National Center for Health Statistics. *Vital Statistics of the US, 1991* 1994; Washington, DC: Public Health Service.

National Research Council. Committee on the Biological Effects of Ionizing Radiation, Board of Radiation Effects, Research Commission on Life Sciences. *Health Effects of Exposure to Low Levels of Ionizing Radiation* 1990; Washington, DC: National Academy Press.

Nemoto T, Patel J, Rosner D et al. Tamoxifen vs adrenalectomy in metastatic breast cancer. *Cancer* 1984; **53**: 1333–5.

Nemoto T, Vana J, Bedwani R et al. Management and survival in female breast cancer. *Cancer* 1980; **15**: 2917–24.

Nicholson RI, McClelland RA, Finlay P et al. Relationship between EGF-R, c-erbB-2 protein expression and k167 immunostaining in breast cancer and hormone sensitivity. *Eur J Cancer* 1993; **29A**: 1018–23.

Nicholson S, Sainsbury JRC, Halcrow P et al. Expression of EGFrs associated with lack of response to endocrine therapy in recurrent breast cancer. *Lancet* 1989; **i**: 182–4.

Nicholson S, Wright C, Sainsbury JRC et al. Epidermal GF receptor as a marker for poor prognosis in node-negative breast cancer patients. Neu and tamoxifen failure. *J Steroid Biochem Mol Biol* 1990; **37**: 811–15.

NIH (National Institutes of Health) Consensus Development Conference Statement: treatment of early stage breast cancer. *JAMA* 1991; **265**: 391–5.

Nolvadex. Adjuvant Trial Organization: controlled trial of tamoxifen as a single adjuvant agent in management of early breast cancer. Analysis at eight years by the Nolvadex-Adjuvant Trial Organization. *Br J Cancer* 1988; **57**: 608–11.

Norton L, Day R. Potential innovations in scheduling of cancer chemotherapy. In Devita VT Jr, Hellman S, Rosenbrg SA (eds) *Important Advances in Oncology* 1991, pp 57–72; Philadelphia, PA: Lippincott.

O'Connell DL, Hulka BS, Chambless LE et al. Cigarette smoking, alcohol consumption and breast cancer risk. *J Natl Cancer Inst* 1987; **78**: 229–34.

Olsson H, Moller TR, Ranstam J. Early oral contraceptive use and breast cancer among premenopausal women: final report from a study in S. Sweden. *J Natl Cancer Inst* 1989; **81**: 1000–1004.

Osborne CK, Hamilton B, Nover M. Receptor binding and processing of EGF by human breast cancer cells. *J Clin Endocrinol Metab* 1982; **55**: 86–93.

Osborne CK, Monaco ME, Lippman ME et al. Correlation among insulin binding, degradation, and biological activity in human breast cancer cells in long-term tissue culture. *Cancer Res* 1978; **38**: 94–102.

Osborne CK, Wiebe NJ, McGuire WL et al. Tamoxifen and the isomers of 4-hydroxytamoxifen in tamoxifen-resistant tumors from breast cancer patients. *J Clin Oncol* 1992; **10**: 304–10.

Osborne CK. Effects of estrogens and antiestrogens on cell proliferation: implications for the treatment of breast cancer. In Osborne CK (ed.) *Endocrine Therapies in Breast and Prostate Cancer* 1988, pp 111–29; Boston, MA: Kluwer Academic.

Paffenbarger RS Jr, Kampert JB, Chang HG. Characteristics that predict risk of breast cancer before and after menopause. *Am J Epidemiol* 1980; **112**: 256–68.

Page DL, Dupont WD. Are breast cysts a premalignant marker? *Eur J Clin Oncol* 1985; **21**: 635–6.

Paik S, Hazan R, Fisher E et al. Pathologic findings from the National Surgical Adjuvant Breast and Bowel Project: Prognostic significance of erb-B2 protein overexpression in primary breast cancer. *J Clin Oncol* 1990; **8**: 103–12.

Palmer JR, Rosenberg L. Cigarette smoking and risk for breast cancer. *Epidemiol Rev* 1993; **15**: 145–56.

Parazzini F, La Vecchia C, Negri E. Spontaneous and induced abortions and risk of breast cancer. *Int J Cancer* 1991; **48**: 816–20.

Paul C, Skegg DG, Spears GFS. Oral contraceptive and risk for breast cancer. *Int J Cancer* 1990; **46**: 366–73.

Pekonen F, Partanen S, Makinen T et al. Receptors for EGF and IGF-I and their relation to steroid receptors in human breast cancer. *Cancer Res* 1988; **48**: 1343–7.

Peres R, Betsholtz C, Westermark B et al. Frequent expression of GFS for mesenchymal cells in human mammary carcinoma cell lines. *Cancer Res* 1987; **47**: 3425–9.

Peters MV. The effect of pregnancy in breast cancer. In Forrest APM, Kunkles PB (eds) *Prognostic Factors in Breast Cancer* 1968, pp 65–89; Baltimore, MD: Williams & Wilkins.

Peto J. Oral contraceptive and breast cancer: is the CASH study really negative? *Lancet* 1989; **1**: 552.

Petru E, Schmahl D. On the role of additive hormone monotherapy with tamoxifen, medroxyprogesterone acetate and aminoglutethimide in advanced breast cancer. *Klin Wochenschr* 1987; **65**: 959–66.

Peyrat JP, Bonneterre J, Hondermarck H et al. Basic fibroblast GF (bFGf) mitogenic activity and binding sites in human breast cancer. *J Steroid Biochem Mol Biol* 1992; **43**: 87–94.

Picard O, Rolland Y, Poupon MF. Fibroblast dependent tumorigenicity of cells in nude mice. Implications for implantation of metastases. *Cancer Res* 1986; **46**: 3290–94.

Pike MC, Henderson BE, Krailo MD et al. Breast cancer in young women and use of oral contraceptives: possible modifying effect of formulation and age at use. *Lancet* 1983; **2**: 926–30.

Pike MC, Henderson BG, Casagrande JT et al. Oral contraceptive use and early abortion as risk factors for breast cancer in young women. *Br J Cancer* 1981; **43**: 72–6.

Pollei SR, Mettler FA Jr, Bartlow SA et al. Occult breast cancer: prevalence and radiographic detectability. *Radiology* 1987; **163**: 459–62.

Powles TJ, Hardy JR, Ashley SE et al. A pilot trial to evaluate the acute toxicity and feasibility of tamoxifen for prevention of breast cancer. *Br J Cancer* 1989; **60**: 126–31.

Powles TJ, Tillyer CR, Jones AL et al. Prevention of breast cancer with tamoxifen: an update on the Royal Marsden Hospital pilot programme. *Eur J Cancer* 1990; **26**: 680–4.

Prentice RL, Sheppard L. Dietary fat and cancer: consistency of the epidemiologic data, and disease prevention that may follow from a practical reduction in fat consumption. *Cancer Causes Control* 1990; **1**: 81–97. Erratum, Cancer Causes Control 1990; **1**: 253.

Press MF. Estrogen and progesterone receptors in breast cancer. *Adv Pathol* (in press).

Pubesgaard T, vonEyben E. Bilateral optic neuritis evolved during tamoxifen treatment. *Cancer* 1986; **58**: 383–6.

Pyrhonen S, Valavaara R, Vuorinen J et al. High dose toremifene in advanced breast cancer resistant to or relapsed during tamoxifen therapy. *Breast Cancer Res Treat* 1994; **29**: 223–8.

Pyrhonen S. Phase III studies of toremifene in metastatic breast cancer. *Breast Cancer Res Treat* 1990; **16**(suppl): S14–46.

Remeick LI. Induced abortion as cancer risk factor: a review of epidemiologic evidence. *J Epidemiol Commun Health* 1990; **44**: 256–64.

Ribeiro G, Swindell R. The Christie Hospital adjuvant tamoxifen trial. Status at 10 years. *Br J Cancer* 1988; **57**: 601–60.

Rieche K. Die bee influssung der funkbouellen antithrombin III in plasma durch tamoxifen und aminoglutethemid. *Krebs Medizin* 1986; **7**: 60–3.

Rissanen PM. Carcinoma of the breast during pregnancy and lactation. *Br J Cancer* 1968; **22**: 663–8.

Rohan TE, Howe GR, Friedenreich CM et al. Dietary fiber, vitamins A, C, and E and risk of breast cancer: a cohort study. *Cancer Causes Control* 1993; **4**: 29–37.

Rohan TG, McMichael AJ. Oral contraceptive agents and breast cancer: a population based case control study. *Med J Aust* 1988; **149**: 520–26.

Romieu I, Willet WC, Colditz GA et al. Prospective study of oral contraceptive use and risk of breast cancer in women. *J Natl Cancer Inst* 1989; **81**: 1313–21.

Roos WK, Oeze L, Loser R et al. Antiestrogenic action of 3-hydroxytamoxifen in human breast cancer cell line MCF-7. *J Natl Cancer Inst* 1983; **71**: 55–9.

Rose C, Andersen KW, Mouridsen HT et al. Beneficial effect of adjuvant tamoxifen therapy in primary breast cancer patients with high estrogen receptor values. *Lancet* 1985; **1**: 16–19.

Rose C, Mouridsen HT. Treatment of advanced breast cancer with tamoxifen. Recent results. *Cancer Res* 1984; **91**: 230–42.

Rosen P, Groshen S, Kinne D et al. Factors influencing prognosis in node-negative breast cancer. Analysis of 767 T1N0M0/T2N0M0 patients with long term F/U. *J Clin Oncol* 1993; **11**: 2090–100.

Rosenberg L, Metzger LS, Palmer JR. Alcohol consumption and risk of breast cancer: A review of the epidemiologic evidence. *Epidemiol Rev* 1993; **15**: 133–44.

Rosenberg L, Miller DR, Kaufman DW et al. Breast cancer oral contraceptive use. *Am J Epidemiol* 1984; **119**: 167–76.

Rushton L, Jones DR. Oral contraceptive use and breast cancer risk: a meta-analysis of variations with age at diagnosis, parity and total duration of oral contraceptive use. *Br J Obstet Gynaecol* 1992; **99**: 239–46.

Rutqvist LE, Cedermark B, Glas V et al. The Stockholm Trial on adjuvant tamoxifen in early breast cancer. Correlation between estrogen receptor level and treatment effect. *Breast Cancer Res Treat* 1987; **10**: 255–66.

Rutqvist LE, Johansson H, Signomklao T et al. Adjuvant tamoxifen therapy for early stage breast cancer and second primary malignacies. *J Natl Cancer Inst* 1995; **87**: 645–51.

Sainsbury JRC, Farndon JR, Needham GK et al. Epidermal-growth factor receptor status as predictor of early recurrence of and death from breast cancer. *Lancet* 1987; **i**: 1398–1402.

Salomon DS, Zwiebel JA, Bano M et al. Presence of TGFs in human breast cancer cells. *Cancer Res* 1984; **44**: 4069–77.

Santen RJ. Clinical use of aromatase inhibitors in human breast carcinoma. *J Steroid Biochem Mol Biol* 1991; **40**: 247–53.

Santen RJ. Clinical use of aromatase inhibitors: current data and therapeutic perspectives. *J Enzym Inhib* 1990; **4**: 79–99.

Saphner T, Tormey DC, Gray R. Venous and arterial thrombosis in patients who received adjuvant therapy for breast cancer. *J Clin Oncol* 1991; **9**: 286–94.

Sawka CA, Pritchard KI, Paterson AHG et al. Role and mechanism of action of tamoxifen in premenopausal women with metastatic breast carcinoma. *Cancer Res* 1986; **46**: 3152–6.

Scarff RM, Toroui H. *Historical Typing of Breast Tumors* 1968, pp 510–13; Geneva: WHO.

Schally AV, Redding TW, Cumaru-Schally AM. Potential use of analogues of luteinizing hormone-releasing hormones in the treatment of hormone-sensitive neoplasm. *Cancer Treat Rep* 1984; **68**: 281–9.

Schiff I, Tulchinsky D, Cramer et al. Oral medroxyprogesterone in the treatment of postmenopausal symptoms. *J Am Med Assn* 1988; **244**: 1443–5.

Schoultz E, Johansson H, Wilking N et al. Influence of prior and subsequent pregnancy on breast cancer prognosis. *J Clin Oncol* 1995; **13**: 430–34.

Segna RA, Dottino PR, Deligdisch L et al. Tamoxifen and endometrial cancer. *Mt Sinai J Med* 1992; **59**: 416–18.

Sellers TA, Kushi LH, Potter JA et al. Effect of family history, body-fat distribution and reproductive factors on the risk of postmenopausal breast cancer. *N Engl J Med* 1992; **326**: 1323–9.

Seoud MA, Johnson J, Weed JC Jr. Gynecologic tumors in tamoxifen treated women with breast cancer. *Obstet Gynecol* 1993; **82**: 165–9.

Silberhorn EM, Glanert HP, Robertson LW. Carcinogenicity of polyhalogenated biphenyl: PCBs and PBBs. *Crit Rev Toxicol* 1990; **20**: 440–96.

Slamon DJ. Studies of the HER-2/neu proto-oncogene in human breast cancer. *Cancer Invest* 1990; **8**(2): 253.

Slattery ML, Kerber RA. A comprehensive evaluation of family history and breast cancer risk. *JAMA* 1993; **270**: 1563–8.

Smart CR, Hendrick RE, Rutledge JH III et al. Benefit of mammography screening in women aged 40–49: current evidence from randomized control trials. *Cancer* 1995; **75**: 1619–26.

Smith HS, Lu Y, Deng G et al. Molecular aspects of early stages of breast cancer progression (review). *J Cell Biochem* 1993; **17G**(suppl): 144–52.

Sporn MB, Roberts AB, Wakefield LM et al. TGF-beta: biological function and clinical structure. *Science* 1986; **233**: 532–4.

Sporn MB, Roberts AB. Role of retinoids in differentiation and carcinogenesis. *Cancer Res* 1983; **43**: 3034–40.

Sporn MB, Torado GJ. Autocrine secretion and malignant transformation of cells. *N Engl J Med* 1980; **303**: 878–80.

Sporn MB. Approaches to prevention of epithelial cancer during the preneoplastic period. *Cancer Res* 1976; **36**: 2699–2702.

Sporn MB. Carcinogenesis and cancers: different perspectives on the same disease. *Cancer Res* 1991; **51**: 6215–18.

Stadel BV, Rubin GL, Webster LA et al. Oral contraceptive and breast cancer in young women. *Lancet* 1985; **2**: 970–73.

Stadel BV, Schlesselman JJ. Oral contraceptive and breast cancer (letter). *Lancet* 1986; **2**: 922–3.

Stamberger RJ, Rukoneva E, Longfield AK et al. Antioxidants and cancer: selenium in the blood of normal and cancer patients. *J Natl Cancer Inst* 1973; **50**: 863–70.

Stebbings JH, Lucas HF, Stehney AF. Mortality from cancer of major sites in female radium dial workers. *Am J Intern Med* 1984; **5**: 435–59.

Storm HH, Anderson M, Boice JD Jr et al. Adjuvant radiotherapy and risk of contralateral cancer. *J Natl Cancer Inst* 1992; **84**: 1245–50.

Sutherland RL, Murphy LC, Foo MS et al. High affinity antiestrogens binding site distinct from the estrogen receptor. *Nature* 1980; **288**: 273–5.

Sutton R, Buzdar A, Hortobagyi G. Pregnancy and offspring after adjuvant chemotherapy in breast cancer patients. *Cancer* 1990; **75**: 847–50.

Swanson CA, Jones DY, Schatzkin A et al. Breast cancer risk assessed by anthropometry in the NHANES I epidemiological follow-up study. *Cancer Res* 1988; **48**: 5363–7.

Tabar L, Duffy SW, Kruseino VB. Detection method, tumor size, and node metastases in breast cancer diagnosed during a trial of breast cancer screening. *Eur J Cancer Clin Oncol* 1987; **23**: 959–62.

Tabar L, Faberberg G, Day NE et al. What is the optimum interval between screening examinations? An analysis based on the latest results of the Swedish two-county breast cancer screening trial. *Br J Cancer* 1987; **55**: 547–51.

Tabar L, Faberberg G, Duffy SW et al. Update of the Swedish two-county program of mammographic screening for breast cancer. *Radiol Clin North Am* 1992; **30**: 187–210.

Tandon AK, Clark GM, Chamness GC et al. Cathepsin D and prognosis in breast cancer. *N Engl J Med* 1990; **322**: 297–302.

Tannenbaum A. The genesis and growth of tumors: effects of a high fat diet. *Cancer Res* 1942; **2**: 468–75.

Tarone RE, Chu KC. Implications of birth cohort patterns in interpreting trends in breast cancer rates. *J Natl Cancer Inst* 1992; **84**: 1402–10.

Tavani A, Negri E, Franceshi S et al. Oral contraceptive and breast cancer in N. Italy: final report from a case-control study. *Br J Cancer* 1993; **68**: 568–71.

Thomas DB, Noonan EA. Risk of breast cancer in relation to use of combined oral contraceptive near the age of menopause. WHO collaborative study of neoplasia and steroid contraceptives. *Cancer Causes Control* 1991; **2**: 389–94.

Thomas DB, Persing JP, Hutchinson WB. Exogenous estrogens and other risk factors for breast cancer in women with benign breast disease. *J Natl Cancer Inst* 1982; **69**: 1017.

Thomas DB. Oral contraceptive and breast cancer: review of the epidemiologic literature. *Contraception* 1991; **43**: 597–642.

Thompson EA, Siiteri PK. The involvement of human placental microsomal cytochrome P-450 in aromatization. *J Biol Chem* 1974; **249**: 5373–8.

Thompson HJ, Herbst EJ, Meeker LD. Chemoprevention of mammary carcinogenesis: a comparative review of the efficacy of a polyamine antimetabolite, retinoids and selenium. *J Natl Cancer Inst* 1986; **77**: 585–98.

Todaro GJ, Fryling CM, Delarco JE. Transforming growth factors produced by certain human tumor cells: polypeptides that interact with epidermal growth factor receptors. *Proc Natl Acad Sci USA* 1980; **77**: 5258–62.

Tokunaga M, Land CE, Yamamoti T et al. Breast cancer in Japanese A-bomb survivors. *Lancet* 1982; **2**: 924.

Toniolo PG, Levitz M, Zeleniuch-Jacquott A et al. A prospective study of endogenous estrogens and breast cancer in postmenopausal women. *J Natl Cancer Inst* 1995; **87**: 190–97.

Turken S, Siris E, Seldin D et al. Effects of tamoxifen on spinal bone density in women with breast cancer. *J Natl Cancer Inst* 1989; **81**: 1086–8.

UK National Case Control Study Group. Breast feeding and risk of breast cancer in young women. *Br Med J* 1993; **307**: 17–20.

UK National Case-Control Study Group. Oral contraceptives and breast cancer risk in young women. *Lancet* 1989; **6**: 973–82.

Ursin G, Aragaki CC, Paganini-Hill A et al. Oral contraceptive and premenopausal bilateral breast cancer: a case control study. *Epidemiology* 1992; **3**: 414–19.

Van Noord PAH, Mass MJ, Van der Tweel et al. Selenium and risk of postmenopausal breast cancer in the DOM study. *Breast Cancer Res Treat* 1993; **25**: 11–19.

Van Veelen H, Willemse PIHB, Tjabbes T et al. Oral high dose medroxyprogesterone acetate vs tamoxifen: a randomized crossover trial in postmenopausal patients with advanced breast cancer. *Cancer* 1986; **58**: 7–13.

Vessey MP. The involvement of estrogen in the development and progression of breast disease: epidemiological evidence. *Proc Roy Soc Edinb* 1989; **95B**: 35–48.

Vogel CL, Shemano I, Schoenfelder J et al. Multicenter phase II efficacy trial of toremifene in tamoxifen-refractory patients with advanced breast cancer. *J Clin Oncol* 1993; **11**: 345–50.

Vojtesek B, Lane DP. Regulation of p53 protein expression in human BC cell lines. *J Cell Sci* 1993; **105**: 607–12.

Wakeling AE, Dukes M, Bowler J. A potent specific pure antiestrogen with clinical potential. *Cancer Res* 1991; **51**: 3861–73.

Wattenberg LW. Chemoprevention of cancer. *Cancer Res* 1985; **45**: 1–8.

Weinstein AL, Mahoney MC, Nasca PC et al. Breast cancer risk and oral contraceptive use: results from a large case-control study. *Epidemiology* 1991; **2**: 353–8.

Weinstein IB. Cancer prevention: recent progress and future opportunities. *Cancer Res* 1991; **51**: 5080–85s.

Welsch CW. Hormones and murine mammary tumorigenesis: an historical view. In Lenug BS (ed.) *Hormonal Regulation of Mammary Tumors* 1982, pp 1–29; Montreal: Montreal Press.

Westin JB, Richter E. The Israeli breast cancer anomaly. *Ann NY Acad Sci* 1990; **609**: 269–79.

White E. Projected changes in breast cancer incidence due to the trend towards delayed childbearing. *Am J Public Health* 1987; **77**: 495–7.

WHO Collaborative Study of Neoplasia and Steroid Contraceptives. Breast cancer and combined oral contraceptive results from a multinational study. *Br J Cancer* 1990; **6**: 110–19.

Wiebe VJ, Osborne CK, McGuire WL et al. Identification of estrogenic tamoxifen metabolites in tamoxifen-resistant human breast tumors. *J Clin Oncol* 1992; **10**: 990–4.

Wile AG, Opfell RW, Marigileth DA. Hormone replacement therapy in previously treated breast cancer patients. *Am J Surg* 1993; **165**: 372–5.

Willet WC, Browne ML, Bain C et al. Relative weight and risk of breast cancer among premenopausal women. *Am J Epidemiol* 1985; **122**: 731–40.

Willet WC, Hunter DJ, Stampfer MJ et al. Dietary fat and fiber in relation to risk of breast cancer. An 8 year follow-up. *JAMA* 1992; **268**: 2037–44.

Willet WC, Stampfer MJ, Colditz GA et al. Dietary fat and the risk of breast cancer. *N Engl J Med* 1987; **316**: 22–8.

Wingo PA, Layde PM, Lee NC et al. The risk of breast cancer in postmenopausal women who have used estrogen replacement therapy. *JAMA* 1987; **257**: 209–15.

Wingo PA, Lee NC, Ory HW et al. Age specific differences in the relationship between oral contraceptive use and breast cancer. *Obstet Gynecol* 1991; **78**: 161–70.

Wolff MS, Toniolo PG, Lee EW et al. Blood levels of organochlorine residues and risk of breast cancer. *J Natl Cancer Inst* 1993; **85**: 648–52.

Wooster R, Neuhausen SL, Mangion J et al. *Science* 1994; **265**: 2088–90.

Wyshak G, Frisch RE. Evidence for a secular trend in age of menarche. *N Engl J Med* 1982; **306**: 1033–5.

Wysowski DK, Comstock GW, Helsing KJ et al. Sex hormone levels in serum in relation to the development of breast cancer. *Am J Epidemiol* 1987; **125**: 791–9.

Yoshimoto Y, Kato H, Schull WJ. Risk of cancer among children exposed in utero to A-bomb radiation, 1950–84. *Lancet* 1988; **2**: 665–9.

Yuan JM, Yu MC, Ross RK et al. Risk factors for breast cancer in Chinese women in Shanghai. *Cancer Res* 1988; **48**: 1949–53.

Appendices of Drugs in Development, Including Marketed Drugs

Appendices of Drugs in Development, Including Marketed Drugs

These Appendices attempt to provide a broad-based, useful collection of drugs in development for women and women's diseases. The editor acknowledges that the status of drugs is constantly in flux. Their phase of development, market status, including potential withdrawals from research and the market, happens daily. The editor would be interested in obtaining comments from companies and updates as they become publicly available to assist in updating this list for further editions.

Drug Development for Women. Edited by V.V. Ragavan. © 1998 John Wiley & Sons Ltd.

APPENDIX A: CONTRACEPTION

Oral Contraceptives

Chemical	Company/co-licensees	Phase of development	Comments
Cyproterone + estradiol valerate	Leiras	Marketed in Northern Europe	Femilar: biphasic contraceptive for women 40+ years who cannot tolerate ethinyl estradiol
Cyproterone acetate + ethinyl estradiol (150/30)	Schering AG	Marketed in Europe	Diane; monophasic
Desogestrel + ethinyl estradiol (150/30)	Organon/Ortho/Johnson & Johnson	Marketed in Europe and USA	Marvelon, Desogen, Ortho-Sept; monophasic
Desogestrel + ethinyl estradiol (150/20)	Akzo/Organon	Marketed in Europe	Mercilon; monophasic, lower dose estrogen
Dienogest + ethinyl estradiol	Schering AG/Jenapharm	Marketed in Germany	Certostat; Certostat 30; Dienogest is a progestin developed by Jenapharm, now a part of Schering AG
Ethinyldiol diacetate + ethinyl estradiol	Searle	Marketed	Demulen; monophasic
Gestodene + ethinyl estradiol	Wyeth-Ayerst/Lederle	Marketed in Europe	Tri-Minulet; triphasic
Gestodene + ethinyl estradiol (75/30)	Schering AG	Marketed in Europe	BiNovum, TriNovum, Meliane; biphasic
Gestodene + ethinyl estradiol (75/20)	Wyeth-Ayerst/Lederle	Marketed in Europe	Harmonet; monophasic
Gestodene + ethinyl estradiol (75/20)	Schering AG	Marketed in Europe	Femidene; monophasic
Levonorgestrel + ethinyl estradiol (100/20)	Wyeth-Ayerst/Lederle	Marketed in USA	Alesse; low dose 20 μg ethinyl estradiol-containing pill
Levonorgestrel + ethinyl estradiol (100/20)	Wyeth-Ayerst/Lederle	Marketed in Europe	Leios; low dose EE/LNG
Levonorgestrel + ethinyl estradiol	Wyeth-Ayerst/Lederle	Marketed	Triphasil, Triphasil 28; triphasic
Levonorgestrel + ethinyl estradiol	Berlex	Marketed	Tri-Levlen, Tri-Levlen 28; triphasic

Composition	Company	Status	Notes
Levonorgestrel + ethinyl estradiol (150/35)	Berlex	Marketed	Levlen, Levlen 28; monophasic
Norgestimate – ethinyl estradiol	Ortho (Johnson & Johnson)	Marketed	Cilest, Ortho Cyclen, Ortho Tri-Cyclen; triphasic. Also approved for acne
Norgestrel + ethinyl estradiol	Wyeth-Ayerst/Lederle	Marketed	Lo-Ovral/Lo-Ovral-28; monophasic
Norgestrel + ethinyl estradiol	Wyeth-Ayerst/Lederle	Marketed	Ovral/Ovral-28; monophasic
Norethindrone + ethinyl estradiol	Ortho	Marketed	Ortho 7/7/7; triphasic
Norethindrone + ethinyl estradiol (0.5/35)	Ortho	Marketed	Modicon 21; Modicon 28
Norethindrone acetate + ethinyl estradiol	Parke-Davis	Marketed	Estrastep; variable estrogen and progestin components
Norethindrone acetate + ethinyl estradiol	Parke-Davis	Marketed	Loestrin/Loestrin Fe; monophasic
Norethindrone + ethinyl estradiol	Bristol-Myers Squibb	Marketed	Ovcon
Norethindrone + ethinyl estradiol	Warner-Chilcott/Various Generic	Marketed	Generic—various brands
Gestodene + ethinyl estradiol	Yamanouchi/Schering AG	Preregistration in Japan	
Levonorgestrel – ethinyl estradiol (100/20)	Schering AG/Wyeth	Submitted in Europe	Loette/Leios; low dose EE/LNG
Levonorgestrel – ethinyl estradiol (100/20)	Schering AG/Wyeth	Submitted in Europe	Low dose
Desogestrel + ethinyl estradiol-bridging regimen (150/20 + bridging)	Organon	Phase III	Mercilon Plus—5 days of low estrogen—prevent ovulation
Drospirenone + ethinyl estradiol	Schering AG	Phase III	Progestin; anti-aldosterone properties; may decrease blood pressure, weight gain; oral
Gestodene + ethinyl estradiol (60/50)	Schering AG	Phase III in Europe	
Norethisterone ethinyl estradiol + Norinyl T28	Daiichi	Phase III in Japan	Oral contraceptive
CTR 25	Organon	Phase III	
CTR 99/77	Organon	Phase III	
Desogestrel and ethinyl estradiol	Organon/R.W. Johnson/Ortho	Not approved	Tri-phasic; High Pearl index. Tri-Desogen; Ortho-Tricept; OrthoCept

Chemical	Company/co-licensees	Phase of development	Comments
CI-1001	Parke-Davis	Phase II	
Norgestimate/ethinyl estradiol (cyclophasic)	R.W. Johnson Pharmaceutical Research Institute	Phase II	Not marketed in USA
Estrogen-priming oral contraceptive: same as above	Bio-Technology General/ Akzo/Bristol-Myers Squibb	Phase II	
Cyclodiol + ethinyl estradiol	Schering AG	Phase I	
Progestin Only			
Norethindrone acetate	Ortho-J&J	Marketed in USA	Minipill
Nomogesterol acetate	Theramex	Marketed in France	Synthetic non-androgenic progestin administered daily; anti-estrogenic activity
ST1435	Population Council	Phase I	Bracelet transdermal system
ST1435	Population Council	Phase I	Topical cream delivery/easily absorbed
Gestodene	Schering AG	Phase I	Transdermal only
Contraceptive Implants			
Levonorgestrel Norplant	Leiras Oy/Wyeth-Ayerst/ Population Council	Marketed	6 Silicon capsules implanted in forearm; releases 30μg/day; Norplant
Norplant II	Population Council; Wyeth-Ayerst	Approved in USA and UK	2 Capsules implanted in the forearm; 3-year duration
3-ketodesogestrel Implanon	Organon/Akzo	Phase III	Releases 40 mg 3-ketodesogestrel a day; 3-year duration; Implanon
ST1435 Nestorone	Population Council	Phase III	Single implant; 2-year duration
Estrogen + progestin; GnRH analog	Balance/Endocon	Preclinical	Bioerodable implants contain GnRH analog
GnRH implant	Endocon	Preclinical	For contraception

Injectables

Name	Company	Status	Description
Depo-medroxyprogesterone acetate	Pharmacia/Upjohn	Marketed	
Norethindrone enanthate + estradiol valerate	Schering AG	Marketed in Mexico; Phase III worldwide	1-Month duration; estrogen, progestogen action; inhibits follicle maturation, ovulation and corpus luteum formation
Mesigyna			
Cyclo-provera	Pharmacia/Upjohn	Phase III	
Leuprolide + estrogen + progesterone	Royal Marsden Hospital/Balance/UCLA	Phase I	Injectable contraceptive may reduce possibility of breast cancer
Anordin	Shanghai Pharmaceuticals	Preclinical	Anti-estrogenic; 1-Month duration
Progestin	Population Council	Preclinical	1-Month duration

IUDs

Name	Company	Status	Description
Progestasert system	Alza	Marketed	
Levonorgestrel, Levonova, Mirena	Pharmacia/Population Council/Leiras	Marketed in Europe	Releases 20 mg/day; 5-year duration
FlexiGard (copper)	Ortho	Marketed in USA	

Barrier/Vaginal Contraceptives

Name	Company	Status	Description
Progesterone	Population Council	Phase III	Vaginal ring for lactating women; 6-month duration
Levonorgestrel (Femring)	Roussel-Uclaf/Galen Ltd./WHO	Phase III preregistration	Vaginal ring, 3-month duration
Prevecon	Biosyn	Phase II/III	Spermicide
3-Ketodesogestrel + ethinyl estradiol	Organon	Phase II	Vaginal ring, worn 3/4 weeks of cycle and then removed for 1 week for menstruation
Estradiol + norethindrone	Population Council	Phase II	Vaginal ring, 1-month duration

Chemical	Company/co-licensees	Phase of development	Comments
Progesterone	Watson	Phase II	Vaginal insert
Progestin ST1435 + ethinyl estradiol	Population Council	Phase II	Vaginal ring; 6-month duration, may be extended to 12- or 24-month duration
Vaginal ring	Akzo Nobel	Phase II	Combination vaginal ring
Norethisterone + ethinyl estradiol	Population Council	Phase II	Vaginal ring, 1-year duration
Antihormones: Antiprogestins, Anti-estrogen, Abortifacients			
Anti-estrogen (Centchroman) antihormones	Central Drug Research Institute/Novo Nordisk	Marketed in India	Used as a twice a week (?) contraceptive in India; being developed by Novo Nordisk for anti-estrogen properties
Mifepristone RU-486; Mifegyne; RU-38486; RU-4866	Roussel Uclaf/Population Council/Hoechst Marion Roussel	Marketed in Europe; registration in USA	Abortifacient in France, Sweden & UK in combination with a prostaglandin
Mifepristone RU-486; Mifegyne; RU-38486; RU-4866	Roussel Uclaf/Population Council/Hoechst Marion Roussel	Phase II	Potential as daily oral contraceptive; changes endometrium
Antiprogestin; Onapristone	Schering AG	Phase III; suspended development	Possible use as abortifacient; Phase III for oral contraceptive
Anti-estrogen CDRI 85287	Central Drug Research Institute/Novo Nordisk	Preclinical	Binds to estradiol receptors, prevents implantation; anti-estrogen; block estradiol–receptor complex formation
Antiprogestin Org-31710	Akzo	Preclinical	Proof of concept studies
Antiprogestin CBD 2914	Research Triangle Institute/NIH	Preclinical	Postcoital emergency contraception
Antiprogestin (several)	Schering AG	Preclinical	Prevents endometrial receptivity, but not ovulation; contraception will not disturb menstrual cycle and will not harm a previous implanted fertilized egg or fetus; possible low dose daily use

Progestin antagonists and agonists (several)	Johnson & Johnson	Preclinical	Contraception will not disturb menstrual cycle and will not harm a previous implanted fertilized egg or fetus; possible low-dose daily use

Vaccines

hCG vaccine	National Institute of Immunology, India	Phase II	1 Year duration
hCG vaccine	WHO	Phase II	Antibodies to immunogenic hCG-b last for up to 6 months
hCG-b vaccine 84/246	Central Drug Research Institute	Phase II	b-hCG + b chain of ovine LH; conjugated with either tetanus or diphtheria toxoid
hCG-b vaccine	WHO/Aphton	Phase II	Neutralized hCG vaccine; 12–18 month duration
hCG-β subunit fragment vaccine	WHO/Aphton?	Phase II	Biodegradable polymer spheres; reversible type of contraception
Praneem vilci	National Institute of Immunology, India	Phase II	Antibacterial and antiviral compound causes local cell-mediated immunity
Antisperm vaccine	Connecticut University	Preclinical	Reversible immunity to sperm protein PH 20
Antisperm vaccine YAL 198	Population Council	Preclinical	Reversible immunity to sperm protein YWK-II
Antisperm vaccine	Virginia University/Ortho	Preclinical	Reversible immunity to sperm proteins
hCG vaccine	Zonagen	Preclinical	Peptide-based hCG vaccine
Zona pellucida vaccine	Zonagen	Preclinical	Antibodies to zona pellucida proteins; locally active contraceptive
Zona pellucida vaccine	Zonagen/Schering AG/ Reproductive Biotechnologies	Preclinical	Zona proteins A and/or B; reversible
Antisperm vaccine	Zonagen	Preclinical	Possible use in males as a contraceptive
ImmuMax	Zonagen	Preclinical	Improves antibody response to vaccines
Cucumariosid	Laboratory of Biological Active Substances	Preclinical	Modulator of immune system; site of action not clear
FSH vaccine	Population Council	Preclinical	α and β chains obtained from pituitary glands of sheep

Chemical	Company/co-licensees	Phase of development	Comments
Transdermal Contraceptives—Combination Estrogen/Progestin			
Estrogen	Schering AG	Preregistration, Phase III	Transdermal estrogen
Progestin	Population Council	Phase II/III	DT 1435—transdermally active progestin
Estrogen + progestin	Pharmetrix	Preclinical	Transdermal estrogen + progestin
Transdermal contraceptive	Cygnus/Ortho	Preclinical	
Other/Miscellaneous/Antisperm Vaginal Agents			
Nonoxynol-9, various spermicides, OTC	Various	Marketed	Foams, gels, suppositories, films
Libian	Yamanouchi	Phase III in Japan	
Prevecon	Biosyn	Phase II/III	Spermicide
Anteovine	Institute of Obstetrics and Gynecology, Russia	Phase II	Prevents secretion of gonadotropins and sex hormones from the basal peri-ovulatory region
85/83	Central Drug Research Institute	Preclinical	Prevents trophoblasts from maturing
CaRest M3	Cell Research/Russian Immunology Institute	Preclinical	Breaks down glycoprotein coat of fertilized egg, inducing immune response
Estrogen receptor ligands	Wyeth-Ayerst/Ligand	Preclinical	
Inhibin	Biotech Australia/Roche	Preclinical	Recombinant human inhibin results in lower FSH levels; initiates sperm and ova production; possible contraceptive for males or females
Lead compound of pyridazine derivatives	Johnson & Johnson	Preclinical	
Progesterone receptor ligands	Wyeth-Ayerst/Ligand	Preclinical	Progestins/antiprogestins
rP4	Repligen	Preclinical	Platelet factor inhibitor

Meiosis-inhibiting substance MIP	Novo-Nordisk	Preclinical	Meiosis-activating sterols; naturally occurring antagonists may be hormone-free
Alzamer polymers	Alza	Preclinical	Sustained release bio-erodible polymers
LHRH antagonists	Abbott	Preclinical	Suppress ovulatory cycle; will need hormone replacement
Yissum Project No. B-0829	Yissum	Preclinical	Possible contraceptives and abortifacient development; inhibits angiogenesis

APPENDIX B: REPRODUCTIVE DISEASES

Endometriosis

Steroidal Products

Chemical	Company/co-licensees	Phase of development	Comments
Danazol	Sanofi	Marketed	Danacrine; oral dosing
Danazol	Barr Labs	Marketed	Generic

Synthetic Gonadorelin Agonists (LHRH Agonists)

Chemical	Company/co-licensees	Phase of development	Comments
Nafarelin	Searle/Recordati	Marketed	Synarel, Samynarel; intranasal twice a day
Goserelin acetate	Zeneca	Marketed	Zoladex; monthly implant delivery system
Leuprolide acetate	Abbott/Takeda/Lederle	Marketed	Lupron; monthly injectable
Buserelin	Hoechst	Marketed in Europe	Intranasal delivery
Triptorelin	Debiopharm/Pharmacia-Upjohn/Beaufour-Ipsen/Tecnofarma	Marketed in Europe	Decapeptyl; once a month injectable
Leuprolide acetate	Abbott/Takeda/Lederle	Marketed	Lupron; once every 3 month injectable
Deslorelin: Somagard	Salk Institute/Roberts/Theramex	Marketed in UK for endometriosis	Gonadorelin superagonist
Histrelin	Roberts	Phase II	Supprelin
Buserelin	Hoechst	Phase II	Injectable delivery system; 3.6 mg
Meterelin	Asta-Medica/Meiolanum/Pharmascience	Phase I	9-Amino acid peptide
Agonist	Pharmavene	Preclinical	

LHRH Antagonists

Drug	Company	Phase	Notes
Cetrorelix	Asta-Medica/Shionogi	Phase III	Injectable formulation
Cetrorelix	Asta-Medica/Shionogi	Phase II	Depot formulation under development
Antide	Serono	Phase II	LHRH antagonist for infertility
Ganirelix	Roche	Phase I	Discontinued LHRH antagonist
Antarelix	Asta-Medica	Phase I	Preclinical for infertility
Org 30850	Organon	Phase I	Inhibits ovulation for endometriosis
A 76154	Abbott/Takeda	Preclinical	Octapeptide
HOE 2013	Hoechst	Preclinical	Discontinued polymer implant degradable by human body for sustained release
Atrigel-LHRH	Atrix/Roche	Preclinical	Based on LHRH receptor
Orally active molecules	Alanex	Preclinical	Studies in endometriosis pending
Anti-GnRH immunogen	Aphton	Preclinical	

Progestins

Drug	Company	Phase	Notes
Gestrinone	Roussel-Uclaf	Marketed outside USA	Progestin with long action
Nomegestrol acetate; Lutenyl	Theramex	Marketed outside USA	Synthetic non-androgenic progestin, administered daily
Dienogest; Dienogestril	Schering AG/Jenapharm	Marketed in Europe Endometriosis—phase III in Europe	Marketed as a contraceptive in Germany (with ethinyl estradiol)
Progesterone suppository	Watson	Phase II (Infertility)	Continue treatment 13 weeks after implantation

Antiprogestins

Drug	Company	Phase	Notes
Mifepristone; RU 486	Roussel Uclaf/Population Council	Phase I/II for endometriosis	Potential treatment for endometriosis
Antiprogestin; Onapristone	Schering AG	Phase II	Discontinued
Org-31710	Akzo	Preclinical	Proof of concept studies

Chemical	Company/co-licensees	Phase of development	Comments
RU-46556	Roussel Uclaf	Preclinical	Mifepristone derivative may not have antiglucocorticoid activity
RU-49295	Roussel Uclaf	Preclinical	Mifepristone derivative may not have antiglucocorticoid activity
LG 1147	Ligand	Preclinical	Non-steroidal compound from seaweed
LG 1447	Ligand	Preclinical	
Antiprogestin	Ligand Pharmaceuticals	Preclinical	Proof of concept studies
Aromatase Inhibitors			
NKS 01	Nippon Kayaku	Phase II	Non-androgenic and non-estrogenic
YM 511	Yamanouchi	Phase I	Non-steroidal compound locally inhibits ovarian aromatase
ORG 33201	Organon	Preclinical	Substituted imidazoylethylphenalene inhibits human placental aromatase
RU-54115	Roussel Uclaf	Preclinical	Discontinued; inhibitor of human placental aromatase
Anti-estrogens			
Raloxifene	Lilly	Phase II	Approved for osteoporosis in USA
Anti-estrogens	Ligand Pharmaceuticals	Preclinical	Proof of concept studies
Other			
Tibolone	Akzo/Kanebo	Marketed in Europe/ Phase III for HRT	Synthetic steroid; being studied with LHRH analogs to prevent hypo-estrogenism
Basic Research Stage	Wyeth-Ayerst/Affymax	Preclinical	Product for endometriosis under development
Basic Research Stage	Zonagen	Preclinical	Product for endometriosis under development

5-aminolevulinic acid; 5-ALA PDT	Deprenyl Research/ Medicis/Draxis	Phase I	Photodynamic therapy; non-laser light source; phase I for endometriosis
Tin ethyl etiopurpurin SnET2	PDT/Pharmacia	Preclinical	Photodynamic therapy; laser light source

Infertility

Follicle-stimulating Hormones (FSH)

Fertinex	Serono	Marketed	Highly purified; non-recombinant natural pure FSH preparation
Metrodin	Serono	Marketed	FSH first generation
ORG 33408; Puregon	Organon	Registered	Highly purified; non-recombinant natural pure FSH preparation
FSH	Serono	Phase III	Recombinant human follicle-stimulating hormone
FSH; Follegon	Organon	Phase III	Recombinant human follicle-stimulating hormone
FSH	Akzo/Cell Genesys	Preclinical	Recombinant follicle-stimulating hormone

Luteinizing Hormone (LH)

LH	Serono	Phase III	Recombinant human luteinizing hormone

Gonadotropins (Combination)

FSH + gonadotropin; Perganol	Serono	Marketed	Human gonadotropin enriched with FSH for treatment of menopausal symptoms and infertility
Menotropin; Humegon	Organon	Marketed	Menopausal gonadotropin
rhHMG + rhFSH	Serono	Phase II/III in Europe	Human recombinant hMG and FSH
Somatotropin	Novo-Nordisk	Phase II/III	Recombinant human somatotropin; treatment of infertility

Chemical	Company/co-licensees	Phase of development	Comments
hCG			
Various generic hCG; Ovidrel	Generic	Marketed	Extracted human chorionic gonadotropin
	Serono	Phase III	Recombinant human chorionic gonadotropin
Antiprolactins			
Bromocriptine	Sandoz	Marketed	Short- and long-acting formulations
Dopamine agonist; lisuride hydrogen maleate	VUFB/Schering AG/ Galena	Marketed outside USA	Treatment for hyperprolactinemia; lowers prolactin levels
Dopamine agonist; Terguride, Dironyl, Terulon	Spofa/Sandoz/Schering AG	Marketed outside USA	'Ergoline derivative'
Dopamine D2 receptor agonist; Cabergoline	Pharmacia/Kissei	Marketed outside USA	Treatment for hyperprolactinemia
Metergoline	Pharmacia	Marketed outside USA	Treatment for hyperprolactinemia
Quinagolide; Norprolac	Sandoz	Marketed outside USA	Treatment for hyperprolactinemia with relatively few side-effects
Tyrosine + phenylpropanolamine; IP-401	Interneuron	Preclinical	Treatment for hyperprolactinemia
Progesterone			
Uterogestan	Besins-Iscovesco	Marketed in Europe	Oral and vaginal formulation
Progesterone; Crinone	Columbia Labs/Wyeth-Ayerst	Registered in Europe; phase III in USA	Vaginal progesterone; ovum donation studies in USA
Progesterone suppository	Watson	Phase II	
Progesterone	Effik	Preclinical	Treatment 13 weeks after implantation
Progestogen	Institute of Obstetrics and Gynecology	Preclinical	Easily absorbed progesterone formulation

Vaccines

LHRH analogs	Proteus International	Preclinical	Synthetic vaccine
LHRH implant	Endocon	Preclinical	Subcutaneous implant
LHRH vaccine; Sterovac 92	Proteus Molecular Design	Preclinical	Analog produces immune response to LHRH

Other

TJ-23	Tsumura	Marketed	Raises concentration of estrogen and hypothalamic and cortical acetylcholine receptors
ORG 32489	Organon	Phase III	
Troglitazone; CI-991	Warner-Lambert	Phase III	
Prostaglandin E2 agonist	Cayman Chemical	Clinical trials	
Activin	Roche	Preclinical	Reproductive system regulation; could treat both male and female infertility
E-TRANS	Alza	Preclinical	
Erythroid differentiation factor	Ajinomoto	Preclinical	EDF from human leukocytes (may later be cloned) stimulates ovaries
Estradiol + progestin	Effik	Preclinical	Treatment of infertility
Melatonin receptor antagonist; IP-101	Interneuron	Preclinical	Treatment for chronobiological irregularities, enhances fertility

Uterine Myomas

Goserelin	Zeneca	Marketed in Europe	Marketed for endometriosis; studied for bleeding of fibroids
Leuprolide	Abbott/Takeda/Lederle	Marketed in Europe; awaiting marketing approval for fibroids	Lupron; marketed for endometriosis; suppresses bleeding in uterine fibroids
Levonorgestrel (IUD)	Leiras/Organon	Marketed in Europe	Could be effective treatment for bleeding

Chemical	Company/co-licensees	Phase of development	Comments
Triptorelin	Debiopharm/Pharmacia/Upjohn	Marketed in Europe	Decapeptyl
LHRH antagonist; Cetrorelix	Kayaku Asta/Shionogi	Phase II	Long-lasting action; potential therapy for uterine fibroids
Mifepristone; RU-486	Roussel Uclaf/Population Council	Phase II	Treatment for endometriosis; potential for fibroids
Antiprogestin; LG 1147	Ligand	Preclinical	Non-steroidal compounds from seaweed
Antiprogestin; LG 1127	Ligand	Preclinical	Non-steroidal compounds from seaweed
Antiprogestin; LG 1447	Ligand	Preclinical	Non-steroidal compounds from seaweed
Hirsutism/Polycystic Ovarian Disease			
Rilutamide	Hoechst	Marketed outside USA / Registered in USA / Preregistration in Europe	Non-steroidal anti-androgen
Bicalutamide	Zeneca	Marketed in UK, Ireland / Registered in France, Finland / Preregistration worldwide	Anti-androgen for use with LHRH analogs
Osaterone	Teikoku Hormone	Preregistration in Japan	Anti-androgen; phase II for treatment of osteoporosis
Progesterone	Dekk-Tec/Schering AG/Pharmachemie	Phase III	Pessary for PCO
Finasteride	Merck	Phase II/III	5-α Reductase inhibitor
Troglitazone	Parke-Davis	Phase II	Decreases peripheral insulin resistance
Cioteronel; cyoctol; X-andron	Chantal/Upjohn	Phase II in USA and Europe	Anti-androgen
WIN 49596	Sanofi	Phase II in USA	Steroidal androgen receptor antagonists
Zanoterone	Sanofi	Phase II in USA	Steroidal androgen receptor antagonist; shows no steroid hormone agonist activity

RU-58841	Roussel Uclaf	Phase II	Non-steroidal androgen; for androgen-related hirsutism
MK 0434	Merck	Phase I in USA and Belgium	5-α Reductase inhibitor
Inocoterone; RU 882, RU 38882	Hoechst/Roussel Uclaf	Phase I	Topical preparation, easily metabolized; anti-androgen
Anti-androgen	Imperial Pharmaceutical Services	Clinicals available for licensing in Europe; unavailable for licensing in USA	Oral anti-androgen
L 651580	Merck	Preclinical in USA; discontinued worldwide	Anti-androgen
I 23	Maryland University/Research Corporation Technologies	Preclinical; discontinued	5-α Reductase and 17-α hydroxylase/C17,20 lyase inhibitor; impedes production of testosterone and dihydrotestosterone
LY 191704	Lilly	Preclinical	5-α Reductase inhibitor may be effective treatment for hirsutism
Anti-androgens	Ligand	Preclinical in USA	Androgen receptor antagonists
Anti-androgen	Schering Plough/Laval University	Preclinical in USA and Canada	Topical anti-androgen
ICI 192779	Zeneca	Preclinical in UK; suspended worldwide	

Dysmenorrhea/Amenorrhea

Levonorgestrel IUD	Leiras/Pharmacia	Marketed outside USA	Reducing menstrual bleeding and symptoms
Cyproterone + estradiol valerate	Leiras	Marketed outside USA	Reduces dysmenorrhea
Uterogestan	Besins-Iscovesco	Marketed in Europe	Oral and vaginal formulations
Prometrium	Schering-Plough	Marketed	Oral micronized progesterone, approved for secondary amenorrhea
Crinone	Columbia/Wyeth-Ayerst	Approved for secondary amenorrhea	Vaginal progesterone
Nomegestrol acetate	Theramex	Marketed outside USA	Treatment of menstrual symptoms

Chemical	Company/co-licensees	Phase of development	Comments
Misoprostol; Cytotec	Monsanto/Searle	Marketed in USA	Prostaglandin E1 agonist
Progesterone	Columbia Labs/Wyeth Ayerst	Approved in USA and various countries for secondary amenorrhea	Crinone; UK approved for dysmenorrhea; USA approved for secondary amenorrhea
Progesterone; Prometrium	LaSalle/Schering Plough	Approved in USA and various countries for secondary amenorrhea	Oral formulation for uterine bleeding and amenorrhea
Diclofenac Potassium	Ciba Geigy	Marketed in USA	Oral tablets
Etodolac	American Home Products/Nippon Shinyaku/Eastman Kodak/Marion Merrell Dow/Almirall	Marketed in USA	Marketed as an anti-inflammatory, may have use for dysmenorrhea
Flupirtine	Asta Medica/Carter-Wallace	Marketed outside USA	Analgesic, muscle relaxant
Progesterone	Dekk-Tec/Pharmachemie	Phase III	Pessary for amenorrhea and uterine bleeding
5-Aminolevulinic acid	Deprenyl Research/Medicis	Phase II	Can be used in place of surgery for women with menorrhagia
IP-401	Interneuron	Preclinical	Menstruation disorders
Lead compound of pyridazine derivatives	Johnson & Johnson	Preclinical	Menstruation disorders

APPENDIX C: SEXUALLY TRANSMITTED DISEASES

Vaginitis: Candidiasis

Chemical	Company/co-licensees	Phase of development	Comments
Tioconazole	Pfizer/Schering AG	Marketed in USA and elsewhere	Treatment for vaginal candidiasis
Terconazole	Johnson & Johnson	Marketed in and outside USA	Antifungal treatment for vaginal candidiasis and mycotic vaginitis
Ketoconazole; Nizoral 2% cream	Janssen/Orion-Farmos/ Esteve/Kyowa Hakko	Marketed in and outside USA	Treatment of recurrent vaginitis
Itraconazole; R 51211	Janssen/Senosiain/Esteve/ Lafrancol/Beta/Isdin/ Dispert/Silesia/Kyowa Hakko/Orion/ Litepharma/Liomont/ Sintyal/Procaps	Marketed in and outside USA	Active both orally and topically to treat mycosis
Terconazole	Johnson & Johnson	Marketed in and outside USA	Antifungal treatment for vaginal candidiasis and mycotic vaginitis
Fluconazole	Pfizer	Marketed in USA	Antifungal treatment for life-threatening infections in AIDS patients; also treatment for vaginal candidiasis
Butoconazole	Roche/Roussel Uclaf	Marketed in USA	Cream
Econazole nitrate	Johnson & Johnson/ Taiho/Otsuka	Marketed in USA	Lotrimin cream, lotion and solution
Clotrimazole	Barre-National	Marketed in USA	Cream
Clotrimazole	Schering	Marketed in USA	Lotrimin cream, lotion and solution
Clotrimazole	Miles	Marketed in USA	Mycelex; Mycelex-7 cream, solution, inserts, tablets
Clotrimazole	Taro	Marketed in USA	Cream
Miconazole	Janssen	Marketed in USA	Monistat I.V.
Miconazole nitrate	Barre-National	Marketed in USA	Cream and suppositories

Chemical	Company/co-licensees	Phase of development	Comments
Miconazole nitrate	Taro	Marketed in USA	Vaginal cream
Miconazole nitrate	Ortho	Marketed in USA	Monistat Dual-Pak; Monistat 3 vaginal suppositories
Butoconazole nitrate	Syntex	Marketed in USA	Femstat; Femstat prefill
Flutrimazole	Uriach/KV	Marketed in Spain	Vaginal candidiasis; mycosis
Sertaconazole	Ferrer/SmithKline Beecham/Roberts	Marketed in Spain	Topical antifungal for candidiasis and vaginal infections
Propenidazole	Farmochimica	Marketed in Italy	Antifungal used to treat *Trichomonas vaginalis* and vaginal candidiasis
Oxiconazole	Roche/Siegfried/Glaxo/ Kaken/Tanabe	Marketed in and outside USA	
Alteconazole	Knoll	Preclinical in Germany; discontinued	Topical and oral treatment against *Candida albicans*; cured vaginitis caused by *C. albicans*
MDL 63766	Lepetit	Developmental status unclear	Against *Candida albicans* vaginitis
A-19009	Department of Pharmaceutical Technology & Biochemistry, Technical University of Gdansk	Developmental status unclear	Anticandidal activity; some slight activity against *Trichomonas vaginalis*
N-MGP	Polfa	Phase I in Poland; present development status unclear	Active against *Trichomonas vaginalis* and mixed *Candida albicans* and *T. vaginalis*
Miconazole	Biosert/KV	Clinical trial in USA	Vaginal yeast infection cured
Antifungal bispecific antibody	Medarex	Preclinical	Treatment of vaginal candidiasis
HBD-9107FG	Jean-Paul Martin	Preclinical in France; discontinued	
Alteconazole	Knoll	Preclinical in Germany; discontinued	Topical and oral treatment against *Candida albicans*; cured vaginitis caused by *C. albicans*

Neocopiamycin-A	Dept of Antibiotics, Research Institute for Chemobiodynamics, Chiba University, Japan	Preclinical in Japan	Against *Candida albicans* and range of yeast and fungi
UR-9746	Uriach	Preclinical in Spain and UK	Vaginal candidiasis
SDZ-89-485	Sandoz	Preclinical in Switzerland	Vaginal candidiasis
Jasplakinolide	Roche	Preclinical in USA; discontinued	Antifungal against vaginal candidiasis
1,6-Dihydroxy-2-chlorophenazine	Schering Plough	Preclinical in USA; discontinued	Antibiotic treatment for *Candida albicans* infection
PR-988-399FB	Fisons	Preclinical in USA; discontinued	Vaginal candidiasis
Sch-31153	Schering Plough	Preclinical in USA; discontinued	Topical treatment against vaginal *C. albicans*
Zinoconazole	Monsanto	Preclinical in USA; discontinued	Topical treatment against vaginal candidiasis
Jasplakinolide; Jaspamide	University of California	Preclinical in USA	Treatment for vaginal *C. albicans* infections
LY-303366	Lilly	Preclinical in USA	Treatment of vaginal candidiasis
MSI-751	Magainin	Preclinical in USA	Vaginal fungal infections topical cream
MSI-753	Magainin	Preclinical in USA	Vaginal candidiasis and prevention of STDs
Perillyl alcohol	Non-industrial source: Center for Research for Anti-infectives and Biotechnology	Preclinical in USA	Possible treatment for vaginal bacterial and yeast infections; cream/suppository forms possible
Bay-1-9139	Bayer	Preclinical in USA and Germany; discontinued	Possible treatment for vaginal candidiasis
ICI-153066	Zeneca	Preclinical in UK; discontinued	Treatment of vaginal candidiasis

HIV Drugs

Retrovir	Glaxo-Wellcome	Marketed	
Crixivan	Merck	Marketed	Proteinase inhibitor

Chemical	Company/co-licensees	Phase of development	Comments
Daunorubicin citrate liposome	NeXstar Pharmaceuticals	Marketed	DaunoXome: HIV/Kaposi's sarcoma
Ritonavir	Abbott	Marketed	Norvir
Nevirapine	Roxane	Marketed	Viramune
Lamivudine	Glaxo-Wellcome	Marketed in Europe	Epivir
Stavudine	Bristol-Myers-Squibb	Marketed in Europe	Zerit
Delaviridine mesylate	Ortho Dermatologic	Approved in USA	Rescriptor
Nelfinavir	Aguron	Approved in USA	Viracept
Forvade	Gilead Sciences	Awaiting approval	Acyclovir resistent herpes associated with AIDS
Paxene	Ivax	Awaiting approval	AIDS-related Kaposi's sarcoma
Retrovir	Glaxo-Wellcome	Awaiting approval	Reducing risk of mother-to-fetus transmission
Mitoguazone	Ilex	Awaiting approval	
Lithium gammalinolenate; EF 13	Scotia	Preregistration in UK, Ireland and Denmark	Specifically destroys cells with high HIV-producing capability
Abacavir-1592U89	Glaxo-Wellcome	Phase III	
Adefovir dipivoxil (GS 840)	Gilead Sciences	Phase III	
Advantage 24	Columbia Labs	Phase III	Prevention of HIV; nanoxynyl-9-containing spermicide
Alferone N	Interferon Sciences	Phase III	
Crixivan	Merck	Phase III	HIV in children
Epivir and Retrovir	Glaxo-Wellcome	Phase III	
Imreg-1	Imreg Inc	Phase III	
Indinavir; Indinavir sulfate	Merck & Co	Phase III in USA, Europe and Brazil	Proteinase inhibitor; alone or in combination with zidovudine
Norvir and Invirase combination	Abbott	Phase III	
Oxandrin	BioTechnology General	Phase III	Androgenic hormone for severe AIDS wasting
Remune	Immune Response Corp	Phase III	HIV in adults
Thymopentin	Johnson & Johnson	Phase III	
Timunox	Immunobiology Research Inst	Phase III	Asymptomatic HIV

Name	Company	Phase	Description
Testoderm	Alza	Phase III	Androgen patch for AIDS wasting
VX-478 with Retrovir and Epivir	Vertex	Phase III	
Saquinavar	Roche	Phase III in USA	HIV proteinase inhibitor
Imiquimod	3M/Daiichi	Phase III in USA	HIV treatment; also effective against HSV types 1 and 2
Docosanol; behenyl alcohol	Lidak/CTS/Boryung/Yamanouchi	Phase III in USA	Antiviral treatment of types 1 and 2 herpes virus infections; may be useful against HIV
Sporidin G	GalaGlen	Phase II/III	
Thalidomide	Andrulis	Phase II/III	AIDS-associated canker sores
Tretinoin	Aronex	Phase II/III	Kaposi's sarcoma
Videx in combination with Retrovir and Zerit	Bristol-Myers-Squibb	Phase II/III	
ABT-378	Abbott	Phase II	
AD 439 and AD 519	Tanox BioSystems	Phase II	In vitro stops HIV-1 replication
AIDS gene therapy	Cell Genesys	Phase II	
Ampligen	Hemispeherix	Phase II	
Anticort	Steroidogenesis Inhibitors	Phase II	
Ateviridine mesylate	Pharmacia and Upjohn	Phase II	
Benzimidivir	Glaxo-Wellcome	Phase II	
Diethylhomspermine (DEHOP)	SunPharm	Phase II	
DMP-266 in combination with Crixivan	DuPont	Phase II	
GEM-91	Hybridon	Phase II	
Genetically modified T cells	Cell Genesys	Phase II	
HBY 097	Hoechst Marion Roussel	Phase II	
HBY 1293A	Hoechst Marion Roussel	Phase II	
HIV-IG	Nabi	Phase II	
HIV-IT	Chiron	Phase II	
Inavirase with Norvir, Crixivan and ViraSept	Hoffmann-LaRoche	Phase II	AIDS in children
Letrazuril	Johnson & Johnson	Phase II	
Loviride	Johnson & Johnson	Phase II	

412

Chemical	Company/co-licensees	Phase of development	Comments
Memantine	Neurobiological Technologies	Phase II	Neuropathic pain associated with AIDS
Proleukin	Chiron Vaccines	Phase II	HIV vaccine
Protovir	Protein Design Labs	Phase II	
Remune with Retrovir and Videx	Immune Response	Phase II	
Remune with Retrovir, Epivir and Crixivan	Immune Response	Phase II	
Retrovector	Viagene	Phase II	
S-1090	Shionogi	Phase II	Infections related to HIV
Thymoctonon	Pharmacia-Upjohn	Phase II	
Testosterone Patch	TheraTech	Phase II	AIDS wasting, sexual function
Tucaresol	Glaxo-Wellcome	Phase II	
VIMRxyn	VIMRx	Phase II	
VX-478	Vertex	Phase II	
WinRho SD	Cangene	Phase II	Monotherapy
Reticulon	Advanced Viral Research	Phase II outside USA; applications for US marketing approval were withdrawn without prejudice when the FDA indicated they would not be approved	Possible treatment of hepatitis A and B and AIDS; used to treat herpes zoster and herpes gestationis; antiviral; immunostimulant
α-Trichosanthin, compound Q	UCSF/Genelabs	Phase II in USA	Treatment of HIV; alone or with zidovudine
Vaccine, MN gp 160 vaccine, AIDS	Immuno	Phase II in USA	Glycosylated gp 160 antigen for both prophylactic and treatment
Niravoline	Roussel Uclaf	Phase II in Europe	Treatment for AIDS

Drug	Company/Institution	Phase	Notes
Soluble T4 rs CD4	Columbia University/Biogen/Genentech/DuPont Merck/Progenics/SmithKline Beecham/Invitron	Phase II in USA; discontinued	HIV treatment
L697661	Merck & Co	Phase I/II in USA and Europe; discontinued	HIV treatment discontinued because virus quickly becomes resistant
Hematopoietic stem cell transplants	SyStemix	Phase I/II	
MDX-240	Medarex	Phase I/II	
MKC-242	Triangle	Phase I/II	
Monophosphoryl (MPL) adjuvant	RibiImmunoChem	Phase I/II	
Perthon	Advanced Plant Pharmaceuticals	Phase I/II	
PMPA	Gilead	Phase I/II	
Scriptine	Ivax, SS Pharmaceuticals	Phase I/II	
SPC3	Columbia Labs	Phase I/II	
Sulfasim	Cortech	Phase I/II	
Activated cellular therapy	Neoprobe	Phase I	
Androvir	Paracelsian	Phase I	Dietary supplement
Bathucuprione disulfonic acid copper (PC1250)	ProCyte	Phase I	
CI-1012/1013	Parke-Davis	Phase I	
FddA	US BioScience	Phase I	
Isis 5320	Isis	Phase I	
Lentinan	AJI Pharma	Phase I	
PNU 16090	Pharmacia-Upjohn	Phase I	
PRO 2000	Procept	Phase I	
Remune	Immune Response	Phase I	HIV in children
RG-201	RiboGene	Phase I	AIDS-related pneumocystii carinii
RP400c	Repligen	Phase I	

Chemical	Company/co-licensees	Phase of development	Comments
U-103017	Pharmacia-Upjohn	Phase I	
Gene therapy, HIV-1 ribozyme	Immusol/Pfizer	Phase I in USA	Gene analysis to develop new drugs
Adenosine-regulating agents	Gensia Scicor	Preclinical	
BB-10010	British Biotech PLC	Preclinical	
β-LFd4C	Vion Pharmaceuticals	Preclinical	
Capsid-targeted viral inactivation gene therapy	Avigen	Preclinical	
GS 1278	Gilead	Preclinical	
GS 2992	Gilead	Preclinical	
GS 3333	Gilead	Preclinical	
Interleukin 10	Schering Plough	Preclinical	
MSI-1436	Magainin	Preclinical	
Multikline	Cel-Sci	Preclinical	
Naked DNA vaccine	Vival Inc/Merck	Preclinical	
Oragen	Hemispherx	Preclinical	
PMPA	Gilead	Preclinical	
PRO 367	Progenics	Preclinical	
PRO 542	Progenics	Preclinical	
SPI-119	Sequus	Preclinical	
TNF-α-converting enzyme	Immunex/Wyeth-Ayerst	Preclinical	
Reverse transcriptase inhibitor n-pentyl-DvFc	Kaken/Shin-Etsu Chemical	Preclinical in Japan and Sweden	Anti-HIV agent
Chemically-degraded heparin; ORG 31733	Organon	Preclinical in Netherlands and Belgium	Therapeutic and preventive agent to be developed
Sulfated bacterial glycosaminoglycan; ORG 31581	Organon	Preclinical in Netherlands and Belgium	Therapeutic and preventive agent to be developed
Anti-HIV peptides	New York Blood Center/ Proteus International	Preclinical in USA; discontinued	Impedes attachment of HIV infection to cell
Anti-HIV agent, vaginal microbicide	Biosyn	Preclinical in USA	Antibiotic; preventive measure against STDs, particularly against AIDS

Compound	Company	Status	Indication
FddA; reverse transcriptase inhibitor	National Institutes of Health/US BioScience	Preclinical in USA	HIV treatment
Apoptosis inhibitors	National Research Council/Receptagen	Preclinical in USA	HIV treatment
Zidovudine; CDS zidovudine	Pharmos/Florida University	Preclinical in USA	
Transcription factor regulators	Signal	Preclinical in USA	Treatment to control herpes and AIDS
Cyclobut G	Abbott/Bristol-Myers-Squibb	Preclinical in USA	HIV treatment; potential against herpes simplex 1 and 2
Cyclobut A	Abbott/Bristol-Myers-Squibb	Preclinical in USA	HIV treatment; potential against herpes simplex 1 and 2

Herpes Simplex: Genital

Compound	Company	Status	Indication
Valaciclovir hydrochloride; aciclovir valine ester	Glaxo-Wellcome/Hoechst/Theraplix	Marketed in UK, Ireland and Switzerland	Treatment for herpes zoster (shingles); suppression of recurrent genital herpes in HIV-infected patients is being studied; genital herpes simplex treatment
Famvir	SmithKline Beecham	Awaiting approval	
Forvade	Gilead Sciences	Awaiting approval	Acyclovir-resistant herpes associated with AIDS
Monophosphyl adjuvant	RibiImmuno	Phase III	Vaccine
Lidakol	Lidak	Phase III	
Virend (SP-303)	Shaman	Phase III	
Viropump	Flamel Technologies, SA	Phase III	
Docosanol; behenyl alcohol	Lidak/CTS/Boryung/Yamanouchi	Phase III in USA	Antiviral treatment of types 1 and 2 herpes virus infections; may be useful against HIV
Vaccine, herpes simplex virus gB2 and gD2 antigens + MF59 vaccine HSV-2	Biocine = Chiron	Phase III in USA	
Lithisil	Scotia	Phase II	
Virend in combination with acyclovir	Shaman	Phase II	

Chemical	Company/co-licensees	Phase of development	Comments
Acyclovir Geomatrix	Genta	Phase II	
Thymoctonon	Pharmacia-Upjohn	Phase II	
Visitide	Gilead	Phase I/II	Recurrent genital herpes
Herpes Simplex DISC	Cantab	Phase I	
Cyclocreatine	Amira	Phase I in USA; discontinued	Potential in herpes simplex virus and cytomegalovirus
Acyclovir	TheraTech	Preclinical	Alternative delivery
Anti-herpes antibody	Protein Design Lab	Preclinical	Neonatal and genital herpes
Transcription factor regulators	Signal	Preclinical in USA	Treatment to control herpes and AIDS
Reticulon			
Cyclobut G	Abbott/Bristol-Myers-Squibb	Preclinical in USA	HIV treatment; potential against herpes simplex 1 and 2
Cyclobut A	Abbott/Bristol-Myers-Squibb	Preclinical in USA	HIV treatment; potential against herpes simplex 1 and 2

Human Papilloma Virus

Chemical	Company/co-licensees	Phase of development	Comments
Podofilox; Condylox	Oclassen	Marketed	Topical treatment of genital warts
Trichloroacetic acid		Marketed	
5-FU; fluorouracil		Marketed	
Alfa-n3; Alferone N Injection	Purdue Fredrick	Marketed	Intralesional injection
AccuSite	Matrix	Awaiting approval	Intralesional injection; 5-FU formulation in collagen matrix
TA-GW	Cantab	Phase II	
Lithisil	Scotia	Phase II	
Forvade	Gilead	Phase I/II	
MEDI-504 HPV-18	MedImmune	Preclinical	
HYV-101400	Hybridion	Preclinical	
IFN-α2b; Intron A			Genital warts associated with AIDS

Chlamydia

Name	Company	Status	Description
Vaccine	Antex Biologics	Preclinical	
Chlamydia gene-based vaccine-naked DNA	Vical	Preclinical in USA	*Chlamydia* antigen is encoded by plasmid
Vaccine, *Chlamydia trachomatis*	Microcarb	Preclinical in USA	Antibodies produced attack the M-selectins present on the bacterial membranes

Trichomonas

Name	Company	Status	Description
Metronidazole gel	Curatek	Marketed in USA	Vaginal gel
Metronidazole; Protostat	Ortho	Marketed in USA	Treatment of trichomoniasis
Metronidazole compressed tablets	Par Pharmaceutical	Marketed in USA	Generic
Metronidazole; Flagyl IV	SCS	Marketed in USA	Injection
Metronidazole; Flagyl	Searle	Marketed in USA	Trichomoniasis
Propenidazole	Farmochimica	Marketed in Italy	Antifungal used to treat *Trichomonas vaginalis* and vaginal candidiasis
N-MGP	Polfa	Phase I in Poland; present developmental status unclear	Active against *Trichomonas vaginalis* and mixed *Candida albicans* and *T. vaginalis*
EU-11100	Euroresearch	Preclinical in Italy; present developmental status unclear	Active against *Candida albicans* and *Trichomonas vaginalis*
A-19009	Department of Pharmaceutical Technology & Biochemistry, Technical University of Gdansk	Developmental status unclear	Anticandidal activity; some slight activity against *Trichomonas vaginalis*
G-1549	Glaxo	Preclinical in UK; discontinued	Possible treatment of *Trichomonas vaginalis*

Chemical	Company/co-licensees	Phase of development	Comments
Bacterial Vaginosis			
Amoxicillin; Amoxil	SmithKline Beecham	Marketed in USA	
Metronidazole gel	Curatek	Marketed in USA	
Metronidazole Redi-Infusion	Elkins-Sinn	Marketed in USA	
Metronidazole; Protostat	Ortho	Marketed in USA	Anaerobic bacterial infections
Metronidazole compressed tablets	Par Pharmaceutical	Marketed in USA	
Metronidazole; Flagyl	Searle	Marketed in USA	For trichomoniasis; anaerobic bacterial infections
Mycosis			
Amphotericin B lipid complex	Liposome Company	Marketed in UK and Luxembourg; preregistration in USA	Systemic fungal infections in immunocompromised patients in UK and Luxembourg; in USA for cancer chemotherapy or bone marrow transplant patients with infections
Other			
Levofloxacin; Ofloxacin	Daiichi/Johnson & Johnson/Hoechst	Marketed outside USA; preregistration in USA	Antibiotic; treatment of STDs
Meropenem	Sumitomo/Zeneca/Yuhan	Marketed outside USA; preregistration in USA	Gynecological infections
Cefpodoxine proxetil; Cefpodoxime	Sankyo/Roussel Uclaf/Upjohn/Glaxo-Wellcome/Alfarma/Luitpold/Biochemie	Marketed in USA	Antibiotic; oral tablet and suspension forms; sexually transmitted disease treatment

Azithromycin	Pliva/Funk/Sigma Tau/Farma/Pfizer/Fabre/Procaps/Legrand	Marketed in the USA	Antibiotic; treatment of sexually transmitted infections; bacterial infection; also used to treat malaria; also treatment of simple sexually transmitted infections caused by *Chlamydia trachomatis*
Clopinazole	VUFB	Phase II in Czech Republic; present developmental status unclear	Antifungal gynecological agent; treat mycotic colpitis
Temafloxacin	Abbott/Tanabe/Zeneca/Dainabot	Withdrawn; had been approved and marketed previously	Antibiotic; withdrawn due to toxicity problems
RU-64004	Roussel Uclaf	Preclinical in France	Antibiotic; treatment for STDs
MSI 420	Magainin	Preclinical in USA	Topical antibacterial formulation; treatment for STDs
Vaccine, STDs	Zonagen	Preclinical in USA	Female prophylactic vaccines

APPENDIX D: PREGNANCY

Chemical	Company/co-licensees	Phase of development	Comments
Inhibition of Pre-term Labor			
Hexoprenaline sulfate; Delaprem	Altana, Inc./Savage Labs	Marketed outside USA; preregistration in USA	β-blocker
Ritodrine HCl	Abbott Labs	Marketed	β-blocker
Magnesium sulfate	Astra	Used but not approved	
Terbutaline	Marion Merrell Dow	Used but not approved	β-blocker
Nifedipine	Generic	Used but not approved	Calcium channel blocker
Rolipram	Schering AG/Meiji Seika	Phase III	
Atosiban	Johnson & Johnson	Phase III	Oxytocin antagonist
Carbetocin	Ferring	Phase II	Oxytocin antagonist; oxytocin analog
HSR-81	Hokuriku Seiyaku/Tokyo Tanabe	Phase II	Inhibits premature labor contractions
Transdermal nitroglycerin	Schwarz	Preclinical	Labor inhibition
Tocolytics	Adeza Biomedical/ Hamamatsu University	Preclinical	
CR-1701	Rotta	Preclinical	Oxytocin antagonist
L-366948	Merck	Preclinical	Oxytocin antagonist
L-366517	Merck	Preclinical	Oxytocin antagonist
L-156373	Merck	Preclinical	Oxytocin antagonist
L-366254	Merck	Preclinical	Myometrial relaxant
L-365209	Merck	Preclinical	Oxytocin antagonist
L-368899	Merck	Preclinical	Oxytocin antagonist
L-367773	Merck	Preclinical	Oxytocin antagonist
L-366509	Merck	Preclinical	Oxytocin antagonist
L-366682	Merck	Preclinical	Oxytocin antagonist
Prostaglandin E2 agonist; AH-13205	Glaxo	Preclinical	Inhibits premature labor contractions

Intravaginal prostaglandin	Trimel	Preclinical in USA and Canada	Labor inhibition; delivers prostaglandins directly to cervix
Induction of Labor			
Hydrogel polymer prostaglandin; prostaglandin E2 pessary	Strathclyde University/Forest/Zeneca/Ferring/Pharmasciences	Marketed in UK; received approval in USA	Labor induction
Dinoprostone	Pharmasciences/Forest Labs	Marketed	Pessary dilates cervix, facilitating childbirth
Progesterone receptor antagonist; mifepristone	Roussel Uclaf	Marketed in Europe/application submitted in USA	Oral formulation; abortifacient, contraceptive, labor inducer; treatment for endometriosis
KB-60	Kanebo	Phase III	Sodium prasterone sulfate suppository makes uterus more sensitive to oxytocin
Relaxin	Genetech/Mitsubishi Kasei	Phase I	Synthetic peptide hormone makes pelvic ligaments more elastic
RU-52562/RU-51996/RU-43044/RU-39973	Roussel Uclaf	Preclinical; discontinued	Labor induction
Other			
Evening Primrose Oil	Scotia	Marketed in Europe	May be of use in toxemia of pregnancy
Rh_0 (D) immune globulin; intravenous human	Univax Biologics	Application submitted	Rh_0 isoimmunization during pregnancy
Carbetocin	Ferring Labs	Phase III	Post-partum blood loss in cesarean section patients
Sufentanil; sufenta	Janssen	Phase III	Treatment of labor and delivery pain

APPENDIX E: MENOPAUSE

Vasomotor Symptoms
Oral HRT

Chemical	Company/co-licensees	Phase of development	Comments
Conjugated estrogens + medroxyprogesterone	Wyeth-Ayerst/American Home Products	Marketed worldwide; phase III for osteoporosis and cardiovascular	Prempro, Premphase, oral HRT for treatment of menopausal symptoms and osteoporosis; Prempro—continuous combined; Premphase—cyclic therapy
Estradiol + norethisterone	Novartis	Marketed outside USA	HRT tablets: 16 contain estradiol valerate and 12 contain estradiol valerate and norethisterone
Estradiol valerate + levonorgestrel	Schering AG	Marketed outside USA	Nuvelle; HRT tablets for menopausal symptoms
Estradiol + dydrogesterone	Solvay	Marketed in Europe	Femoston
Estradiol valerate + medroxyprogesterone acetate	Orion-Farmos/ Organon-Azko Nobel	Marketed outside USA	Divitren; 91-day HRT for osteoporosis and menopausal symptoms: estradiol valerate for 70 days, estradiol valerate + medroxyprogesterone for 14 days, no treatment for 7 days, causes less withdrawal bleeding than similar formulations
Estradiol valerate + medroxyprogesterone acetate	Orion-Farmos/Klimalet	Marketed outside USA	Divina; 28-day HRT for osteoporosis and menopausal symptoms: estradiol valerate for 11 days, estradiol valerate + medroxyprogesterone for 10 days, no treatment for 7 days
Estradiol + norethindrone acetate	Novo Nordisk/RPR	Marketed outside USA; phase III in USA	Kliogest; continuous combined
Estradiol + norethindrone acetate p	Novo Nordisk	Marketed outside USA	Trisequens—cyclic

Drug	Company	Status	Trade name / comments
Ethinyl estradiol + norethindrone acetate	Warner-Lambert	Phase III	
Ethinyl estradiol and gestodene	Schering AG	Phase III	Meliane
Dionegest + estradiol valerate	Jenapharm	Phase III	Treatment of osteoporosis and menopausal symptoms
Trimegestone + estradiol	Roussel Uclaf	Phase III in Europe	HRT
Medroxyprogesterone acetate/Estropipate	Upjohn	Phase III	Provera/Ogen
RPR 106522	Rhone-Poulenc Rorer	Phase III	
ORG 2812	Organon	Phase III	
Cyclophasic HRT	R.W. Johnson Pharmaceutical Research Institute	Phase II	
Estradiol valerate and drospirenone	Schering AG	Phase I	Antimineralocorticoid progestogen

Estrogen Alone

Drug	Company	Status	Trade name / comments
Conjugated estrogens	Wyeth-Ayerst	Marketed worldwide	Premarin; estrogen alone, several doses available
Conjugated estrogens	Solvay	Marketed worldwide	Presomen
Estradiol	Bristol-Myers-Squibb	Marketed worldwide	Estrace
Estropipate			Ogen
Estratab	Solvay	Marketed in USA	Esterified estrogens
Menest	SmithKline Beecham		Micronized estradiol
Zumenon	Solvay		
Estring	Pharmacia-Upjohn		Vaginal ring

Progestins

Drug	Company	Status	Trade name / comments
Medroxyprogesterone acetate	Pharmacia-Upjohn	Marketed	Provera
Medroxyprogesterone acetate	Wyeth-Ayerst	Marketed	Cycrin

Chemical	Company/co-licensees	Phase of development	Comments
Nomegestrol acetate	Solvay	Marketed in Europe	Lutenyl
Dydrogesterone	Schering AG	Marketed in Europe	Duphaston
Cyproterone acetate	Roussel Uclaf	Phase II/III	Anti-androgen
Trimegestone			
Progesterone	Effik	Preclinical	HRT easily absorbed progesterone formulation; delivery system not specified
Progesterone	Schering/Solvay	NDA review	Prometrium, micronized progesterone
Progesterone agonists	Ligand	Preclinical	HRT for menopausal symptoms

Other Miscellaneous Steroids/Products

Chemical	Company/co-licensees	Phase of development	Comments
Synthetic steroid, Tibolone	Akzo/Kanebo/Organon	Marketed in Europe; phase III in USA	Livial; treatment of endometriosis, HRT and osteoporosis, 2.5 mg/day, oral estrogenic, androgenic, progestogenic steroid
Esterified estrogens + methyltestosterone	Solvay	Marketed worldwide	Estrogen + androgen combination
Estradiol gel	Akzo Nobel/Organon	Phase III	Divigel, Sandrena; menopausal symptoms
Org 32818	Akzo Nobel	Phase III	Menopausal symptoms
Estradiol gel	Besims/Scovesco/Solvay	Phase III	
Estradiol	Pharmos/Florida University	Phase II	Vasomotor symptoms; estradiol can pass through blood–brain barrier with Pharmos Chemical Delivery System
Estradiol	Hisamitsu	Preclinical	Treatment for menopausal symptoms; delivery system not specified
Estradiol + progestin	Effik	Preclinical	HRT enhances fertility and treats menopausal symptoms
Somatomedin B; insulin-like growth factor 2 (IGF-2)	Llorente	Preclinical	HRT
STS-386	Jenapharm	Preclinical	HRT delivery system not specified

Transdermal HRT

Estradiol	Ciba Geigy/Alza	Marketed	Estraderm: reservoir transdermal HRT patch
Estradiol	Noven/Rhone-Poulenc Rorer/Ciba Geigy/Novartis	Marketed	Menorest, Vivelle 3–4 day transdermal HRT patch
Estradiol	Schering AG/3M	Marketed	Climara, 7-day transdermal HRT patch
Estradiol	Johnson & Johnson	Marketed	Cystem, Evorel, System, 0.1 mm thick transdermal HRT matrix patch, releases 50 mg of estradiol per day
Estradiol	Cilag	Mark ted	Transdermal patch
Estradiol	Pharmacia/Leiras Oy	Marketed	Low doses of 17-β estradiol released by intravaginal ring
Estradiol + norethisterone P	Alza/Ciba Geigy	Marketed	Transdermal HRT patches: 4 estrogen patches worn for 2 weeks and 4 progesterone patches worn for next 2 weeks
Estradiol	Procter & Gamble; TheraTech	Marketed	HRT patch
Estradiol	Cygnus Research/Elf Sanofi/Warner-Lambert	Approved in the USA	Fempatch, transdermal HRT patch for osteoporosis and menopausal symptoms
Estradiol	Merck KGaA	Phase III in USA	Estrogen replacement; 7-day HRT patch Fem 7
Estradiol	Fournier	Phase III in USA; marketed in Europe	Transdermal HRT patches: 6 estradiol patches worn for 3 weeks, no treatment 4th week
Estradiol	Noven Pharmaceuticals/Rhone-Poulenc Rorer/Ciba Geigy	Phase III	12-day Transdermal HRT patch for osteoporosis and menopausal symptoms
Estradiol	Pierre Fabre	Phase III	Transdermal HRT patch
Estradiol	Rotta Research	Phase III	Transdermal HRT patch for osteoporosis and menopausal symptoms
Estradiol + norethisterone	Ethical Pharmaceuticals/Solvay/Il-Yang	Phase III	Fematrix; transdermal HRT patch for osteoporosis and menopausal symptoms
Estrogen + progestogen, RPR 106522	Rhone-Poulenc Rorer	Phase III	HRT combination patch for postmenopausal symptoms

Chemical	Company/co-licensees	Phase of development	Comments
Estrogen/progestogen	E Merck/Solvay	Phase III	7-Day transdermal estradiol + levonorgestrel
Estropipate + norethindrone	Johnson & Johnson	Phase III	Ortho-EST Plus
Norethisterone	Ethical/Pierre Fabre	Phase III	3–4 Day transdermal HRT patch
Norethisterone	Ethical Pharmaceuticals	Phase III	14-Day treatment of transdermal norethisterone to be administered with estradiol in HRT
Estradiol/norethisterone acetate patch	R.W. Johnson Pharmaceutical Research Institute	Phase III	7-Day transdermal HRT patch
Estradiol + progestin	Procter & Gamble/TheraTech	Phase I	
Estradiol	Ethical Pharmaceuticals/Searle	Phase II/III	Transdermal estrogen for osteoporosis and menopausal symptoms
Estradiol, TSH-01	Teijin	Phase II	2-Day transdermal HRT patch
Estradiol	Pharmed	Phase II	HRT transdermal
Estrogen + progestin combi-patch	Rhone-Poulenc Rorer/Noven	Phase II	
Estradiol	Hercon	Phase I	Transdermal HRT patch
Estradiol	Pharmetrix	Phase I	Transdermal HRT patch
Estradiol	Teikoku Hormone/Nitto Denko	Phase I	Alcohol-free transdermal HRT for reduced irritation
Estradiol + norethisterone	Pierre Fabre	Phase I	Transdermal HRT patch
Estrogen + progestin	Fournier	Phase I	Transdermal HRT patch
ph-923	Pharmed	Phase I	Transdermal HRT patch
Norethisterone + estradiol	Ethical	Phase I	Transdermal HRT patch
Progestogen/estrogen	Noven Pharmaceuticals/Rhone-Poulenc Rorer	Phase I	Transdermal HRT patch for osteoporosis and menopausal symptoms
Estradiol	Biosearch	Preclinical	Transdermal HRT patch
Estradiol + progestin	Cygnus Research/Elf Sanofi	Preclinical	Transdermal HRT patch for osteoporosis and menopausal symptoms

Compound	Company	Status	Description
Estradiol + progestogen	Pharmetrix	Preclinical	Transdermal HRT patch
Estrogen	Cygnus Research/American Home Products	Preclinical	7-Day transdermal HRT patch
Estrogen + progesterone	Cygnus Research/American Home Products	Preclinical	7-Day transdermal HRT patch
Estrogen + progestin	Sano	Preclinical	Combination patch
Estrogen + progestin	Hercon	Preclinical	Transdermal HRT patch
Estradiol + testosterone patch	TheraTech	Phase I	Combination patch for menopausal symptoms
Testosterone patch	TheraTech/Procter & Gamble	Phase II	Used in combination with oral estrogen
IP1112	Shire	Preclinical	
IP1162	Shire	Preclinical	
IP1163	Shire	Preclinical	
IP1164	Shire	Preclinical	
Progestogen	Noven	Preclinical	Transdermal

Alternative Delivery Systems

Compound	Company	Status	Description
Estring	Pharmacia-Upjohn	Marketed	Estrogen vaginal ring
Femring	Roussel-Uclaf/Galen	Phase III	Intravaginal ring may be used to administer estrogen for HRT
IUTS progesterone	Alza	Phase III	Intra-uterine therapy
Estradiol	Pharmos	Phase II	Sublingual estradiol formulation for hot flashes and endometriosis
Estrasorb	Novavex	Phase II	
Estradiol	Condos/University of Lund	Phase I	Vaginal ring for atrophic vaginitis, vasomotor symptoms
Estradiol	Nastech	Preclinical	Intranasal formulation
Estradiol + cyclodextrin	Biotechnology General	Preclinical	Sublingual formulation

Chemical	Company/co-licensees	Phase of development	Comments
Atrophic Vaginitis			
Premarin Cream	Wyeth-Ayerst	Marketed	Vaginal cream
Estrace Cream	Bristol-Myers-Squibb	Marketed	Vaginal cream
Estrone	Organon	Marketed in Europe	Ovestin; vaginal cream and tablets
Estradiol	Novo Nordisk	Marketed in Europe; phase III in USA	Vagifem; vaginal tablets
Estradiol	Condos/University of Lund	Phase I	Vaginal ring for atrophic vaginitis, vasomotor symptoms
HBD-91070S	Jean-Paul Martin	Preclinical	Treatment for atrophic vaginitis
Urinary Incontinence			
Desmopressin; KW 8008	Ferring/Kyowa Hakko/ Rhone-Poulenc Rorer/ IBAH	Marketed	
Estradiol	Kabi/Pharmacia	Marketed	Vaginal ring
Midodrine; midodrine hydrochloride; Metligene; Midon	Nycomed/Il Yang/ Taisho/Roberts/Boots	Marketed in Europe	
Propiverine, P-4; Mictonorm; BUP-4	VEB Apogepha/Taiho	Marketed	Anticholinergic spasmolytic
Tolterodine; KABI 2234	Pharmacia/Kissei	Marketed	Anticholinergic
Cystrin CR	PenWest Pharmaceuticals Group; Leiras/Oy	Awaiting approval	Urinary incontinence and pediatric vesico-urethral reflux
Detrusitol	Pharmacia-Upjohn	Awaiting approval	Urinary incontinence
Vamicamide, FK 176	Fujisawa	Preregistration	Anticholinergic; treatment for instability of bladder muscle
Amantine	Roberts	Phase III	Urinary incontinence
Alfuzosin	Fujosawa	Phase III	Urinary incontinence
NS 21	Nippon Shinyaku	Phase III	Anticholinergic; calcium antagonist

Compound	Company	Development phase	Properties / Indication
Terodiline; TD 758; Mictrol; Bicor	Pharmacia/Forest/Rhone-Poulenc Rorer	Phase III	Antispasmodic
TTS Oxybutynin	Alza	Phase II/III	Transdermal oxybutynin; urge urinary incontinence
Darifenacin	Pfizer	Phase II	Anticholinergic; muscarinic antagonist
Duloxetine	Lilly/Shionogi	Phase II	Noradrenaline re-uptake inhibitor
FK 584	Fujisawa	Phase II	
NS 49	Synthelabo/Nippon Shinyaku	Phase II	Derived from phenylethanolamine; α-adrenergic antagonist
Terflavoxate	Nippon Shinyaku/Recordati/Dainippon	Phase II	Derived from flavone; calcium antagonist; antispasmodic
YM 934	Yamanouchi	Phase I	Activates potassium channel
S-butynin	Sepracor	Phase I	Urinary incontinence
ZD169	Zeneca	Phase I	Urinary incontinence
Hylan B	Biomatrix/Bard	Phase I; discontinued	Cicatrizant
JO 1870	Jouveinal	Phase I	Opiate agonist
NC 1800	Nippon Chemiphar	Clinical trials	
Lanperisone; lanperisone hydrochloride	Nippon Kayaku	Preclinical	
5HT4, human neuroreceptor	Synaptic	Preclinical; discontinued	
Adospine	Menarini	Preclinical	Spasmolytic properties
Bladder and urethral patch	Organogenesis	Preclinical	Bladder and urethral repair
Bladder neck suspension string	Organogenesis	Preclinical	Urinary stress incontinence
Collagen injectable	Organogenesis	Preclinical	Urge incontinence and pediatric vesico-urethral reflux
CR 1467	Rotta	Preclinical	Potential spasmolytic
FR 75513	Fujisawa	Preclinical	Treatment for patients with overactive detrusor muscle
HSR 175	Hokuriku	Preclinical	α-adrenergic antagonist
UR 8225	Uriach	Preclinical	Activates potassium channel
Urinary antispasmodic	Marion Merrell Dow/Scios Nova	Preclinical	Muscarinic antagonist; anticholinergic
Urinary antispasmodic agent	Sepracor	Preclinical	
ZD 6169	Zeneca	Preclinical	Derived from terodoline

APPENDIX F: OSTEOPOROSIS

Chemical	Company/co-licensees	Phase of development	Comments
Antiresorptive Agents			
Estrogen and progestins: detailed listing of products can be found under the Menopause listings. Although not all estrogens are approved specifically for osteoporosis, they are used as such.			
Partial Agonists/Antihormones			
Raloxifene; LY 1394811, LY 156758; keoxifene	Eli Lilly	Marketed	Tissue-specific anti-estrogen, Evista®
Toremifine	Schering Plough/Orion-Farmos	Approved for breast cancer	Under study for osteoporosis
Droloxifene	Klinge/Pfizer	Phase III for breast cancer; phase II for osteoporosis	Under study for osteoporosis
Osaterone acetate; TZP 4238, TZP 5258	Teikoku Hormone	Preregistration in Japan; Phase II (as anti-osteporotic)	Chlormadinone acetate (CMA) derivative; developed as an anti-androgen; has possible anti-osteoporotic properties
Idoxifene; CB-7432, CB-7386	Institute of Cancer Research/SmithKline Beecham/British Technology	Phase II for breast cancer	Under study for osteoporosis
Ormeloxifene	Central Drug Research Institute/ZymoGenetics	Preclinical	L-enantiomer of centrochroman
NNC-46-0200	Karo Bio/Novo Nordisk	Preclinical	Partial estrogen receptor antagonist
Estrogen agonists	Ligand Pharmaceuticals/Pfizer	Preclinical	Tissue-specific estrogenic product; positive effects (no harm to bone or heart) of estrogen without greater breast cancer or uterine cancer risks
Estrogen analogs	Hoechst Marion Roussel	Preclinical	Local estrogenic activity on bone tissue

Compound	Company/Institution	Status	Comments
FC 1217	Orion-Farmos	Preclinical	Toremifene derivative with anti-estrogenic and estrogenic properties
Centrochroman; Centron	Central Drug Research Institute/Novo-Nordisk	Preclinical	Marketed as an oral contraceptive; being developed by Novo Nordisk as an osteoporotic agent

Bisphosphonates

Compound	Company/Institution	Status	Comments
Alendronate sodium; Fosamax®	Merck & Co/Gentili/Teijn/Sigma-Tau/Neopharmed/Wyeth-Ayerst	Marketed in USA and in Europe	Fosamax; daily oral formulation inhibits resorption and increases bone density
Clodronate disodium	Gentili/Boehringer Mannheim/many other companies	Marketed in Europe	Bonefos; Clastoban; drug substance off patent
Disodium pamidronate; Avedia®	Henkel/Ciba-Geigy/Almirall/Chiron	Marketed	Hypercalcemia of malignancy in the USA; drug substance off patent
Etidronate disodium; Didronel®	Procter & Gamble	Marketed for Paget's worldwide/osteoporosis ex-USA	Didrocal, Didronel
APD disodium 3-amino-1-(hydroxypropylidine)-1,1-diphosphonate; Avedia®	Novartis	Marketed	i.v. injectable
Risedronate sodium/risedronic acid; NE 58095	Procter & Gamble/Hoechst Marion Roussel/Takeda/Ajinomoto	Phase III in USA; clinical trial (Japan)	Intravenous, subcutaneous and oral formulations under development
Tiludronic acid/tiludronate disodium; SR 41319B, ME 3737	Sanofi/Meiji Seika	Marketed	Paget's disease
Ibandronic acid	Boehringer Mannheim/Rhone-Poulenc Rorer	Phase III for osteoporisis; marketed for hypercalcemia	Third generation bisphosphonate

Chemical	Company/co-licensees	Phase of development	Comments
YM-175; Incadronate	Yamanouchi/Glaxo	Phase III	Oral liquid form/injection, bisphosphonate
EB-1053	Leo Denmark	Phase III	Oral/intravenous formulation under development. In animals, it is 50 times more potent than APD and 10 times more potent than dimethyl-APD
Phosphonic acid, bis-, disodium salt (CAS)	Yamanouchi/Glaxo Wellcome	Preregistration/preclinical	Oral formulation in liquid form (phase II/injection formulation; 10 times more potent than pamidronate
YM-529	Yamanouchi/Hoechst	Phase II/III	Derived from YM-175, oral and intravenous formulations; possibly less toxicity than YM-175
Aminohexane diphosphate; AHDP	Gentili/Shire	Phase II	Hypocalcemic agent
Mildronic acid	Gador	Phase II	Inhibits bone resorption
Olpadronic	Gador	Phase II	
Zoledronic acid; CGP-42446	Novartis	Phase I	Diphosphonate anti-osteoporotic agent, animal studies show 100 times greater efficacy at increasing mineralized bone tissue than disodium pamidronate; may also be less inhibitive of bone formation than other antiresorptive agents
Bisphosphonic acid derivative	Leiras Oy	Preclinical	
Neridronic acid	Gentili/Shire	Preclinical	
Biophosphonates, Yissum	Yissum	Preclinical	Anticalcification properties, treat Ca metabolism irregularity, may treat osteoporosis, renal calculi, hypercalcemia, etc.
Bisphosphonic acid; BM-211182	Boehringer Mannheim	Preclinical	High oral bioavailability, long duration; back-up for BM-210955
Etidronate disodium i.v.	MGI Pharma	Preclinical	

Phosphonate carboxylate derivatives	Procter & Gamble	Preclinical	Treatment of calcium metabolism disorders; impedes bone tissue resorption/reduces chance of bone mineralization
SR-2013	Symphar	Preclinical	Anti-oxidant
Thionaphene-2-carboxylic lysine salt; TNLY	MacroChem	Preclinical	
Thionaphene carboxylic acid; TNCA	MacroChem	Preclinical	Also a possible development for hypercalcemia of malignancy

Calcitonin

Calcitonin; Salmon HC 581, RG-83630	Rhone-Poulenc Rorer/ Asahi Chemical/ Hisamitsu/Innothera/ Hafslund Nycomed/ Merck/Ferrer/CEPA/ SmithKline Beecham/ Chong Kun Dang	Marketed in Europe	Calcimar; Calsynar; Elcatonin; Calcin; Dompe; Prontocalcin; intranasal and parenteral calcitonin; improved bone mineral content without affecting bone formation markers, serum alkaline phosphatase or osteocalcin and minimal local side-effects
Calcitonin; salmon	Novartis	Marketed in USA	Micalcin injection; intranasal and injectable salmon calcitonin
Calcitonin; salmon	Novartis	Marketed in USA	Cibalcin injection; injectable salmon calcitonin
Calcitonin; human	Novartis	Marketed in USA	Micalcin injection
Calcitonin	Novartis	Marketed	Cibacalcin; intranasal calcitonin formulation
Calcitonin; salmon	Teikoku Hormone	Marketed in Japan	Synthetic injectable salmon calcitonin
Calcitonin; salmon	Rhone-Poulenc Rorer	Awaiting approval	Calcimar intranasal
Calcitonin; modified recombinant chicken calcitonin MCI-536	Mitsubishi Kasei/Fujirebio	Phase III	Avicatonin
Calcitonin; salmon	Pharma Bissendorf	Phase III	
Calcitonin	Cortecs/Osteometer Biotech	Phase II	Oral salmon calcitonin formulation; Macromol delivery system

Chemical	Company/co-licensees	Phase of development	Comments
Calcitonin; STH 32	Teijin	Phase II	Intranasal salmon calcitonin
Calcitonin; SUN 8577; human calcitonin; hCT	Suntory	Phase II	Intranasal recombinant human calcitonin
Calcitonin	Beaufour-Ipsen	Phase II	Sustained-release salmon calcitonin; described as useful in bone metabolism disorders
Calcitonin-salmon	Inhale Therapeutics	Phase I	Aerosol formulation
Calcitonin-salmon	Druamed	Phase I	Spiros
Calcitonin	IBAH	Phase I	Rectal suppository of micro-emulsion calcitonin
Calcitonin	Pharmos/Hebrew University	Clinical trials	'Submicron emulsion formulation' helps to cause higher bioavailability
Calcitonin; ACT 15	Chugai/Asahi Chemical	Preclinical	Chimeric mixture of human and salmon calcitonin
Calcitonin, Vicalcins	Vical	Preclinical	Synthetic peptide analogs to human, salmon, eel calcitonin
Calcitonin	Cygnus	Preclinical; suspended	Transdermal formulation
Calcitonin	Emisphere	Preclinical	Oral formulation
Calcitonin	Pharmaceutical Development Associates	Preclinical	Oral formulation
Calcitonin	Protein Delivery	Preclinical	PROTEIMER polymer delivery system; route of administration unknown
Calcitonin	TheraTech	Preclinical	Buccal oral transmucosal formulation
Calcitonin	Unigene	Preclinical	Oral formulation under development; may be discontinued
Calcitonin	Yissum	Preclinical	Delivery system is intra-uterine (or transendometrium)
Calcitonin gene	Transkaryotic Therapies	Preclinical	Gene therapy; development of recombinant hormones
Calcitonin	Fidia	Preregistration in Italy	Hyaluronic acid microsphere sustained-release vaginal delivery system; salmon

Calcitonin	Peptide Technology	Preregistration in Europe	Intranasal salmon calcitonin
Calcitonin	Liposome Technology	Development status unclear	Oral formulation

Fluorides

Monofluorophosphate	Rotto Research	Marketed in Europe	
Sodium fluoride; Neosten®	Mission Pharmacal	Application submitted	
EMD-59976	E Merck (Germany)	Phase III	
Fluoride, Osteo-F	Hoyt Labs	Phase III	
Sodium monofluorophosphate	Colgate-Palmolive	Phase III	
Fluoride, calcium and vitamin D3 supplement	Merck KGaA	Phase II/III	Salt combination containing fluoride

Vitamin D and Vitamin D Analogs

Calcitriol	Roche	Phase III; marketed for renal osteodystrophy	Rocaltrol
Vitamin D3 derivative; hexafluorovitamin D3 ST 630	Taisho/Sumitomo	Phase III (Japan); preclinical (USA)	Hypercalcemic, 5–10 times as osteogenic as natural Vitamin D3 in animal studies; increases bone metabolism/reduces calcium resorption
Vitamin D2 analog; One-alpha-D2	Bone Care International/Draxis Health/Deprenyl Research	Phase II	Anti-osteoporotic, also treat secondary hyperparathyroidism; does raise calcium levels at tested doses
Vitamin D2 derivative; TSA 870	Bone Care International/Draxis	Phase II	Osteogenic compound less likely to produce kidney stones
Vitamin D3 derivative; K-DR	Kureha Chemical/Sankyo	Phase II	Osteogenic compound promotes 'normal' bone growth
Vitamin D analog; EL-715	Elan	Developmental status not clear	Not much information
Bonealpha	Teijin		
Vitamin D3 analog; LR 108	Lunar	Phase II	Vitamin D3 precursor should not hyperstimulate dietary Ca^{+2}

Chemical	Company/co-licensees	Phase of development	Comments
Vitamin D3 agonists	Karo Bio	Preclinical	Designer molecule based on studies of structure of the vitamin D receptor
Vitamin D3 analog; ED-71	Chugai	Preclinical	Promotes intestinal calcium absorption and bone formation
Vitamin D3 analog; NOF 002	NOF Corporation	Preclinical	
Parathyroid Hormones			
Teriparatide	Asahi Chemical	Marketed	Active fragment of parathyroid hormone; induced bone formation activity and minimized osteopenia in rats; may cause mild hypotension and headache
Parathyroid hormone; ALX1-11	Allelix	Phase III	Recombinant human PTH increases calcium absorption and significantly promotes bone growth
Parathyroid hormone analog; RS 66271	Roche Bioscience	Phase III	
Parathyroid hormone	Lilly	Phase IV	
Parathyroid hormone	Wellcome	Phase I/II	
PTH	Astra AB	Phase I	Inhalent/injection
PTH analog	Hemisphere	Preclinical	Oral formulation
PTH fragment	Takeda	Preclinical	Cell adhesion inhibitors; potential anti-osteoporotic; stimulated osteogenesis by 7 times cf. control in cell culture
Parathyroid hormone analog	Allelix/Glaxo	Preclinical	Based on ALX1-11
Parathyroid hormone analog	Karo Bio	Preclinical	
Parathyroid hormone; rhPTH	Chugai	Preclinical	Recombinant human PTH
Parathyroid hormone fragment	Boehringer Mannheim	Preclinical	
Parathyroid hormone; PTH 1-34	Karo Bio	Suspended	
Parathyroid hormone; PTH 1-84	Karo Bio	Suspended	

Growth Factors

Drug	Company	Status	Description
Mecasermin	Fujisawa	Marketed for insulin-resistant diabetes/growth hormone-resistant dwarfism; may have use in osteoporosis	Recombinant somatomedin-1, may treat bone diseases
Somatotropin	Serono	Marketed for growth hormone deficiency; clinical trials	Recombinant human growth hormone
Somatotropin	Novo-Nordisk	Marketed for growth hormone deficiency	Recombinant human somatotropin under study for osteoporosis and infertility
Somatrem	Genentech	Marketed for growth hormone deficiency	Protropin; recombinant human growth hormone
Somatomedin-C, IGF-1; mecasermin	Llorente/Pharmacia	Approved in Sweden for growth hormone sensitivity	Insulin-like growth factor-1; being investigated for osteoporosis treatment
Somatomedin-C; CGP 35126	Cephalon Incorporate/Chiron/Kyowa Hakko	Phase III; preregistration for ALS	Oral and subcutaneous recombinant somatomedin-C
Somatomedin-C	Fujisawa	Phase III	Recombinant somatomedin-C from *E. coli*
TGF-β_2	Celtrix Pharmaceuticals/Enzon/Santen	Phase III	Recombinant TGF-β_2
TGF-β_2; Fovalin, BetaKine	Celtrix/Santen/Genzyme	Phase III	Promotes angiogenesis; role in osteoporosis unclear
Fibroblast growth factor	Scios Nova/Kaken	Phase II in Japan for osteoporosis	Recombinant human basic fibroblast growth factor
Somatomedin-1 and somatomedin-2; CGP 35126	Chiron/Cephalon Incorporated/Kyowa Hakko	Phase II from NMDW94	Recombinant somatomedin-1 and somatomedin-2 grown in yeast
Examorelin, Hexarelin	Europeptides	Phase II	Hexapeptide growth hormone releasing hormone analog
Growth hormone releasing factor; MK 677, L 692429	Merck & Co.	Phase II	GHRP-6 analog (growth hormone-releasing hexapeptide)

Chemical	Company/co-licensees	Phase of development	Comments
Somatomedin-C	Biogen	Phase II	Recombinant somatomedin-C grown in *E. coli* and yeast
Somatomedin-C	Genentech	Phase II	Recombinant somatomedin-C
β-FGF; Fiblast	Scios Nova/E Merck/Kaken	Phase II	Basic fibroblast growth factor
Growth hormone releasing factor	Cambridge Biotech/BioNebraska/R & C Enterprises	Phase I	
Growth hormone releasing peptides; GPA 748, KP-102	Kaken Pharmaceuticals/Wyeth-Ayerst	Phase I	Orally active growth hormone releasing agent
Somatomedin-C	Nikken	Phase I	Recombinant somatomedin-C
Somatotropin (Humatrope)	Lilly		Same as natural hormone; recombinant DNA technology is used
Somatotropin human	Celltech		Recombinant DNA technology is used
Somatomedin-2; IGF-2	British Bio-Technology	Possibly preclinical	Possibly bone-promoting growth factor
Growth hormone releasing factor; Sermorelin	Salk Institute/Ares Serono/Bachem	Preclinical	Marketed for in vivo diagnostic
Polyethylene glycol TGFβ-2	Enzon/Celtrix	Preclinical	Growth factor—possible local action
Somatomedin-1; insulin-like growth factor	GeneMedicine	Preclinical	IGF-1 gene (non-viral administration)
Somatomedin-1; insulin-like growth factor	BioGrowth	Preclinical	IGF-1 gene (non-viral administration)
Somatomedin-B; IGF-2	Llorente	Preclinical	Bone-promoting growth factor
Somatomedin-C	GeneMedicine	Preclinical	Bone-promoting growth factor
Somatomedin-C + binding protein; IGF-BP3; SomatoKine	Celtrix/Green Cross	Preclinical	Recombinant IGF-1 bonded to BP3, injected daily

Bone-forming Factors

Chemical	Company/co-licensees	Phase of development	Comments
Bone morphogenetic protein-2; YM 484	Wyeth-Ayerst/Genetics Institute/Yamanouchi/Sofamor Danek	Phase II	Recombinant BMP-2 promotes formation of bone and cartilage

Osteogenic and anti-resorptive drugs; TEI 3313	Teijin	Phase II; discontinued	Causes minerals to form for osteoblast cells; slows loss of bone
SC 116	Scotia	Phase II	Osteogenic triglyceride
Bone proteins	Xoma	Phase I	Show enhanced bone formation
Osteogenic and antiresorptive drugs, bone-inducing compound, BIC	Ossacur/Merck	Phase I	May work by increasing angiogenesis
Osteogenic peptides	Telios Pharmaceuticals/Lilly	Preclinical	Synthetic peptides with RGD (arginine, glucine, aspartic acid); integrin receptors binding
Bone morphogenetic protein-1(PHAR); osteogenic protein-1(IPUR)	Creative BioMolecules/Stryker	Preclinical	Recombinant human osteogenic protein
ALX 2-1	Allelix/Glaxo-Wellcome	Preclinical	Suspended drug increases bone density
Bone growth factor genes	Transkaryotic Therapies	Preclinical	Gene therapy
Bone growth factors	Orquest	Preclinical	Biocompatible collagen matrix for bone growth
Bone morphogenetic protein-52; MP 52	BIOPHARM/Hoechst	Preclinical	Recombinant protein
Bone morphogenetic proteins	Biomet	Preclinical	Bone morphogenetic protein-2 and bone morphogenic protein-7 heterodimer
Bone morphogenetic proteins	Xoma	Preclinical	
Cartilage growth factors	Orquest	Preclinical	Biocompatible collagen matrix for cartilage growth
Osteoblast-stimulating factor	Hoechst	Preclinical	Recombinant OSF
Osteoblast-stimulating factor	Innogenetics	Preclinical	Isolation of endogenous substances stimulating osteogenesis
Osteogenesis inducers	Hoechst Marion Roussel	Preclinical	Stimulates bone formation
Osteogenic and anti-resorptive drugs TEI 7457	Teijin	Preclinical	Boron amino acid analogs increase osteoblast activity and decrease resorption
Osteogenic and anti-resorptive drugs	Boron Biologicals	Preclinical	Peptidic and non-peptidic anti-osteoporotics
Osteogenic and anti-resorptive drugs	Dompe	Preclinical	

Chemical	Company/co-licensees	Phase of development	Comments
Osteogenic and anti-resorptive drugs	Oncogene Science/Wyeth-Ayerst	Preclinical	Gene products
Osteogenic factors	Dompe	Preclinical	Treatment of severe osteoporosis; lead compounds under analysis
Osteogenic growth peptide	Yissum	Preclinical	Potentially anti-osteoporotic. Can be suitable for administration by non-invasive routes
Osteogenic peptides	Procyte	Preclinical	Early research on copper peptides
Osteogenic pyridazine derivatives	Johnson & Johnson	Preclinical	Pyridazine-derivative progestin agonists and antagonists
Osteogenin	Genentech/Roche	Preclinical	Discontinued osteogenic compound
Osteoinductive factor + growth factor β-2	Collagen	Preclinical	Osteogenic compound
Osteopoietin, OPO	Metra Biosystems	Preclinical	Osteogenic proteins isolated from human urine; triggered undifferentiated cells to become osteoblasts in cell culture
Osteoporotics	Wyeth-Ayerst/Panlabs	Preclinical	
Noggin	Regeneron	Preclinical	Bone growth disorders

Other Possible Anti-osteoporotics

Chemical	Company/co-licensees	Phase of development	Comments
Ipriflavone	Chinoin/Chiesei/Takeda/Kukje/Sintyal/Therabel/Somerset Labs/Sanofi/Draxis	Marketed in Europe and Asia	Anti-osteoporotic with few side-effects, 600 mg/day; greater bone density; less pain/demineralization; fewer fractures
Vitamin K2, Vitamin K2 or D3 derivative menatetrenone; Grakay	Eisai	Marketed for Vitamin K deficiency/awaiting approval in Japan for osteoporosis	Prevents bone loss in ovariectomized rats; oral formulation, marketed for blood-clotting disorder
Gallium nitrate; NSC 15200	Sloan Kettering Institute/Fujisawa/Lilly	Marketed for hypercalcemia of malignancy early phase for osteoporosis	Inhibits nitric oxide synthase; used in hypercalcemia if malignancy

Drug	Company	Phase	Description
Livial	Akzo Nobel	Phase III in Europe & USA; phase II in Japan	
System patch	R.W. Johnson Pharmaceutical Research Institute	Phase III	
Norethindrone acetate + ethinyl estradiol; CI-376	Warner-Lambert	Phase III	
HP 228	Houghten	Phase II	
EF 40	Scotia	Phase II	Oral formulation for long-term use; found to increase Ca absorpton from the diet, reduce Ca urinary excretion, increase Ca uptake into bones
SC-116	Scotia Pharmaceuticals	Phase II in UK	Improves calcium absorption and inhibits calcium removal
KB-889	Kanebo	Phase II	Calcium metabolism regulator
Norcalcin	NPS Pharmaceuticals, Kirin Brewery	Phase II	Calcium receptor stimulant; works on PTH cells, may also work on bone cells
Osteogenic and anti-resorptive drugs; S-12911	Servier	Phase II	Strontium salt
S-12911	Servier	Phase II	Antiresorptive strontium salt
SB 205179	SmithKline Beecham	Phase II	Possible treatment for osteoporosis; mechanism unknown
Osteogenic drugs; Zeolite A	Whitby Pharmaceuticals	Phase I	A stimulator for bone formation. Sodium aluminosilicate raises concentration of Si (but not Al) in blood plasma
N 2749	Nisshin Flour Milling/ Teikoku Hormone	Phase I; suspended	Possible treatment
Osteogenic pyridazine derivatives	Johnson & Johnson	Preclinical	Progestin agonists and antagonists derived from pyridazine; treatment for osteoporosis and menopausal symptoms
Cathepsin O2 inhibitors	Khepri	Preclinical	Inhibit enzyme involved in osteoclast activity
CT 1	Osteopharm	Preclinical	Synthetic anti-osteoporotic peptide
CT 2	Osteopharm	Preclinical	Recombinant anti-osteoporotic peptide

Chemical	Company/co-licensees	Phase of development	Comments
Cytokine leukaemia inhibitory factor—recombinant form	Amrad (Australia)/Merck & Co		Being studied for osteoporosis
Computer-aided drug design	Karo Bio/Novo Nordisk	Preclinical	Products for treating and preventing of osteoporosis
SRC inhibitor	Ariad/Hoechst Marion Roussel	Preclinical	
MPI; metalloproteinase inhibitors	British Biotech	Preclinical	Discontinued worldwide; orally-active matrix metalloprotease inhibitors that treat arthritis and inflammatory diseases; may be anti-osteoporotic
Boron analogs	Boron Biologicals	Preclinical	Inhibition of bone and fibroblast cells
Boron analogs of amino acids	Boron Biologicals	Preclinical	Greater calcium absorption by bones and proline absorption into collagen; more loss of calcium and hydrolyzing of collagen
Carbonic dehydratase inhibitor; Polyacrylic acid	Research Corporation Technologies	Preclinical	Carbonic hydrase inhibitor binds to a substance associated with the bone mineral hydroxyapatite less bone mass reduction
Collagenase inhibitor	Boron Biologicals	Preclinical	Inhibit aryl sulfatase, cathepsin, serine protease, elastase, acid phosphatase in osteoporotic cells
Genes involved in osteoporosis	Sequana Therapeutics/Corange	Preclinical	Joint research to locate genes related to osteoporosis
Halystatin	Takeda	Preclinical	Platelet aggregation inhibitor; has potential in treating metabolic bone diseases
Human mesenchymal stem cell regulators	Houghten/Osiris	Preclinical	Proof of concept studies
Integrin antagonists	Hoechst/Genentech	Preclinical	Contain RGD sequence of amino acids
Ion channel activator	Sphinx Pharmaceuticals/ICAgen	Preclinical	Affects osteoporotic cells
Isoflavanone; WS 7528	Fujisawa	Preclinical	
KCA 098	Kissei	Preclinical	Coumestrol derivative inhibits resorption and promotes growth

Agent	Company	Phase	Description
Lactol oligopeptides	Takeda	Preclinical	For use as cathepsin-L inhibitors
Matrix metalloproteinase inhibitors	New York State University Research Foundation/Collagenex	Preclinical	Non-antibiotic, may prove useful for long-term use
Matrix metalloproteinase inhibitors	British Biotech/SmithKline Beecham	Preclinical; discontinued	
MP-52	Biopharm GmbH (Germany)/Hoechst Marion Roussel	Preclinical	Recombinant bone morphogenetic protein increased growth of chrondocytes and osteoblasts, improved bone tissue formation in rat cells
NOF 003	NOF Corporation	Preclinical	Acid analog of eicosapentaenic
Osteoclast calcimimetic	SmithKline Beecham/NPS	Preclinical	Oral formulation blocks parathyroid calcium receptors and prevents secretion of osteoclast proteins and enzymes
Osteopontin	Innogenetics	Preclinical	Treatment of bone fractures
Osteoporosis therapies	Hoechst Marion Roussel	Preclinical	Estrogenic effects on bone
Parathyroid cell calcilytic	NPS/SmithKline Beecham	Preclinical	Blocks calcium receptor on parathyroid cells
Cellular adhesion protein	Genetics Institute/American Home Products	Preclinical	Cellular adhesion protein which affects movement of white blood cells out of bloodstream; can treat osteoporosis, inflammation and a variety of others
Bone resorption suppressive agent	Ariad	Preclinical	Interacts with signal transduction pathway to interfere with excessive bone resorption
Prostaglandin delivery agent	Merck & Co	Preclinical	Effective delivery agents of prostaglandins
Signal transduction control	Ariad	Preclinical	Control intracellular signal transduction; also potential treatment of asthma, rheumatoid, etc.
Sulfonate and carbamate derivatives	Lilly	Preclinical	Under investigation for osteoporosis
Proteinase nexin-1; PN-1	Incyte	Preclinical	Inhibits osteoclast enzymes
RCT Project No. 242-1430	Research Corporation Techonologies	Preclinical	Bone-targeted carbonic anhydrase inhibitors treat menopausal osteoporosis

444

Chemical	Company/co-licensees	Phase of development	Comments
Signal transducing agent; AP 448	Ariad	Preclinical	Binds to Src protein, blocking osteoclast activity
TAN-1756A; TAN-1756B	Takeda	Preclinical	Epoxysuccinic acid derivative; inhibits cathepsin B and L
TNCA; CP-2569; TNLY; thionaphthenecarboxylic acid	MacroChem	Preclinical	TNLY, fewer side effects, better oral bioavailability; inhibition of calcium absorption
Wortmannin analog; 17β-hydroxywortmannin	Lilly	Preclinical	Slows down bone resorption in vitro by inhibiting osteoclasts
Vitronectin receptor antagonist	ICRT	Preclinical	Osteoclast vitronectin receptor antagonists and antibodies
ZM 230487	Zeneca	Preclinical	May inhibit bone resorption by acting through 5-lipoxygenase inhibitor
Cancer therapy	Sugen; Toyama Prefectural University	Preclinical for cancer treatment	Inhibition of tyrosine kinase, tyrosine phosphatases, and related molecules; possible use in osteoporosis
C/EBPβ inhibitors; signal	Signal Pharmaceuticals	Preclinical	Inhibit factors stimulating osteoclast formation
PC-1250	Procyte	Preclinical	Primarily for HIV inhibition, may also treat osteoporosis

APPENDIX G: BREAST CANCER

STEROIDAL AGENTS

Chemical	Company/co-licensees	Phase of development	Comments
Anti-estrogen—Partial Estrogen Agonist			
Tamoxifen	Zeneca	Marketed worldwide	Anti-estrogen, prototype, approved for adjuvant therapy after primary treatment and in metastatic disease
Toremifene; FC 1157A; NK622	Farmos/Nippon Kayaku/Asta Medica/Schering Plough/Orion-Farmos/Pharmacia	Marketed/approved in USA	Fareston, Tremifen; anti-estrogenic tamoxifen derivative for postmenopausal breast cancer, marketed in Europe
Droloxifene; FK-435; K-060; K-21060; RP 60850	Kling (Fujisawa)/Pfizer	Phase III	Tamoxifen analog
Centrochroman; 6720-CDR; Centron; Choice-7, Saheli	Central Drug Research Institute, India/Zymogenetics	Phase II/III	Anti-estrogen; marketed in India as a contraceptive; phase I or II for breast cancer
ICI-182780	Zeneca	Phase II	Injectable anti-estrogen
Idoxifene; CB-7386, CB-7432	British Technology Group/Bristol-Myers-Squibb/SmithKline Beecham	Phase II	Anti-estrogen, similar action to tamoxifen, a prototype anti-estrogen
TAT-59; DP-TAT-59	Taiho	Phase II	Anti-estrogen derived from triphenylethylene
Non-steroidal anti-estrogens	Endorecherche, Schering-Plough	Phase I	
Panomifene; EGIS-5650; GYKI-13504	EGIS/Fujimoto/Institute for Drug Research (Budapest)	Phase I	Anti-estrogen; triphenylethylene derivative
Exemestane/FCE-24304	Pharmacia (Farmatalia Carlo Erba)/Upjohn	Phase II/III; possibly discontinued	Anti-estrogen

Chemical	Company/co-licensees	Phase of development	Comments
Estrogen agonists and antagonists			
Estrogen antagonist	Karo Bio	Preclinical	Anti-estrogen
	Research Corporation Technologies/MGI Pharma	Preclinical	Anti-estrogen
MDL-103323; MDL-104890; MDL-104931	Merion Merrell Dow	Preclinical	Anti-estrogen
Progestin and estrogen antagonists	Ligand Pharmaceuticals	Preclinical	Anti-estrogen
RU-58668	Roussel Uclaf	Preclinical	Anti-estrogen
RU-58668	Roussel Uclaf	Preclinical	Anti-estrogen; useful for tumors resistant to tamoxifen
WS-7528	Fujisawa	Preclinical	Anti-estrogen injection
LG2716	Ligand	Preclinical	Anti-estrogen
ZK-119010	Schering AG	Preclinical	Anti-estrogen
Progestins/Antiprogestins			
Medroxyprogesterone acetate	Upjohn/Generic	Marketed	Used in refractory cancer
Megesterol acetate	Bristol-Myers-Squibb	Marketed	Used in refractory cancer
Onapristone/ZK-98299	Schering AG	Phase II	Antiprogestin—no longer under study
Mifepristone/RU-38486/ Mifegyne/RU486	Roussel Uclaf	Preclinical	Antiprogestin and glucocorticoid receptor antagonist, under study for breast cancer
Org-31710; Org-31806	Azko	Preclinical	Antiprogestin
ZK-112993	Schering AG	Preclinical	Antiprogestin; may work well with vinblastine
Anti-androgens			
Osaterone acetate/TZP-4238	Teikoku Hormone	Registered	Anti-androgen derived from clormadinone acetate
Androgen antagonists	Ligand Pharmaceuticals	Preclinical	

Aromatase Inhibitors

Compound	Company	Status	Notes
Fadrozole; CGS-16949a, CGS-20287	Novartis	Marketed in 2–3 countries	Second line therapy
Formestane; 4-HAD; 4-OHA; CGP-32349; Lentaron	Novartis	Approved in some countries	Second line therapy
ICI-D1033; ZD-1033; IDI-D-1033/Arimidex	Zeneca	Approved worldwide	Second line therapy
Letrozole; CGS-20267	Novartis	Close to approval	Fadrozole analog
Fadrozole	Novartis	Phase III	
Vorozole/R-76713; R-83842/Rivizor	Janssen	Phase III	Fadrozole analog; non-steroidal
Atamestane/SH-489/ZK-95639	Schering AG	Phase II	Fadrozole analog
Rogletimide; pyrido-glutethimide	British Technology Group/US BioScience/Schering-Plough	Phase II	Fadrozole analog amino-glutethimide derivative
FCE-27993	Pharmacia (Farmatalia Carlo Erba)	Phase I	Aromatase inhibitor; steroidal; irreversible
YM-511	Yamanouchi	Phase I	Aromatase inhibitor; improved specificity for aldosterone inhibition as compared to fadrozole
CGP-47465; CGP-52653	Novartis	Preclinical	Aromatase inhibitor; derived from fluoro and methyl compounds
Diphenylalkyl imidazole derivatives/aromatase inhibitor	Orion-Farmos	Preclinical	Aromatase inhibitor; derived from diphenylalkyl imidazole
RU-54115; RU-56562	Roussel Uclaf	Preclinical	Aromatase inhibitor
SEF-19; SAE-9; SEF-32	Zenyaku Kogyo	Preclinical	Aromatase inhibitor
YM-553	Yamanouchi	Preclinical	Aromatase inhibitor

NON-STEROIDAL AGENTS

LHRH Agonists

Chemical	Company/co-licensees	Phase of development	Comments
Triptorelin, Avecap, Decapeptyl, AY-25650; BIM-21003; WY-42422 decapeptyl CR	Tulane University/Debiopharm/Ferring/Noristan/Beaufour-Ipsen/Organon	Marketed in Europe	Injectable long-acting gonadotropin-releasing hormone analog
Buserelin	Hoechst	Marketed in Europe	Intranasal gonadotropin-releasing hormone analog
Goserelin acetate implant; ICI 118630; Zoladex	Zeneca	Marketed in Europe; approved for pre-menopausal breast cancer	Gonadotropin-releasing hormone agonist suppresses ovarian function and endogenous estrogen use in premenopausal women only
Nafarelin/RS-94991/RS-94991-298/Synarel	Syntex/Recordati/Johnson & Johnson	Marketed for endometriosis	Gonadotropin-releasing hormone analog/nasal; developing microencapsulated formulation
Leuprolide/Lupron	Abbott/Lederle/Takeda	Marketed for endometriosis; Phase III for Takeda	Injectable long-acting gonadotropin-releasing hormone analog
Deslorelin; analog/Somagard	Monmouth (Roberts)/Theramex; Salk Institute	Registered	Subcutaneous daily-dose gonadotropin-releasing hormone analog
rhl-11/Neumega Buserelin/Suprefact	Genetics Institute/Hoechst	Phase II	Gonadotropin-releasing hormone agonist; suppresses ovarian function and endogenous estrogen use in premenopausal women only
Meterelin	Europeptides	Phase I	Gonadotropin-releasing hormone agonist; suppresses ovarian function and endogenous estrogen use in premenopausal women only
Leuprolide + estrogen + progesterone ED 950116	Royal Marsden Hospital/Balance/UCLA	Phase I	Injectable contraceptive may reduce possibility of breast cancer
LHRH implant	Endocon	Preclinical	Subcutaneous implant for breast cancer
LHRH vaccine	Proteus International	Preclinical	Vaccine against LHRH to suppress ovarian function

LHRH Antagonists

Antide/ORF-23541	Serono	Phase II	Gonadotropin-releasing hormone antagonist; suppresses ovarian function without initial stimulation; use in premenopausal women
Cetrorelix; SB 75, SB 075	Veterans Administration Medical Center/Asta Medica/Shionogi/ KAYAKU ASTA Medica/Tulane U School of Medicine	Phase II	As above
Ganirelix/RS-26306	Syntex/Searle	Phase II	As above
Antarelix; EP 25332	Europeptides (Mediolanum/ Pharmascience)	Phase I	As above
Meterelin; EP 23904	Europeptides (Mediolanum/ Pharmascience)	Phase I	As above

Growth Hormone Antagonists

Octreotide/SMS-201-995/ Sandostatin	Sandoz/Sankyo/ Italfarmaco	Marketed for VIPoma	Analog of somatostatin/growth hormone antagonist
Lanreotide; BIM 23014, BIM 23014C, DC 13116; Somatuline	Tulane University/ Beaufour-Ipsen/ Neoprobe	Phase III	Somatostatin analog marketed for acromegaly
Vapreotide; BMY-41606; RC-160; Octastain	Prof AV Schally, Tulane U School of Medicine/ Debiopharm	Phase II; Phase III (NS)	Octapeptide growth hormone antagonist/non-specific growth suppressor
Growth hormone antagonist	Sensus/Edison Animal Biotechnology Center, Ohio	Phase I	

Chemical	Company/co-licensees	Phase of development	Comments
Microtubule Inhibitors			
Paclitaxel	Bristol-Myers-Squibb	Marketed worldwide	Inhibits microtubule growth
Vinorelbine/KW-23071; Navelbine	Pierre Fabre/Kyowa Hakko/Wellcome/ Boehringer/Ingelheim/ Pasteur Merieux/ Rhone-Poulenc Rorer/ Gedeon Richter	Marketed (NS)	Semisynthetic vinca alkaloid/tubulin antagonist
Docetaxel/taxotere/ NSC-628503; RP-56976	Rhone-Poulenc Rorer/ Chugai; NIH	Marketed	Microtubule inhibitor
Oncocase/P-30	Alfacell/NIH	Phase II	Inhibition of microtubules
Rhizoxin/FR-900216; NSC-332598; WF 1360	Fujisawa/Institute of Microbiology, U Tokyo; EORTC; NCi	Phase I	Acts against tubulin
DNA Inhibitors			
Gemcitabine; LY-188011; Gemzar	Eli Lilly	Phase III	Difluoro-nucleoside agent; DNA synthesis inhibitor
KRN-8602; MX-2; MY-5; NSC-619003	Kirin Brewery/Japanese Foundation for Cancer Research & Inst. of Microbial Chemistry, Japan	Phase II	Series of anthracycline anticancer antibiotics/ DNA antagonists
Tallimustine/FCE-24517	Pharmacia	Phase II	DNA antagonist/derived from distamycin A/ for progressed cancers/solid tumors
5-gluor pyrimidine	Sparta	Preclinical	

RNA Inhibitors

Drug	Company	Status	Description
Idarubicin/Zavedos	Pharmacia	Marketed	RNA synthesis inhibitor; Daunorubicin derivative
Pirabucin; THP-doxorubicin/1609RB/Pinorubin; Therprubicine; Therarubicin	Meiji Seika/Institute of Microbial Chemistry, Japan; Nippon Kayaku; Rhone-Poulenc Rorer	Marketed	RNA synthesis inhibitor
Doxorubicin; TLC D-99; TLC-DOX99	Liposome Company/Pfizer; U British Columbia, McGill U	Phase III	RNA synthesis inhibitor; liposomal formulation; for breast cancer resistant to platinum and taxol regimens
Daunorubicin, Vestar/VS-103/DaunoXome	Vestar	Phase III	RNA synthesis inhibitor/liposomal formulation
DMP 840	DuPont Merck	Phase I	Bis-naphthalimide/RNA inhibitor
Doxorubicin-CEA; DOX-CEA	Immunomedics	Preclinical	Antibody conjugate/RNA synthesis inhibitor

Protein Synthesis Inhibitors

Drug	Company	Status	Description
Bispecific MAb/MDX-210	Medarex		Protein synthesis antagonist
Fenretinide, McN-R-1967, HPR	McNeil (Johnson & Johnson)/NCI	Phase II	Protein synthesis antagonist; chemopreventive for breast cancer

Miscellaneous

Drug	Company	Status	Description
Doxorubicin, stealth liposome formulation; DOX-SL	Liposome Technology	Submitted to FDA	
Amifostine/NSC-296961; WR-2721/Ethiofos/Ethyol/Gammaphos	US BioScience/Schering-Plough/SmithKline Beecham/Southern Research Institute	Preregistration	Radio & chemoprotectant; oxygen scavenger

Chemical	Company/co-licensees	Phase of development	Comments
Her-2, monoclonal antibody	Genentech	Phase III	Oncoprotein; immunostimulant; antibody attacks gene for receptor associated with a proportion of breast cancers. HER-2/neu proto-oncogene is responsible for encoding growth factor receptor which appears amplified in 25–35% of primary human breast cancers
Epirubicin/Pharmorubicin	Pharmacia/Kyowa Hakko	Phase III	4'-epimer of doxorubicin
Liarolzole; R-75251	Janssen (Johnson & Johnson)	Phase III	Cytochrome P450 oxidoreductase inhibitor
PIXY-321/PIXYKINE	Immunex/American Cyanamid	Phase III	Fusion molecule
Sargramotism/Interberin; Leukine; Prokine	Immunex/Behringwerke (Hoechst); Roussel Uclaf	Phase III	rhu-GM-CSF
Suramin, NIH	National Cancer Institute/ Warner-Lambert	Phase III	Polymerase inhibitor; RNA-directed DNA
Polyadenylic & Polyuridylic acid; BN-52101, Polyadenur	Beaufour-Ipsen	Phase III	Immune response analog; interferon analog
Topotecan/hycaptamine/ NSC-609699/SK&F-104864	SmithKline Beecham	Phase III	Inhibition of DNA topoisomerase activity
Emitefur/BOF-A2	Otsuka	Phase II	
FCE-24517	Pharmacia (Farmatalia Carlo Erba)	Phase II	Alkylating agent
Anamycin	Aronex	Phase II	Breast cancer resistant to other therapies
rhu-IL-3 (E. coli)	Sandoz	Phase II	
Allovectin-7	Vicl	Phase II	
Trans-retinoic acid	National Cancer Institute	Phase II	
Trimetrexate/CI-898/JB-11/ NSC-249008/NSC-328564/ NSC-352122	Parke-Davis (Warner-Lambert)/US BioScience; Dainippon; NIH	Phase II	Dihydrofolate reductase inhibitor

Drug	Company/Institution	Phase	Description
IL-1 agonist	Yeda; IntePharm (Serono)	Phase II	
EF-13	Scotia Pharmaceuticals (Efamol)/St. Bartholomew's Hospital	Phase II	Stimulates prostaglandin synthase
Losoxantrone/CI-941	Warner-Lambert/DuPont Merck	Phase II	Inhibition of DNA topoisomerase
ZD-1694;ICI-D-1694; Tomudex	Zeneca; British Technology Group	Phase II	Folate analog/thymidylate synthase inhibitor; water soluble
PALA; sparfosate sodium; sparfosic acid/CI-882/ NSC-224131	US BioScience/Schering-Plough/SmithKline Beecham/Parke-Davis (Warner-Lambert)/NCI	Phase II	Aspartate carbamoultransferase inhibitor; improves 5-FU and FU-related drug activity
Adozelesin/U-73975/Adosar	Upjohn/NIH; Yakult Honsha	Phase II	Rachelmycin derivative; P-glycoprotein inhibitor; increases specificity and reduces toxicity
Melphalan IV	National Cancer Institute	Phases I, II and III	
Aastrom Cell Production Systems	Aastrom BioSciences	Phase I	Promotion of recovery of breast cancer patients
Cyclosporin analog/PSC-833	Sandoz	Phase I (NS)	Non-immunosuppressant derivative of cyclosporin/chemotherapy protectant
Pancarcinoma/Re-186 MAb	NeoRx	Phase I (NS)	
Bryostatin-1	Cancer Research Campaign	Phase I	Macrolytic lactone; protein kinase C pathway inhibitor
CM-101	CarboMed	Phase I	Bacterial polysaccharide
D 20453	Asta Medica	Phase I	Discontinued treatment for hormone-sensitive tumors
Mifepristone; RU 486; Mifegyne	Roussel Uclaf/Population Council	Clinical tests	Marketed as an abortifacient
Lentinan; LC-33; YM-09222	Ajinomoto/Roussel-Morishita; Yamanouchi	Clinical	Polysaccharide vaccine agonist
CT-1541	Cell Therapeutics	Preclinical	TNF inhibitor/inhibit Bursten pathway
D-3967	Chiroscience	Preclinical	Isomer compound
Maspin/LXR023	LXR/Dana-Farber Cancer Institute	Preclinical	Apoptosis modulator; metastatic cancer

Chemical	Company/co-licensees	Phase of development	Comments
Pyridazine derivatives/bone formation stimulant	Ortho (Johnson & Johnson)	Preclinical	Pyridazine derivatives/bone formation stimulant/? hypercalcemia if malignancy
Genetic prodrug activating therapy (GPAT)	Hammersmith Hospital	Preclinical	Cytosine deaminase/prodrug enzyme changes 5-FC to 5-FU
Bizelesin	Upjohn/NIH	Preclinical (NS)	Analog of Rachelmycin

Non-hormonal Oncologic Agents

Chemical	Company/co-licensees	Phase of development	Comments
Paclitaxel taxol	Bristol-Myers-Squibb/National Cancer Institute	Marketed for breast cancer	For patients non-responsive to chemotherapy
Onconase	Alfacell	Phase III for pancreatic cancer	Being tested on a variety of tumors including breast cancer
Liposomal daunorubicin; DaunoXome	Vestar	Phase III	
Human interleukin-6, recombinant, E. coli; rhu-il-6	Sandoz	Phase III	
Imagent LN	Alliance Pharmaceutical	Phase III	
ImmuRAID; CEA	Immunomedics	Phase III	
Mitoxantrone in combination with paclitaxel	Immunex	Phase III	
Leuvoleucovorin, Isovorin	Immunex	Phase III	In combination with 5-fluorouracil
Rivizor	Johnson & Johnson	Phase III	Breast cancer relapses
Gemzar	Eli Lilly	Phase III	
Octreotide acetate; Sandostatin LAR	Novartis	Phase III	
BUDR	National Cancer Institute	Phase II/III	
Interferon α	National Cancer Institute	Phase II/III	
Leucovorin calcium	Immunex	Phase II/III	
Leucovorin calcium	Immunex	Phase II/III	In combination with 5-fluorouracil
Altretamine; Hexalen	US Bioscience	Phase II/III	

Drug	Company	Phase	Notes
G-CSF	National Cancer Institute	Phase I/II/III	
GM-CSF	National Cancer Institute	Phase I/II/III	
Onconase	Alfacell	Phase II	
Novantrone	Immunex/Wyeth-Ayers	Phase II	
Difluormethylornithine	Ilex Oncology	Phase II	
Caelyx	Sequus	Phase II	
Anthrapyrazole	DuPont Merck	Phase II	
BMS 182248	Bristol-Myers-Squibb	Phase II	
Catrix	Lescarden	Phase II	
CI-958	Warner-Lambert	Phase II	
CI-980	Warner-Lambert	Phase II	
Detox-B	Ribi ImmunoChem	Phase II	
Fenretinide	R.W. Johnson Pharmaceutical Research Institute	Phase II	
Interleukin-2	National Cancer Institute	Phase II	
IUDR	National Cancer Institute	Phase II	
IV hydroxyurea	National Cancer Institute	Phase II	
Mitoxantrone, Novantrone	Lederle	Phase II	
Taxol/doxorubicin w/G-CSF	National Cancer Institute	Phase II	Combination regimen
Theratope, therapeutic vaccine	Biomira	Phase II	
MDX-210	Medarex	Phase II	HER 2+ cancers
BB-10010	British Biotech	Phase II	Protects stem cells
Xeloda	Hoffman-LaRoche	Phase II	
VX-710	Vertex	Phase II	
Menogaril; Tomosar	Pharmacia/Upjohn	Phase II	
Fenretinide	Johnson & Johnson	Phase II	
C225	ImClone	Phase I/II	
$DAB_{389}EGF$, EGF fusion toxin	Seragen	Phase I/II	
Interleukin-1 alpha	National Cancer Institute	Phase I/II	
LGD 1057	Ligand	Phase I/II	
LGD 1069	Ligand	Phase I/II	
MAb CC-49	National Cancer Institute	Phase I/II	

Chemical	Company/co-licensees	Phase of development	Comments
P587^{99m} technetium peptide	Diatech	Phase I/II	
Recombinant-methionyl human stem-cell factor	Amgen	Phase I/II	
C225	ImClone Systems	Phase I/II	EGF-R+ cancers
MDX-447	Medarex	Phase I/II	
MUC1 tumor antigen	Corixa	Phase I	Vaccine against breast cancer
Sluasterone	Aeson	Phase I	
Gene therapy	Genetic Therapy, Include	Phase I	Protection of blood system of patient with metastatic breast cancer
Neovastat		Phase I	
CAI	National Cancer Institute	Phase I	
Dystamycin	Pharmacia-Adria	Phase I	
Interleukin-6; mutein	ImClone Systems	Phase I	
Lomotrexol	Eli Lilly	Phase I	
LY231514	Eli Lilly	Phase I	
Sulfonylurea	Eli Lilly	Phase I	
Topoisomurase I inhibitor (GG211)	Glaxo	Phase I	
323A3	Centocor	Phase I	Monoclonal antibody-based therapy
Anamycin	Aronex	Phase I	
Gene therapy	Genetic Therapy	Phase I	Bone marrow protection
Muc-1 tumor antigen	Corixa	Phase I	
GF 120918	Glaxo-Wellcome	Phase I	Inhibition of multidrug resistance
Multiple drug resistance gene transfer	Rhone-Poulenc Rorer	Phase I	
E1A-RGG0853	Rgene Therapeutics/Fournier	Phase I	
E1A-Gene therapy tgDCC-E1A	Targeted Genetics	Phase I	
Thalidomide	EntreMed/Bristol-Myers-Squibb/National Cancer Institute	Phase I	

Muc-1	Therion	Phase I	Vaccine against breast cancer
Pan-Her antagonist	Sugen/Astra Medica	Phase I	
Suramin	Cell Genesys	Preclinical	
SMART Abl 364 antibody	Protein Design	Preclinical	
Maspin	LXR Biotechnology	Preclinical	Breast cancer suppressor
H-Nuc	Canji	Preclinical	
DOX-CEA	Immunomedics	Preclinical	
AR102	Aronex	Preclinical	
Oncostatins	Bristol-Myers-Squibb	Preclinical	Prevent growth of cancer cells; no effect on normal cell growth
Breast cancer immunoconjugate	ImmunoGen	Preclinical	
EGF RTK antagonist	Sugen	Preclinical	
HER2 antagonist	Sugen	Preclinical	
Her2/Neu tumor peptides	Corixa	Preclinical	
Muc-1	Therion Biologics	Preclinical	Vaccine
SMART ABL 364	Protein Design Labs	Preclinical	

Index

Page numbers followed by app. refer to the Appendices of Drugs in Development

Index compiled by Anne McCarthy

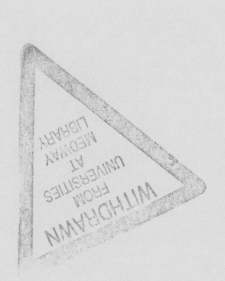

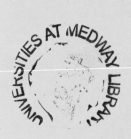